Editors

ASIF M. ILYAS
SHITAL N. PARIKH
SAQIB REHMAN
GILES R. SCUDERI
FELASFA M. WODAJO

ORTHOPEDIC CLINICS OF NORTH AMERICA

www.orthopedic.theclinics.com

October 2015 • Volume 46 • Number 4

ELSEVIER

1600 John F. Kennedy Boulevard • Suite 1800 • Philadelphia, Pennsylvania, 19103-2899.

http://www.orthopedic.theclinics.com

ORTHOPEDIC CLINICS OF NORTH AMERICA Volume 46, Number 4
October 2015 ISSN 0030-5898, ISBN-13: 978-0-323-40094-7

Editor: Jennifer Flynn-Briggs
Developmental Editor: Kristen Helm

Orthopedic Clinics of North America (ISSN 0030-5898) is published quarterly by Elsevier Inc., 360 Park Avenue South, New York, NY 10010-1710. Months of issue are January, April, July, and October. Business and Editorial Offices: 1600 John F. Kennedy Blvd., Suite 1800, Philadelphia, PA 19103-2899. Customer Service Office: 3251 Riverport Lane, Maryland Heights, MO 63043. Periodicals postage paid at New York, NY and additional mailing offices. Subscription prices are $310.00 per year for (US individuals), $596.00 per year for (US institutions), $365.00 per year (Canadian individuals), $727.00 per year (Canadian institutions), $450.00 per year (international individuals), $727.00 per year (international institutions), $150.00 per year (US students), $220.00 per year (Canadian and international students). Foreign air speed delivery is included in all *Clinics* subscription prices. All prices are subject to change without notice. **POSTMASTER:** Send change of address to *Orthopedic Clinics of North America*, **Elsevier Health Sciences Division, Subscription Customer Service, 3251 Riverport Lane, Maryland Heights, MO 63043. Customer Service (orders, claims, online, change of address): Elsevier Health Sciences Division, Subscription Customer Service, 3251 Riverport Lane, Maryland Heights, MO 63043. Tel: 1-800-654-2452 (U.S. and Canada); 314-447-8871 (outside U.S. and Canada). Fax: 314-447-8029. E-mail:** journalscustomerservice-usa@elsevier. com **(for print support);** journalsonlinesupport-usa@elsevier.com **(for online support).**

Reprints. For copies of 100 or more, of articles in this publication, please contact the Commercial Reprints Department, Elsevier Inc., 360 Park Avenue South, New York, NY 10010-1710. Tel.: 212-633-3874; Fax: 212-633-3820; E-mail: reprints@elsevier. com.

Orthopedic Clinics of North America is covered in *MEDLINE/PubMed* (*Index Medicus*), *Cinahl, Excerpta Medica,* and *Cumulative Index to Nursing and Allied Health Literature.*

PROGRAM OBJECTIVE

Orthopedic Clinics of North America offers clinical review articles on the most cutting-edge technologies and techniques in the field, including adult reconstruction, the upper extremity, pediatrics, trauma, oncology, and sports medicine.

TARGET AUDIENCE

Practicing orthopedic surgeons, orthopedic residents, and other healthcare professionals who specialize in orthopedic technologies and techniques for adult reconstruction, the upper extremity, pediatrics, trauma, oncology, and sports medicine.

LEARNING OBJECTIVES

Upon completion of this activity, participants will be able to:

1. Review the indications for and side effects of total joint arthroplasty in the hip and knee.
2. Discuss options in the treatment of adult and pediatric disorders of the upper extremity, such as osteoporosis and trigger finger.
3. Recognize common management strategies of orthopedic traumas such as traumatic dislocations.

ACCREDITATION

The Elsevier Office of Continuing Medical Education (EOCME) is accredited by the Accreditation Council for Continuing Medical Education (ACCME) to provide continuing medical education for physicians.

The EOCME designates this enduring material for a maximum of 15 *AMA PRA Category 1 Credit*(s)™. Physicians should claim only the credit commensurate with the extent of their participation in the activity.

All other health care professionals requesting continuing education credit for this enduring material will be issued a certificate of participation.

DISCLOSURE OF CONFLICTS OF INTEREST

The EOCME assesses conflict of interest with its instructors, faculty, planners, and other individuals who are in a position to control the content of CME activities. All relevant conflicts of interest that are identified are thoroughly vetted by EOCME for fair balance, scientific objectivity, and patient care recommendations. EOCME is committed to providing its learners with CME activities that promote improvements or quality in healthcare and not a specific proprietary business or a commercial interest.

The planning committee, staff, authors and editors listed below have identified no financial relationships or relationships to products or devices they or their spouse/life partner have with commercial interest related to the content of this CME activity:

John Alexander, MD; Mamun Al-Rashid, MD, FRCS (Orth); M. Tyrrell Burrus, MD; Jourdan M. Cancienne, MD; Jacob Coleman, BS; Kurosh Darvish, PhD; Randa DK Elmallah, MD; Simcha G. Fichman, MD; Jennifer Flynn-Briggs; Anjali Fortna; John R. Fowler, MD; Juan M. Giugale, MD; Matthew Gunton, MD, FRCSC; Christina Gutowski, MD, MPH; Jared L. Harwood, MD; Kristen Helm; Asif M. Ilyas, MD; Justin A. Iorio, MD; Andre M. Jakoi, MD; Christopher M. Jones, MD; Aidin Kashigar, BSc, MD; Kevin Klingele, MD; Indranil Kushare, MBBS, DNB; Paul R.T. Kuzyk, MD, MASc, FRCSC; James R. Lachman, MD; Frederic E. Liss, MD; Santiago A. Lozano-Calderón, MD, PhD; Tatu J. Mäkinen, MD, PhD; Laura Matsen Ko, MD; Joel L. Mayerson, MD; Oluseun Olugbode, MS; Shital N. Parikh, MD, FACS; Todd P. Pierce, MD; Paul S. Pipitone, DO; Santha Priya; Dipak B. Ramkumar, MD; Kevin Raskin, MD; Saqib Rehman, MD; Oleg Safir, MD, MEd, FRCSC; Walter Samora, MD; Thomas J. Scharschmidt, MD; Stephen C. Sizer, DO; Venessa Stas, MD; Megan Suermann; Jacob Tulipan, MD; Patrick J. Ward, MD; Felasfa M. Wodajo, MD; Seth R. Yarboro, MD.

The planning committee, staff, authors and editors listed below have identified financial relationships or relationships to products or devices they or their spouse/life partner have with commercial interest related to the content of this CME activity:

Michael C. Ain, MD is on the speakers bureau for Stryker, and receives royalties/patents from Lanx, Inc.

John W. Barrington, MD is on the speakers' bureau for Pacira Pharmaceuticals, is a consultant/advisor for Pacira Pharmaceuticals; Biomet, Inc.; Smith & Nephew, United Surgical Partners International; and Orthosensor Inc.

Walter B. Beaver, MD is a consultant/advisor for DJO, LLC; Orthosensor Inc; Pacira Pharmaceuticals; and Stryker, has research support from DePuy Sythes; DJO, LLC; and Stryker, and receives royalties/patents from Stryker.

Jeffrey J. Cherian, DO is a consultant/advisor for DJO, LLC.

Paul J. Duwelius, MD is on the speakers' bureau for Zimmer Inc, is a consultant/advisor for Signature HealthCARE LLC; Accellero Health; and UniteOR, has stock ownership in UniteOR, and receives royalties/patents from Zimmer Inc.

Roger H. Emerson, Jr, MD is on the speakers' bureau for Biomet, Inc.; Pacira Pharmaceuticals; and Medtronic, has research support from Biomet, Inc. and Pacira Pharmaceuticals, and receives royalties/patents from Biomet, Inc.

Francis J. Hornicek, MD, PhD is a consultant/advisor for Stryker and BioMed Valley Discoveries, Inc., has research support from the National Institutes of Health, and receives royalties/patents from the Cancer Chemotherapy National Service Center.

Scott Lovald, PhD, MBA has stock ownership in Exponent, Inc., research support from Pacira Pharmaceuticals, Inc., and an employment affiliation with Exponent, Inc.

Charles T. Mehlman, DO, MPH is a consultant/advisor for Oakstone Publishing, LLC; WebMD, LLC; and Stryker, has research support from Bracing in Adolescent Idiopathic Scoliosis II trial and the National Institutes of Heath, an employment affiliation with Cincinatti Children's Hospital Medical Center, and receives royalties/patents from Oakstone Publishing, LLC.

Michael A. Mont, MD is a consultant/advisor for DJO, LLC; MCS Med Inc.; Sage Products LLC; Stryker; TissueGene, Inc.; and MicroPort Scientific Corporation; has research support from DJO, LLC; Sage Products Inc; Stryker; TissueGene, Inc.; Micro-Port Scientific Corporation; and Joint Active Symptoms, Inc.; and receives royalties/patents from Stryker and MicroPort Scientific Corporation.

Kevin Ong, PhD, PE has an employment affiliation with and stock ownership in Exponent, Inc., is a consultant/advisor for Pacira Pharmaceuticals; Stryker; Paradigm Spine; Ethicon US, LLC; Medtronic; MAKO Surgical Corp; and Zimmer.

Joseph Schwab, MD, MS is a consultant/advisor for Stryker and Synthes.

Giles R. Scuderi, MD is on speakers' bureau for ConvaTec, Inc., Medtronic, Inc. and Zimmer; is a consultant/advisor for Medtronic, Inc., Pacira Pharmaceuticals, Inc. and Zimmer Inc.; has a research grant from Pacira Pharmaceuticals, Inc., and has royalties/patents from Zimmer Inc.

Heather Watson, PhD has employment affiliation with Exponent, Inc., and is a consultant/advisor for Pacira Pharmaceuticals.

David B. Weiss, MD is on the speakers' bureau for AO North America and DePuy Synthes, has research support from the Orthopedic Trauma Association, and receives royalties/patents from Elsevier Inc.

UNAPPROVED/OFF-LABEL USE DISCLOSURE

The EOCME requires CME faculty to disclose to the participants:

1. When products or procedures being discussed are off-label, unlabelled, experimental, and/or investigational (not US Food and Drug Administration [FDA] approved); and
2. Any limitations on the information presented, such as data that are preliminary or that represent ongoing research, interim analyses, and/or unsupported opinions. Faculty may discuss information about pharmaceutical agents that is outside of FDA-approved labelling. This information is intended solely for CME and is not intended to promote off-label use of these medications. If you have any questions, contact the medical affairs department of the manufacturer for the most recent prescribing information.

TO ENROLL

To enroll in the *Orthopedic Clinics of North America* Continuing Medical Education program, call customer service at 1-800-654-2452 or sign up online at http://www.theclinics.com/home/cme. The CME program is available to subscribers for an additional annual fee of USD 215.

METHOD OF PARTICIPATION

In order to claim credit, participants must complete the following:

1. Complete enrolment as indicated above.
2. Read the activity.
3. Complete the CME Test and Evaluation. Participants must achieve a score of 70% on the test. All CME Tests and Evaluations must be completed online.

CME INQUIRIES/SPECIAL NEEDS

For all CME inquiries or special needs, please contact elsevierCME@elsevier.com.

Contributors

EDITORS

ASIF M. ILYAS, MD – *Upper Extremity*
Program Director of Hand Surgery
Fellowship, Rothman Institute; Associate
Professor of Orthopaedic Surgery,
Jefferson Medical College, Philadelphia,
Pennsylvania

SHITAL N. PARIKH, MD, FACS – *Pediatrics*
Pediatric Orthopaedics and Sports Trauma,
Associate Professor of Orthopaedic Surgery,
Cincinnati Children's Hospital Medical Center,
University of Cincinnati School of Medicine,
Cincinnati, Ohio

SAQIB REHMAN, MD – *Trauma*
Director of Orthopaedic Trauma, Associate
Professor of Orthopaedic Surgery and Sports
Medicine, School of Medicine, Temple
University Hospital, Temple University,
Philadelphia, Pennsylvania

GILES R. SCUDERI, MD – *Adult Reconstruction*
Vice President, Orthopedic Service Line,
Northshore Long Island Jewish Health
System; Fellowship Director, Adult Knee
Reconstruction Lenox Hill Hospital, New York,
New York

FELASFA M. WODAJO, MD – *Oncology*
Musculoskeletal Tumor Surgery, Inova
Fairfax Hospital, Fairfax, Virginia; Associate
Professor, Orthopedic Surgery, VCU School of
Medicine, Inova Campus; Assistant Professor,
Orthopedic Surgery, Georgetown University
Hospital, Arlington, Virginia

AUTHORS

MICHAEL C. AIN, MD
Department of Orthopaedic Surgery, The
Johns Hopkins University, Baltimore,
Maryland

MAMUN AL-RASHID, MD, FRCS (Orth)
Clinical Fellow, Musculoskeletal Oncology,
Orthopaedic Oncology Service, Department of
Orthopaedic Surgery, Massachusetts General
Hospital; Beth Israel Deaconess Medical
Center, Harvard Medical School, Boston,
Massachusetts

JOHN H. ALEXANDER, MD
Department of Orthopaedics, The Ohio State
University, Columbus, Ohio

JOHN W. BARRINGTON, MD
Plano Orthopedic Sports Medicine and Spine
Center, Plano, Texas

WALTER B. BEAVER, MD
OrthoCarolina Hip and Knee Center, Charlotte,
North Carolina

M. TYRRELL BURRUS, MD
Division of Orthopaedic Trauma, Department
of Orthopaedic Surgery, University of Virginia
Health System, Charlottesville, Virginia

JOURDAN M. CANCIENNE, MD
Division of Orthopaedic Trauma, Department
of Orthopaedic Surgery, University of Virginia
Health System, Charlottesville, Virginia

JEFFREY J. CHERIAN, DO
Rubin Institute for Advanced Orthopedics,
Center for Joint Preservation and
Replacement, Sinai Hospital of Baltimore,
Baltimore, Maryland

JACOB J. COLEMAN, BS
Providence Health and Services, Orthopedic
Institute, Portland, Oregon

KUROSH DARVISH, PhD
Department of Mechanical Engineering,
Temple University, Philadelphia, Pennsylvania

PAUL J. DUWELIUS, MD
Orthopedic + Fracture Specialists, Providence
St. Vincent Medical Center, Portland, Oregon

RANDA D.K. ELMALLAH, MD
Rubin Institute for Advanced Orthopedics,
Center for Joint Preservation and
Replacement, Sinai Hospital of Baltimore,
Baltimore, Maryland

ROGER H. EMERSON Jr, MD
Texas Center for Joint Replacement, Plano,
Texas

SIMCHA G. FICHMAN, MD
Division of Orthopaedic Surgery, Mount Sinai
Hospital, Toronto, Ontario, Canada

JOHN R. FOWLER, MD
Department of Orthopaedic Surgery, University
of Pittsburgh, Pittsburgh, Pennsylvania

JUAN M. GIUGALE, MD
Department of Orthopaedic Surgery, University
of Pittsburgh, Pittsburgh, Pennsylvania

MATTHEW GUNTON, MD, FRCSC
Division of Orthopaedic Surgery, Mount Sinai
Hospital, Toronto, Ontario, Canada

CHRISTINA GUTOWSKI, MD, MPH
Department of Orthopaedic Surgery, Thomas
Jefferson University, Philadelphia,
Pennsylvania

JARED L. HARWOOD, MD
Department of Orthopaedics, The Ohio State
University, Columbus, Ohio

FRANCIS J. HORNICEK, MD, PhD
Professor of Orthopaedic Surgery,
Orthopaedic Oncology Service, Department of
Orthopaedic Surgery, Massachusetts General
Hospital, Harvard Medical School, Boston,
Massachusetts

ASIF M. ILYAS, MD
Program Director of Hand Surgery Fellowship,
Rothman Institute; Associate Professor of
Orthopaedic Surgery, Jefferson Medical
College, Philadelphia, Pennsylvania

JUSTIN A. IORIO, MD
Department of Orthopaedic Surgery,
Temple University Hospital, Philadelphia,
Pennsylvania

ANDRE M. JAKOI, MD
Department of Orthopaedic Surgery, Drexel
University, Philadelphia, Pennsylvania

CHRISTOPHER M. JONES, MD
Department of Orthopaedic Surgery, Rothman
Institute, Thomas Jefferson University,
Philadelphia, Pennsylvania

AIDIN KASHIGAR, BSc, MD
Division of Orthopaedic Surgery, Mount Sinai
Hospital, Toronto, Ontario, Canada

KEVIN KLINGELE, MD
Department of Orthopedics, Nationwide
Children's Hospital, Columbus, Ohio

INDRANIL KUSHARE, MBBS, DNB
Department of Orthopedics, Nationwide
Children's Hospital, Columbus, Ohio

PAUL R.T. KUZYK, MD, MASc, FRCSC
Division of Orthopaedic Surgery, Mount Sinai
Hospital, Toronto, Ontario, Canada

JAMES R. LACHMAN, MD
Resident, Department of Orthopaedic
Surgery and Sports Medicine, PGY-3,
Temple University Hospital, Philadelphia,
Pennsylvania

FREDERIC E. LISS, MD
Department of Orthopaedic Surgery, Rothman
Institute, Thomas Jefferson University,
Philadelphia, Pennsylvania

SCOTT LOVALD, PhD, MBA
Exponent, Inc, Menlo Park, California

SANTIAGO A. LOZANO-CALDERÓN, MD, PhD
Instructor of Orthopaedic Surgery, Orthopaedic Oncology Service, Department of Orthopaedic Surgery, Massachusetts General Hospital; Beth Israel Deaconess Medical Center, Harvard Medical School, Boston, Massachusetts

TATU J. MÄKINEN, MD, PhD
Division of Orthopaedic Surgery, Mount Sinai Hospital, Toronto, Ontario, Canada

LAURA MATSEN KO, MD
Orthopedic + Fracture Specialists, Providence St. Vincent Medical Center, Portland, Oregon

JOEL L. MAYERSON, MD
Department of Orthopaedics, The Ohio State University, Columbus, Ohio

CHARLES T. MEHLMAN, DO, MPH
Division of Pediatric Orthopaedic Surgery, Cincinnati Children's Hospital Medical Center, Cincinnati, Ohio

MICHAEL A. MONT, MD
Rubin Institute for Advanced Orthopedics, Center for Joint Preservation and Replacement, Sinai Hospital of Baltimore, Baltimore, Maryland

OLUSEUN OLUGBODE, MS
Texas Center for Joint Replacement, Plano, Texas

KEVIN ONG, PhD
Exponent, Inc, Philadelphia, Pennsylvania

TODD P. PIERCE, MD
Rubin Institute for Advanced Orthopedics, Center for Joint Preservation and Replacement, Sinai Hospital of Baltimore, Baltimore, Maryland

PAUL S. PIPITONE, DO
Associate Professor, Department of Orthopaedic Surgery, Nassau University Medical Center, East Meadow, New York

DIPAK B. RAMKUMAR, MD
Resident, Department of Orthopaedic Surgery, Dartmouth-Hitchcock Medical Center, Lebanon, New Hampshire

KEVIN RASKIN, MD
Assistant Professor of Orthopaedic Surgery, Orthopaedic Oncology Service, Department of Orthopaedic Surgery, Massachusetts General Hospital, Harvard Medical School, Boston, Massachusetts

SAQIB REHMAN, MD
Director of Orthopaedic Trauma, Associate Professor of Orthopaedic Surgery and Sports Medicine, School of Medicine, Temple University Hospital, Temple University, Philadelphia, Pennsylvania

OLEG SAFIR, MD, MEd, FRCSC
Division of Orthopaedic Surgery, Mount Sinai Hospital, Toronto, Ontario, Canada

WALTER SAMORA, MD
Department of Orthopedics, Nationwide Children's Hospital, Columbus, Ohio

THOMAS J. SCHARSCHMIDT, MD
Department of Orthopaedics, The Ohio State University, Columbus, Ohio

JOSEPH SCHWAB, MD, MS
Assistant Professor of Orthopaedic Surgery, Orthopaedic Oncology Service, Department of Orthopaedic Surgery, Massachusetts General Hospital, Harvard Medical School, Boston, Massachusetts

STEPHEN C. SIZER, DO
Rubin Institute for Advanced Orthopedics, Center for Joint Preservation and Replacement, Sinai Hospital of Baltimore, Baltimore, Maryland

VENESSA STAS, MD
Orthopedic + Fracture Specialists, Providence St. Vincent Medical Center, Portland, Oregon

JACOB TULIPAN, MD
Department of Orthopaedic Surgery, Thomas Jefferson University, Philadelphia, Pennsylvania

PATRICK J. WARD, MD
Department of Orthopaedic Surgery, University of Pittsburgh, Pittsburgh, Pennsylvania

HEATHER WATSON, PhD
Exponent, Inc, Menlo Park, California

DAVID B. WEISS, MD
Division of Orthopaedic Trauma,
Department of Orthopaedic Surgery, University
of Virginia Health System, Charlottesville,
Virginia

SETH R. YARBORO, MD
Assistant Professor, Division of Orthopaedic
Trauma, Department of Orthopaedic Surgery,
University of Virginia Health System,
Charlottesville, Virginia

Contents

Adult Reconstruction

The mainstay of treatment of pertrochanteric fractures is internal fixation using a sliding hip screw or a cephalomedullary device. However, in patients with ipsilateral hip osteoarthritis or avascular necrosis of the femoral head, or inflammatory arthritis, arthroplasty should be considered as the primary treatment modality to reduce the likelihood of a secondary procedure. Unstable fracture patterns with concomitant poor bone quality represent a challenge for internal fixation, with high rates of lag screw cut-out and hardware failure. Prosthetic replacement for unstable pertrochanteric fractures has therefore been considered as an alternative primary treatment option. Further prospective randomized trials are required.

Marked blood loss during lower extremity total joint arthroplasties may lead to higher rates of transfusion, which may negatively affect surgical outcomes and yield greater complication rates. It is therefore ideal to identify factors that may increase the likelihood of blood loss, so they can be modified. From this review, it can be concluded that preoperative anemia, older age, multiple comorbidities, increased operative time, and use of postoperative anticoagulation may lead to higher blood loss and transfusion rates, although the influence of other factors remains controversial.

Corrosion of modular components at the femoral neck remains a complication of total hip arthroplasty (THA). The authors have found the iliopsoas sign (pain on resisted flexion of the hip) to be suggestive of femoral component corrosion. These cases represented 8 of 120 revision hip arthroplasties (7%) performed at the authors' institution. After the revisions, all iliopsoas tendonitis symptoms resolved. Based on the authors' experience and the recent literature, they recommend that the iliopsoas sign or presentation of a sterile iliopsoas abscess in a previously well-functioning THA be concern for corrosion of the femoral component of the total hip.

Pain after total joint arthroplasty (TJA) can be severe and difficult to control. A single-dose local analgesic delivers bupivacaine in a liposomal time-release platform. In 2248 consecutive patients with hip and knee arthroplasty, half (Pre) were treated using a well-established multimodal analgesia, including periarticular injection (PAI), and half had the PAI substituted for a liposomal bupivacaine injection technique (Post). Pain scores were significantly lower for patients in the Post group for both hip and knee procedures. A large series of patients who had TJA experienced pain relief after the introduction of liposomal bupivacaine as part of an established multimodal protocol.

Trauma

Knee dislocations are catastrophic injuries that demand emergent evaluation and often require a multidisciplinary approach. Long-term outcome studies are relatively scarce secondary to the variability in any given study population and the wide variety of injury patterns between knee dislocations. Multiple controversies exist with regard to outcomes using various treatment methods (early vs late intervention, graft selection, repair vs reconstruction of medial and lateral structures, rehabilitation regimens). Careful clinical evaluation is essential when knee dislocation is suspected.

Local antibiotics have a role in orthopedic trauma for both infection prophylaxis and treatment. They provide the advantage of high local antibiotic concentration without excessive systemic levels. Nonabsorbable polymethylmethacrylate (PMMA) is a popular antibiotic carrier, but absorbable options including bone graft, bone graft substitutes, and polymers have gained acceptance. Simple aqueous antibiotic solutions continue to be investigated and appear to be clinically effective. For established infections, such as osteomyelitis, a combination of surgical debridement with local and systemic antibiotics seems to represent the most effective treatment at this time. Further investigation of more effective local antibiotic utilization is ongoing.

Percutaneous sacroiliac (SI) screw fixation is indicated for unstable posterior pelvic ring injuries, sacral fractures, and SI joint dislocations. This article provides a review of indications and contraindications, preoperative planning, imaging techniques and relevant anatomy, surgical technique, complications and their management, and outcomes after SI screw insertion.

Pediatrics

Orthopedic surgeons frequently encounter short statured patients. A systematic approach is needed for proper evaluation of these children. The differential diagnosis includes both proportionate and disproportionate short stature types. A proper history and physical examination and judicious use of plain film radiography will establish the diagnosis in most cases. In addition to the orthopedic surgeon, most of these patients will also be evaluated by other specialists, including endocrinologists and geneticists. This article provides an overview of the evaluation of the child with short stature and offers several illustrative examples.

Discoid lateral meniscus is a common abnormal meniscal variant in children. Detailed history and physical examination combined with an MRI of the knee predictably diagnose a discoid meniscus. The clinical presentation varies from being asymptomatic to snapping, locking, and causing severe pain and swelling of the knee. Because of the pathologic anatomy and instability, discoid menisci are more prone to tearing. Treatment options for symptomatic patients vary based on the type of anomaly, the age of the patient, stability, and the presence or absence of a tear. Improvements in arthroscopic equipment and technique have resulted in good to excellent short-term outcomes for saucerization and repair.

Upper Extremity

Although the decision for operative versus nonoperative treatment of distal radius fractures remains subjective and is performed on a case-by-case basis, evaluation and treatment of patients with concomitant osteoporosis requires understanding of the behavior of this injury as a distinct subset of distal radius fractures. Age, infirmity, and osteoporosis affect every aspect of the fracture. Understanding what makes these fractures unique assists surgeons in more effective and efficient treatment. The authors present the current understanding of osteoporotic fragility fractures of the distal radius, focusing on epidemiology, biomechanics of bone healing, and its implication on strategies for management.

Left untreated, scapholunate dissociation can lead to posttraumatic wrist arthritis. Multiple surgical procedures have been designed to reduce the scapholunate interval, restore normal wrist kinematics, and prevent the development of arthritis. Unfortunately, current surgical procedures have not been shown to consistently maintain radiographic alignment at long-term follow-up and result in decreased wrist range of motion and strength compared with the contralateral side. The purpose of this article is to review the current reconstructive options for scapholunate ligament tears without evidence of radiographic arthritis.

Trigger fingers are common tendinopathies representing a stenosing flexor tenosynovitis of the fingers. Adult trigger finger can be treated nonsurgically using activity modification, splinting, and/or corticosteroid injections. Surgical treatment options include percutaneous A1 pulley release and open A1 pulley release. Excision of a slip of the flexor digitorum superficialis is reserved for patients with persistent triggering despite A1 release or patients with persistent flexion contracture. Pediatric trigger thumb is treated with open A1 pulley release. Pediatric trigger finger is treated with release of the A1 pulley with excision of a slip or all of the flexor digitorum superficialis if triggering persists.

The purpose of this study is to investigate the failure sequence of the distal radius during a simulated fall onto an outstretched hand using cadaver forearms and high-speed X ray and video systems. This apparatus records the beginning and propagation of bony failure, ultimately resulting in distal radius or forearm fracture. The effects of 3 different wrist guard designs are investigated using this system. Serving as a proof-of-concept analysis, this study supports this imaging technique to be used in larger studies of orthopedic trauma and protective devices and specifically for distal radius fractures.

Oncology

The current understanding of Paget disease of bone (PDB) has vastly changed since Paget described the first case in 1877. Medical management of this condition remains the mainstay of treatment. Surgical intervention is usually only used in fractures through pagetic bone, need for realignment to correct deformity in major long bones, prophylactic treatment of impending fractures, joint arthroplasty in severe arthritis, or spinal decompression in cases of bony compression of neural elements. Advances in surgical technique have allowed early return to function and mobilization. Despite medical intervention, a small subset of patients with PDB develops Paget sarcoma.

Targeted Chemotherapy in Bone and Soft-Tissue Sarcoma 587

Jared L. Harwood, John H. Alexander, Joel L. Mayerson, and Thomas J. Scharschmidt

Historically surgical intervention has been the mainstay of therapy for bone and soft-tissue sarcomas, augmented with adjuvant radiation for local control. Although cytotoxic chemotherapy revolutionized the treatment of many sarcomas, classic treatment regimens are fraught with side effects while outcomes have plateaued. However, since the approval of imatinib in 2002, research into targeted chemotherapy has increased exponentially. With targeted therapies comes the potential for decreased side effects and more potent, personalized treatment options. This article reviews the evolution of medical knowledge regarding sarcoma, the basic science of sarcomatogenesis, and the major targets and pathways now being studied.

Adult Reconstruction

Preface

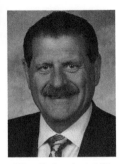

Giles R. Scuderi, MD
Editor

In this issue of *Orthopedic Clinics of North America*, we have several articles that review current topics in joint arthroplasty. In the first article, Dr Mäkinen and coauthors report on total hip arthroplasty for pertrochanteric hip fractures. In patients with hip osteoarthritis, inflammatory arthritis, or osteonecrosis of the femoral head with an unstable ipsilateral pertrochanteric hip fracture, these authors found that total hip arthroplasty appears to be a reliable option when compared with internal fixation.

Realizing that blood management is an important factor in postoperative recovery following total joint arthroplasty, Dr Sizer and coauthors report on predicting blood loss in total knee and hip arthroplasty. Utilizing predictive patient factors with a strict postoperative transfusion protocol, these authors establish a safer and more successful perioperative experience for total joint arthroplasty patients.

Knowing that preoperative evaluation is important for determining the cause of pain and failure following total hip arthroplasty, Dr Coleman reports on iliopsoas irritation as presentation of head-neck corrosion after total hip arthroplasty.

The iliopsoas sign, pain with resisted flexion of the hip, or the presence of a sterile iliopsoas abscess in a previously successful total hip arthroplasty is suggestive of femoral component corrosion. Following revision total hip arthroplasty, all iliopsoas symptoms resolved.

Finally, in the last article in this section, Dr Barrington reports on their multimodal approach with periarticular injections for the management of postoperative pain following total joint arthroplasty. Current multimodal analgesia protocols include periarticular injections with various medications and combination of medications. These authors found improved scores with the introduction of liposomal bupivacaine in their multimodal protocol for total joint arthroplasty.

I hope that surgeons find these articles useful in the treatment of their total joint patients.

Giles R. Scuderi, MD
210 East 64th Street
New York, NY 10065, USA

E-mail address:
gscuderi@nshs.edu

Orthop Clin N Am 46 (2015) xv
http://dx.doi.org/10.1016/j.ocl.2015.07.001
0030-5898/15/$ – see front matter © 2015 Published by Elsevier Inc.

orthopedic.theclinics.com

Arthroplasty for Pertrochanteric Hip Fractures

Tatu J. Mäkinen, MD, PhD*, Matthew Gunton, MD, FRCSC,
Simcha G. Fichman, MD, Aidin Kashigar, BSc, MD,
Oleg Safir, MD, MEd, FRCSC, Paul R.T. Kuzyk, MD, MASc, FRCSC

KEYWORDS

- Pertrochanteric fracture • Unstable hip fracture • Ipsilateral hip osteoarthritis • Hip arthroplasty
- Trochanteric slide osteotomy

KEY POINTS

- The mainstay of treatment of pertrochanteric fractures is internal fixation using a sliding hip screw or a cephalomedullary device.
- Arthroplasty should be considered as a primary treatment modality in patients with ipsilateral hip osteoarthritis or avascular necrosis of the femoral head, inflammatory arthritis, unstable fracture patterns with poor bone quality, or neglected fractures.
- Trochanteric slide osteotomy preserves the abductor mechanism and the posterior structures of the hip.
- Cemented stems with or without calcar replacement, uncemented extensive porous-coated cylindrical stems, or uncemented tapered stems can be used to reconstruct the femur.
- Arthroplasty is associated with higher postoperative blood transfusion rates, but a shorter time to weight bearing and a lower failure rate.

INTRODUCTION

Hip fractures remain a leading cause of morbidity and mortality in an aging population and are projected to reach 289,000 cases/y in the United States by 2030.[1] Hospital and rehabilitation needs and loss of patient mobility and independence account for a significant burden to the health care system. Pertrochanteric fractures account for half of all hip fractures in the elderly. Compared with femoral neck fractures, pertrochanteric fractures tend to occur in older patients with worse baseline function and greater medical comorbidities.[2,3] Approximately 50% to 60% of pertrochanteric fractures are considered unstable, increasing the technical difficulty of internal fixation.[4] Despite significant advances in internal fixation methods and implants there remains a significant failure rate of fixation in unstable pertrochanteric fractures (Fig. 1).[5–8] Failed pertrochanteric fracture fixation is associated with significant loss of mobility with additional morbidity, mortality, and costs. The goals of care for patients with pertrochanteric fractures include expeditious and safe surgical stabilization to enable rapid mobilization and avoidance of medical complications. Arthroplasty may be considered an effective alternate treatment to internal fixation and may be associated with improved early mobilization and lower failure rates.

Disclosure: The authors have nothing to disclose.
Division of Orthopaedic Surgery, Mount Sinai Hospital, 600 University Avenue, Toronto, Ontario M5G 1X5, Canada
* Corresponding author.
E-mail address: tatu.makinen@hus.fi

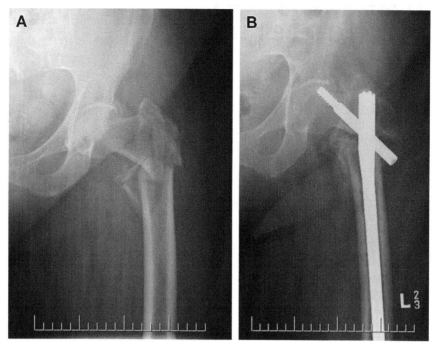

Fig. 1. Preoperative radiograph (*A*) of an unstable pertrochanteric hip fracture (reverse oblique) treated with cephalomedullary nail. Fixation went on to fail with lag screw cut-out (*B*).

INDICATIONS

Arthroplasty should be considered as a primary treatment option in a carefully selected and small patient population with pertrochanteric fractures (**Box 1**). Patients with preexisting hip osteoarthritis, inflammatory arthritis, or avascular necrosis are good candidates for total hip arthroplasty even at younger ages because it reduces the likelihood of subsequent reoperations. In these patients, the diminished range of motion of the hip joint increases the loads at the fracture site, possibly increasing the failure rate of internal fixation. In low-functioning elderly patients (age >75 years) with unstable fracture pattern and poor bone quality, arthroplasty may be particularly useful to avoid the extended periods of protected weight bearing required when there is tenuous internal fixation. Appropriate fracture features include grossly unstable fracture patterns, marked fracture comminution, poor bone quality shown by thin cortices and wide intramedullary canal, and significant fracture displacement indicating a more severe insult to surrounding soft tissue structures.

IDENTIFICATION OF UNSTABLE FRACTURES

Identifying a fracture pattern as unstable is of great importance because these fractures have a high failure rate with internal fixation.[9] Although often impractical in the preoperative setting, an anteroposterior view with internal rotation and gentle traction offers the best assessment of ease of reduction and instability.[4] Computed tomography scan of the hip may provide further information on the number and displacement of fracture fragments. Multiple classifications systems have been devised to guide treatment. Evans[10] (1949) was the first to classify pertrochanteric fractures based on stability. The orthopaedic trauma association (OTA) classification system, based on the arbeitsgemeinschaft für osteosynthesefragen (AO) comprehensive classification, is probably the most commonly used classification for

---

Box 1
Indications for arthroplasty in pertrochanteric fractures

Ipsilateral hip osteoarthritis

Ipsilateral avascular necrosis of the femoral head

Inflammatory arthritis

Unstable fracture pattern with poor bone quality

Complications of internal fixation (ie, lag screw cut-out)

Neglected fractures

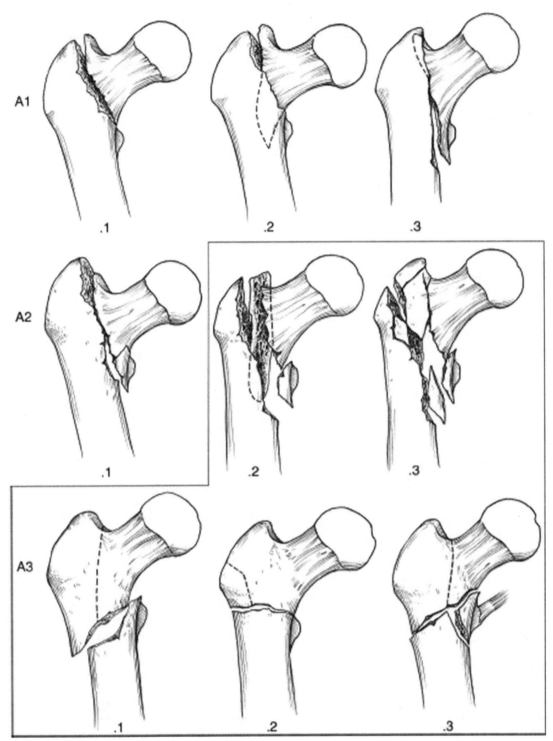

Fig. 2. AO/OTA classification of unstable pertrochanteric hip fractures. Types A2.2, A2.3, A3.1, A3.2, and A3.3 are considered as unstable fractures.

pertrochanteric fractures (**Fig. 2**).[11] This system classifies fractures based on number and orientation of fracture lines but does not account for displacement or fracture alignment. Unstable OTA fracture types are those with extensive posteromedial comminution and reverse oblique or subtrochanteric fracture lines (ie, AO/OTA types A2.2, A2.3, A3.1, A3.2, and A3.3). Other fracture features indicating instability and high rate of internal fixation failure are varus alignment and gross displacement.[9] The hallmarks of poor bone quality in plain radiographs include thin cortices and cylindrical shape of the femoral canal.[12]

SURGICAL TECHNIQUES
Surgical Approach

Surgeon preference and experience as well as fracture pattern are important considerations when deciding on an approach for arthroplasty in the setting of an unstable pertrochanteric fracture. The most commonly used hip arthroplasty approaches, direct lateral (or modified Hardinge) and posterior approaches are acceptable choices and carry the advantage of familiarity to the surgeon.[13] Each of these approaches has its own distinct disadvantages in the setting of an unstable fracture pattern: the direct lateral approach may cause further insult to the injured abductor musculature, whereas the posterior approach may be complicated by postoperative instability. A modified trochanteric slide osteotomy is an alternative approach that is useful when the greater trochanter is fractured, and carries advantages of preserved abductor mechanism and posterior structures.[14] Regardless the approach selected, the patient is positioned in the lateral decubitus position and prepped such that the contralateral knee can be palpated through the drapes to give a reference for leg lengths. Our protocol has been to use a trochanteric slide osteotomy unless the greater trochanter and lateral wall of the femur remains intact (ie, type A1 and A2.1 fractures), in which case we use a transgluteal approach.

Modified Trochanteric Slide Osteotomy

Unstable pertrochanteric fractures with fracture lines running to or below the rough line of the greater trochanter (AO/OTA types A2.2, A2.3, and A3.1–3.3) are particularly amenable to approach with a modified trochanteric slide osteotomy. Popular in revision hip arthroplasty and complex primary hip arthroplasty, a trochanteric slide osteotomy uses existing fracture lines while maintaining the continuity of the abductors, greater trochanter, and vastus lateralis. This technique uses a laterally based approach to the hip with a coronal oriented osteotomy commencing lateral to the insertion of the posterior capsule and external rotators (**Fig. 3**A). In most cases, the trochanter is fractured off as a separate fragment, so an osteotomy may not be required. The piriformis is easily palpated and remains medial to the osteotomy, thereby preserving the external rotators. The osteotomized trochanter with attached glutei and vastus lateralis are retracted anteriorly after reflection of minimus off the hip capsule (see **Fig. 3**B). The remaining femoral shaft is externally rotated and an anterior capsulotomy is performed, providing excellent access to the fractured femoral head and neck (**Fig. 4**A). The femoral head and neck is then removed from the acetabulum by releasing its capsular attachments and the ligamentum teres (see **Fig. 4**B).

Implant Choice

Cemented and uncemented prostheses are available and have both been used with success for unstable pertrochanteric fractures. Cemented implants offer the advantage of immediate stability without the need for bone ingrowth and show acceptable middle-term to long-term results with modern cementing techniques.[15] Cemented stems are recommended in patients with very thin cortical bone in the femoral diaphysis, making insertion of uncemented diaphyseal fitting stems difficult and increasing the risk of periprosthetic fracture (**Fig. 5**A). Comminuted pertrochanteric fractures generally have significant proximal femoral bone loss and therefore we favor a cemented implant with a calcar-replacement option (see **Fig. 5**B).

The major disadvantage of cemented prostheses is bone cement implantation syndrome, which is characterized by perioperative events such as hypotension, hypoxia, and confusion.[16] Cement implantation syndrome occurring in the setting of cemented hemiarthroplasty for pertrochanteric fractures has an intraoperative mortality of 1.6%.[17] Patients with impaired cardiopulmonary function are at particular risk of complications from cementing procedures.[18] Cement fixation also generally adds 20 to 30 minutes to the procedure. Furthermore, healing of the trochanteric fracture or osteotomy may be compromised by the presence of cement within the proximal femur.

Uncemented femoral stems have been used extensively in the treatment of Vancouver B2 and B3 periprosthetic femoral fractures.[19] Uncemented fixation has gained popularity for the treatment of hip fractures in general, and offers the advantage of avoiding cement-related complications in this vulnerable patient population. Other advantages include reduced operative time and blood loss.

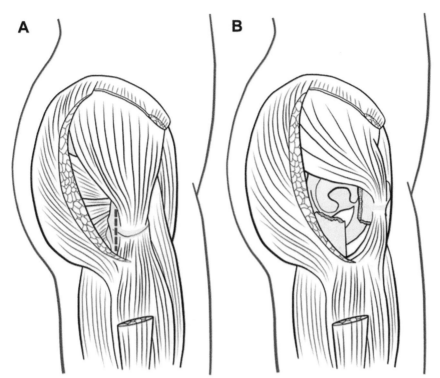

Fig. 3. Trochanteric slide osteotomy with fascia lata and gluteus maximus removed. Osteotomy (*dotted red line*) is performed superficial to the insertion of the piriformis and short external rotators (*A*). The trochanteric osteotomy with attached gluteus medius and vastus lateralis is retracted anteriorly to expose the hip capsule (*B*).

Several recent randomized controlled trials studying intracapsular hip fractures report excellent short-term results and equivalency to cemented hemiarthroplasty with regard to functional outcome, complications, and mortality.[20–22] Common concerns regarding the use of uncemented components in the fracture setting include thigh pain and higher risk of periprosthetic fracture (**Box 2**).[23]

Pertrochanteric fractures may present specific challenges with respect to proximal femoral bone loss because many uncemented prostheses rely on metaphyseal fit. In situations in which the metaphysis is significantly disrupted or unreliable (as is often the case with unstable pertrochanteric fractures), a femoral revision stem is required that relies on diaphyseal fixation. These revision stems are generally either cylindrical (**Fig. 6**) or tapered (**Fig. 7**) in shape. Tapered stems have been shown to have lower rates of stem failure and improved bone on-growth compared with cylindrical stems when used in the revision total hip setting.[24] Modular stems may be considered rather than monoblock stems because these stems allow for impaction of the distal stem until it is stable and then the overall femoral component length, version, and offset maybe adjusted through the proximal body.

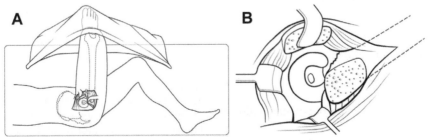

Fig. 4. The leg is externally rotated and placed in a sterile leg bag to provide excellent visualization of the fractured femoral head and neck (*A*). The fractured head and neck may be removed from the acetabulum with the greater trochanter retracted anterior and the femoral shaft retracted posterior (*B*).

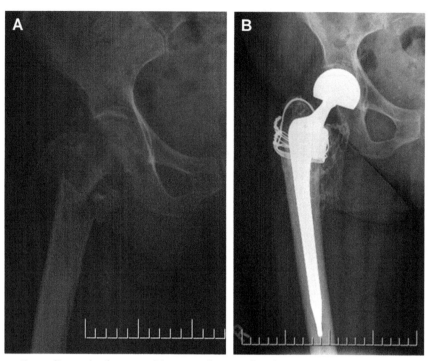

Fig. 5. Preoperative radiograph of an unstable pertrochanteric hip fracture (reverse oblique) with thin femoral cortices (*A*). Postoperative radiograph showing treatment with a cemented calcar replacing femoral stem (*B*). A trochanteric slide osteotomy was used for the approach and the osteotomy was repaired using cerclage wires.

Abductor Mechanism Repair

Cerclage wire or cable fixation of trochanteric fragments or osteotomized bone is suitable when the remaining trochanter is of sufficient size and quality. Alternatively, multiple trochanteric plate options exist, such as a hook plate, but these may be complicated by significant soft tissue irritation and bursitis should nonunion occur. Occasionally, nonabsorbable suture fixation may be required when the bone fragments are too small, comminuted, or osteoporotic for any other type of fixation. Despite efforts to repair the fractured trochanter, trochanteric escape is a frequent complication with both arthroplasty and internal fixation management techniques, but it is well tolerated and often asymptomatic in the elderly, lower functioning hip fracture population.

The decision regarding the use of total hip arthroplasty or hemiarthroplasty depends on the underlying hip joint disorder. If the patient has severe ipsilateral hip osteoarthritis or inflammatory joint disease, a total hip arthroplasty is the preferred option. In geriatric patients without significant acetabular involvement, hemiarthroplasty is usually sufficient. Hemiarthroplasty is also inherently more stable because of the large head size of the articulation.

POSTOPERATIVE CARE

All patients should receive some form of deep vein thrombosis prophylaxis (mechanical and/or pharmacologic) according to the current recommendations.[25] Patients are encouraged to mobilize early with assistance of physiotherapy and are allowed to weight bear as tolerated on postoperative day 1. If a trochanteric slide osteotomy is used, active leg abduction is restricted for 8 weeks to allow for healing of the abductor mechanism. Clinical and radiographic follow-up is maintained at 6-week intervals to assess the union of the osteotomy. Hip precautions are maintained for a total of 3 months.

Box 2
Femoral component options

Cemented stem with or without calcar replacement

Uncemented extensively porous-coated cylindrical stem

Uncemented monoblock tapered stem

Uncemented modular tapered stem

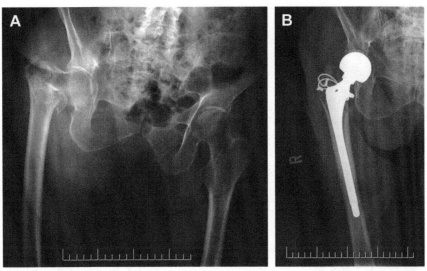

Fig. 6. Preoperative radiograph of an unstable pertrochanteric hip fracture with fairly well-preserved metaphyseal bone and good diaphyseal bone stock (*A*). Postoperative radiograph showing treatment with an uncemented, extensively porous-coated, cylindrical femoral stem (*B*).

OUTCOMES

There is a lack of high-level evidence for the use of arthroplasty for unstable pertrochanteric fractures. Only 2 randomized controlled trials and a limited number of prospective and retrospective comparative studies have been published (**Table 1**).

In terms of randomized controlled trials, Kim and colleagues[26] investigated the use of a cephalomedullary nail with an antirotation screw (Proximal Femoral Nail, Mathys Medical, Bettlach, Switzerland) compared with a long-stem cementless calcar-replacement hemiarthroplasty (Mallory-Head calcar-replacement stem; Biomet, Bridgend, United Kingdom). The patient population was limited to patients aged 75 years or older with a pertrochanteric fracture classified as AO/OTA 31.A2, Evans type III, or Evans type IV. A total of 58 patients were studied, with half of these patients treated using proximal femoral nails and the other half with long-stem cementless calcar-replacement prosthesis. The study showed no

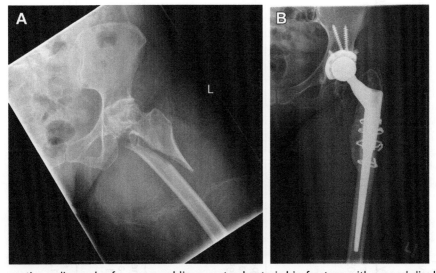

Fig. 7. Preoperative radiograph of a reverse oblique pertrochanteric hip fracture with a good diaphyseal bone stock. The patient had an avascular necrosis of the ipsilateral femoral head (*A*). Follow-up radiograph showing treatment with an uncemented, tapered, modular femoral stem (*B*).

Table 1
Overview of the literature published on arthroplasty for unstable intertrochanteric hip fractures

Study	Study Design	Number of Patients and Inclusion Criteria	Internal Fixation Group	Arthroplasty Group	Outcomes
Kim et al,[26] 2005	Level I Randomized	n = 58 Age >75 y AO 31.A2, Evans III/IV	Proximal femoral nail	Long-stem cementless calcar-replacement prosthesis (Mallory-Head calcar-replacement stem, Biomet)	No significant difference in functional outcomes, hospital stay, time to weight bearing, or general complications Shorter operative time, less blood loss, fewer units of blood transfused, lower mortality, and lower hospital costs with internal fixation
Stappaerts et al,[9] 1995	Level I Randomized	n = 90 Age >70 y AO 31.A2 Nonarthritic hip	Dynamic hip screw	Cemented VDP endoprosthesis	No significant difference in operating time, wound complications, mortalities, functional capacity at time of discharge, mechanical complications, need for reoperation Higher failure rate (redisplacement, total collapse) with internal fixation Higher transfusion rate with arthroplasty
Bonnevialle et al,[30] 2011	Level II Prospective Comparative Multicenter	n = 247 Age >75 y AO 31.A2.2, A3.1, A.3.3	Short or long locking nail (Gamma, Stryker)	Mixture of hemiarthroplasty and arthroplasty prosthesis	No significant difference in mortality Higher mechanical complication rate with internal fixation Better functional outcomes with arthroplasty
Shen et al,[31] 2012	Level II Prospective Comparative	n = 124 Age >70 y AO 31.A2.2/3, A3.1, A3.3	Dynamic hip screw or intramedullary nailing (Smith-Nephew; Weigao)	Bipolar hemiarthroplasty (DePuy/Johnson & Johnson; Union; Weigao)	No significant difference in mortality Shorter operating time, less blood loss and need for transfusion with internal fixation Improved functional outcome with satisfactory reduction, worsened functional outcome with unsatisfactory reduction compared with arthroplasty

Study	Design	Population	Fixation	Arthroplasty	Outcomes
Tang et al,[29] 2012	Level III Retrospective Comparative	n = 303 All intertrochanteric fractures (AO 31.A)	Proximal femoral nail antirotation	Hemiarthroplasty	No significant difference in functional outcome; Shorter operating time, less blood loss, fewer blood transfusions, shorter hospital stay, and lower mortality with internal fixation; Shorter time to weight bearing with arthroplasty
Sinno et al,[28] 2010	Level III Retrospective Comparative	n = 102 Age >70 y AO 31.A2, 31.A3	Dynamic hip screw	Bipolar prosthesis (DePuy International)	No significant difference in mortality; Shorter operating time, less blood transfusion, shorter time to full weight bearing, reduced rate of postoperative complications, and improved functional outcomes with arthroplasty
Broos et al,[32] 1991	Level III Retrospective Comparative	n = 287 Age >70 y AO 31.A2	Dynamic hip screw	Bipolar prosthesis or long spherostem total hip VDP endoprosthesis	No significant difference in operating time, blood loss, mortality, pain, major complications, or functional status
Broos et al,[33] 1989	Level III Retrospective Comparative	n = 157 Age >70 y	Ender nails or angled blade plate	Bipolar prosthesis or long spherostem total hip VDP endoprosthesis	No significant difference in mortality; Shorter operating time, less blood loss with bipolar hemiarthroplasty; Lower mechanical complication rates with arthroplasty
Claes et al,[27] 1985	Level III Retrospective Comparative	n = 168 Age >70 y All intertrochanteric fractures	Ender nails or blade plate (types unknown)	Endoprosthesis (types unknown)	Improved walking ability and reduced mechanical complications with arthroplasty

Abbreviation: VDP, Vandeputte.
Data from Refs.[9,26–33]

significant difference in functional outcome, time to weight bearing, or 1-year mortality. A shorter operative time, less blood loss, and lower 3-year mortality was seen with internal fixation. The finding of reduced 3-year mortality in the fixation group should be treated with caution because some patients were not followed beyond 2 years, cause of death between 1 and 3 years was not given, and there was no significant difference in the 1-year mortality. The study's 2 main limitations are a small sample size and the inclusion of potentially stable hip fractures. As previously discussed, not all fractures classified as 31.A2 are considered unstable; a portion of these fractures (eg, 31.A2.1) are easy to reduce and stabilized using internal fixation.

The second randomized controlled trial, by Stappaerts and colleagues,[9] investigated the use of a compression hip screw compared with a Vandeputte cemented endoprosthesis. A total of 90 patients were recruited, with the inclusion criteria being patients who were 70 years or older with a nonarthritic hip and a fracture that was classified as AO/OTA 31.A2. Forty-seven patients were treated with compression hip screws, whereas 43 underwent the insertion of a cemented endoprosthesis. The study showed no significant difference in mortalities, mechanical complications, or need for reoperation. With arthroplasty, there was a significantly shorter time to weight bearing. This finding is supported by several nonrandomized trials.[27–29] Internal fixation was associated with lower transfusion rate but with higher failure rate (including redisplacement and total collapse). Similar to Kim and colleagues,[26] this study was limited by a small sample size and the inclusion of all 31.A2 fractures, some of which may be considered as stable pertrochanteric fractures. Further, given the age of this study, the treatment option of compression hip screws is no longer considered the optimal method for unstable pertrochanteric fractures.

Parker and Handoll[23] combined the results of the 2 randomized controlled trials in a meta-analysis. There were important differences in interventions used between the 2 studies: cemented versus uncemented femoral stems in the arthroplasty groups and extramedullary versus intramedullary fixation in the fixation groups. Furthermore, the studies were too small to detect clear differences in mortality, morbidity, or function between the two treatments. Parker and Handoll[23] concluded from the pooled data that there was insufficient evidence to determine whether arthroplasty has any advantage compared with internal fixation for extracapsular femoral fractures. They suggested that further randomized controlled trials

were required with follow-up times longer than 2 years.

Apart from the randomized controlled trials, several nonrandomized prospective and retrospective studies have compared prosthesis with internal fixation methods. In a prospective multicenter study, Bonnevialle and colleagues[30] showed higher mechanical complication rates and lower functional outcomes with cephalomedullary nailing. Shen and colleagues[31] performed a prospective study that showed that, when a satisfactory reduction is performed with internal fixation for unstable intertrochanteric fractures in the elderly (ie, short tip-apex distance and similar femoral neck angulation to the contralateral hip), the patients benefit from improved functional outcomes compared with prosthesis.[31] However, it is challenging for the surgeon to determine preoperatively which fractures can be fixed in a satisfactory manner using internal fixation. In a retrospective study, Tang and colleagues[29] found no significant difference in long-term functional outcome or complication rates, reduced operating time, and reduced transfusion rate with cephalomedullary nailing, but a longer time to weight bearing compared with arthroplasty. Sinno and colleagues[28] retrospectively compared prosthesis with compression hip screws and showed a reduced time to weight bearing and improved functional outcome with arthroplasty. Several older studies have also investigated the use of arthroplasty for unstable pertrochanteric fractures, but the internal fixation methods reported in those articles are no longer commonly used for the treatment of these fracture types.[27,32,33]

Overall, there is a paucity of high-level studies in this area. Based on the current literature, compared with internal fixation, arthroplasty is associated with higher postoperative blood transfusion rates, no difference in long-term functional outcomes, but a potentially shorter time to weight bearing and a lower failure rate. Further prospective randomized trials are required in order to compare the functional outcomes of arthroplasty and internal fixation for unstable pertrochanteric fractures, allowing for larger patient sizes, longer follow-up periods, and improved identification of the subgroup of pertrochanteric fractures that would benefit from arthroplasty.

SUMMARY

Unstable pertrochanteric fractures can present a significant challenge to treating surgeons because of the difficulty of achieving stable fixation to allow early weight bearing. Despite adequate reduction and acceptable internal fixation, there still remains potential for hardware failure and need for revision surgery. Arthroplasty is an acceptable primary treatment option for carefully selected unstable intertrochanteric fractures, particularly for elderly patients with a fracture pattern that is unlikely to be reduced satisfactorily using internal fixation techniques. It is also beneficial for younger patients with underlying hip disorders, such as end-stage osteoarthritis, inflammatory arthritis, or avascular necrosis.

We caution that hip arthroplasty in the setting of pertrochanteric hip fracture is technically demanding and should be performed by an experienced arthroplasty surgeon. Surgeon preference, injury pattern, and bone quality help guide the choice of approach and selection of femoral stem for reconstruction. Cemented stems with calcar replacement are a good option for patients with thin femoral cortices, but surgeons must be wary of cement implantation syndrome. Uncemented stems relying on diaphyseal fixation are recommended when there are reasonably thick femoral cortices. Uncemented tapered modular revision stems are particularly useful because they allow for stable diaphyseal fixation with the femoral stem and the ability to easily adjust length, offset, and version through the modular body.

Arthroplasty may allow earlier mobilization and lower failure rates compared with internal fixation for unstable pertrochanteric fractures. Further prospective studies are required to compare these treatments and determine the specific fracture types that are best treated with arthroplasty.

REFERENCES

1. Stevens JA, Rudd RA. The impact of decreasing U.S. hip fracture rates on future hip fracture estimates. Osteoporos Int 2013;24(10):2725–8.
2. Koval KJ, Aharonoff GB, Rokito AS, et al. Patients with femoral neck and intertrochanteric fractures. Are they the same? Clin Orthop Relat Res 1996;(330):166–72.
3. Fox KM, Magaziner J, Hebel JR, et al. Intertrochanteric versus femoral neck hip fractures: differential characteristics, treatment, and sequelae. J Gerontol A Biol Sci Med Sci 1999;54(12):M635–40.
4. Lindskog DM, Baumgaertner MR. Unstable intertrochanteric hip fractures in the elderly. J Am Acad Orthop Surg 2004;12(3):179–90.
5. Zhang B, Chiu KY, Wang M. Hip arthroplasty for failed internal fixation of intertrochanteric fractures. J Arthroplasty 2004;19(3):329–33.
6. Hsu CJ, Chou WY, Chiou CP, et al. Hemi-arthroplasty with supplemental fixation of greater trochanter to treat failed hip screws of femoral intertrochanteric fracture. Arch Orthop Trauma Surg 2008;128(8):841–5.
7. Haidukewych GJ, Berry DJ. Hip arthroplasty for salvage of failed treatment of intertrochanteric hip fractures. J Bone Joint Surg Am 2003;85-A(5):899–904.
8. Kashigar A, Vincent A, Gunton MJ, et al. Predictors of failure for cephalomedullary nailing of proximal femoral fractures. Bone Joint J 2014;96-B(8):1029–34.
9. Stappaerts KH, Deldycke J, Broos PL, et al. Treatment of unstable peritrochanteric fractures in elderly patients with a compression hip screw or with the Vandeputte (VDP) endoprosthesis: a prospective randomized study. J Orthop Trauma 1995;9(4):292–7.
10. Evans EM. The treatment of trochanteric fractures of the femur. J Bone Joint Surg Br 1949;31B(2):190–203.
11. Marsh JL, Slongo TF, Agel J, et al. Fracture and dislocation classification compendium - 2007: Orthopaedic Trauma Association classification, database and outcomes committee. J Orthop Trauma 2007;21(10 Suppl):S1–133.
12. Sah AP, Thornhill TS, LeBoff MS, et al. Correlation of plain radiographic indices of the hip with quantitative bone mineral density. Osteoporos Int 2007;18(8):1119–26.
13. Chechik O, Khashan M, Lador R, et al. Surgical approach and prosthesis fixation in hip arthroplasty world wide. Arch Orthop Trauma Surg 2013;133(11):1595–600.
14. Goodman S, Pressman A, Saastamoinen H, et al. Modified sliding trochanteric osteotomy in revision total hip arthroplasty. J Arthroplasty 2004;19(8):1039–41.
15. Maurer SG, Baitner AC, Di Cesare PE. Reconstruction of the failed femoral component and proximal femoral bone loss in revision hip surgery. J Am Acad Orthop Surg 2000;8(6):354–63.
16. Donaldson AJ, Thomson HE, Harper NJ, et al. Bone cement implantation syndrome. Br J Anaesth 2009;102(1):12–22.
17. Parvizi J, Holiday AD, Ereth MH, et al. The Frank Stinchfield Award. Sudden death during primary hip arthroplasty. Clin Orthop Relat Res 1999;(369):39–48.
18. Herrenbruck T, Erickson EW, Damron TA, et al. Adverse clinical events during cemented long-stem femoral arthroplasty. Clin Orthop Relat Res 2002;(395):154–63.
19. Munro JT, Garbuz DS, Masri BA, et al. Tapered fluted titanium stems in the management of Vancouver B2 and B3 periprosthetic femoral fractures. Clin Orthop Relat Res 2014;472(2):590–8.
20. Figved W, Opland V, Frihagen F, et al. Cemented versus uncemented hemiarthroplasty for displaced

femoral neck fractures. Clin Orthop Relat Res 2009; 467(9):2426–35.

21. Deangelis JP, Ademi A, Staff I, et al. Cemented versus uncemented hemiarthroplasty for displaced femoral neck fractures: a prospective randomized trial with early follow-up. J Orthop Trauma 2012; 26(3):135–40.

22. Taylor F, Wright M, Zhu M. Hemiarthroplasty of the hip with and without cement: a randomized clinical trial. J Bone Joint Surg Am 2012;94(7):577–83.

23. Parker MJ, Handoll HH. Replacement arthroplasty versus internal fixation for extracapsular hip fractures in adults. Cochrane Database Syst Rev 2006;(2):CD000086.

24. Revision Total Hip Arthroplasty Study Group. A comparison of modular tapered versus modular cylindrical stems for complex femoral revisions. J Arthroplasty 2013;28(8 Suppl):71–3.

25. Falck-Ytter Y, Francis CW, Johanson NA, et al. Prevention of VTE in orthopedic surgery patients: Antithrombotic Therapy and Prevention of Thrombosis, 9th ed: American College of Chest Physicians Evidence-Based Clinical Practice Guidelines. Chest 2012; 141(2 Suppl):e278S–325S.

26. Kim SY, Kim YG, Hwang JK. Cementless calcar-replacement hemiarthroplasty compared with intramedullary fixation of unstable intertrochanteric fractures. A prospective, randomized study. J Bone Joint Surg Am 2005;87(10):2186–92.

27. Claes H, Broos P, Stappaerts K. Pertrochanteric fractures in elderly patients: treatment with Ender's nails, blade-plate or endoprosthesis? Injury 1985; 16(4):261–4.

28. Sinno K, Sakr M, Girard J, et al. The effectiveness of primary bipolar arthroplasty in treatment of unstable intertrochanteric fractures in elderly patients. N Am J Med Sci 2010;2(12):561–8.

29. Tang P, Hu F, Shen J, et al. Proximal femoral nail anti-rotation versus hemiarthroplasty: a study for the treatment of intertrochanteric fractures. Injury 2012; 43(6):876–81.

30. Bonnevialle P, Saragaglia D, Ehlinger M, et al. Trochanteric locking nail versus arthroplasty in unstable intertrochanteric fracture in patients aged over 75 years. Orthop Traumatol Surg Res 2011; 97(6 Suppl):S95–100.

31. Shen J, Wang DL, Chen GX, et al. Bipolar hemiarthroplasty compared with internal fixation for unstable intertrochanteric fractures in elderly patients. J Orthop Sci 2012;17(6):722–9.

32. Broos PL, Rommens PM, Deleyn PR, et al. Pertrochanteric fractures in the elderly: are there indications for primary prosthetic replacement? J Orthop Trauma 1991;5(4):446–51.

33. Broos PL, Willemsen PJ, Rommens PM, et al. Pertrochanteric fractures in elderly patients. Treatment with a long-stem/long-neck endoprosthesis. Unfallchirurgie 1989;92(5):234–9.

Predicting Blood Loss in Total Knee and Hip Arthroplasty

Stephen C. Sizer, DO[a], Jeffrey J. Cherian, DO[a],
Randa D.K. Elmallah, MD[a], Todd P. Pierce, MD[a],
Walter B. Beaver, MD[b], Michael A. Mont, MD[a,*]

KEYWORDS

- Blood loss • Total hip arthroplasty • Total knee arthroplasty • Transfusion risk • Tranexamic acid

KEY POINTS

- Preoperative anemia is one of the strongest predictors of postoperative transfusion.
- Older age, an American Society of Anesthesiologists III score or higher, and a Charlson Index greater than 3 have been associated with an increase in intraoperative blood loss as well as increased transfusion rates.
- Men have been shown to have a higher risk for blood loss with no increased risk for receiving a transfusion, likely because of a higher baseline hemoglobin level and greater reserve.
- The risk for bleeding and allogeneic transfusions appears to be complex and multifactorial in nature, and adequate preoperative preparation is necessary.
- The use of blood loss strategies, such as tranexamic acid, may reduce the role these factors play in bleeding and transfusion risk.

INTRODUCTION

Lower extremity total joint arthroplasties (TJA) have gained popularity because of their success in treating knee and hip osteoarthritis (OA); however, they can be extensive procedures that may be associated with substantial blood loss.[1] Moreover, this blood loss can result in complications and cost increases, which may impede the success of the surgery.[2,3] In particular, patients may be subject to longer hospital admissions and worse postoperative rehabilitation.[2] As demand for these surgeries increases secondary to the increasing prevalence of the elderly and obese populations, surgeons are seeking ways to minimize these risks and ensure ongoing success.[3,4]

With substantial blood loss, these patients are also at an increased risk of requiring allogeneic blood transfusions, which are associated with a new plethora of risks and costs,[1] which include longer hospital stays, infectious disease transmission, immunologic reactions, acute lung injury, cardiopulmonary overload, hemolytic and anaphylactic reactions, and increased mortality (**Table 1**).[5] In addition, allogeneic blood transfusions have been shown to modify the role of host macrophages, dampen the normal lymphocytic response to antigens, and produce a decreased ratio of helper to suppressor T cells.[6] As a result of this immunosuppressive effect, patients are placed at a higher risk of periprosthetic joint infection.[7,8]

[a] Rubin Institute for Advanced Orthopedics, Center for Joint Preservation and Replacement, Sinai Hospital of Baltimore, 2401 West Belvedere Avenue, Baltimore, MA 21215, USA; [b] OrthoCarolina Hip and Knee Center, 2001 Vail Avenue, Charlotte, NC 28207, USA
* Corresponding author.
E-mail addresses: mmont@lifebridgehealth.org; rhondamont@aol.com

Orthop Clin N Am 46 (2015) 445–459
http://dx.doi.org/10.1016/j.ocl.2015.06.002
0030-5898/15/$ – see front matter © 2015 Elsevier Inc. All rights reserved.

Table 1
Risks of blood transfusion

Adverse Event	Odds (per Event)
Fever/allergic reaction	1:200
Hemolytic transfusion reactions	1:6000
Fatal hemolytic reactions	1:1,000,000
HIV infection	1:1,900,000
HBV infection	1:180,000
HCV infection	1:1,600,000
Bacterial contamination	1:3000
TRALI	1:50,000
TACO	1:5000
Anaphylaxis	1:50,000

Abbreviations: HBV, hepatitis B virus; HCV, hepatitis C virus; HIV, human immunodeficiency virus; TACO, transfusion-associated circulatory overload; TRALI, transfusion-related acute lung injury.

From Klein HG. How safe is blood, really? Biologicals 2010;38(1):101; with permission.

To minimize these potential dangers, it is important to understand factors that influence blood loss and subsequent transfusions. Predicting blood loss encompasses not only preoperative factors, but intraoperative and postoperative factors as well. By being able to risk-stratify patients, clinicians can limit intraoperative loss and use postoperative protocols to improve patient outcomes.

With the advent of blood management strategies, surgeons may have an opportunity to reduce blood loss and transfusion risk. In particular, tranexamic acid (TXA) has gained popularity in recent literature for significantly reducing bleeding without an increased thromboembolic risk.[3,9] Consequently, the factors that influence perioperative bleeding may eventually come to play a minimal role and TXA may considerably alter transfusion evaluation and practices. However, TXA is yet to be widely adopted in orthopedic practice, and it is thought that it is still important to outline potential predictors of blood loss in lower extremity TJA.[3]

Therefore, in this review, the purpose is to identify preoperative, intraoperative, and postoperative factors that may influence the risk of blood loss and receiving transfusions as well as to delineate the effect of TXA on bleeding and postoperative transfusion rates.

PREOPERATIVE FACTORS

As with any surgery, the most important first step is a thorough history and physical examination. Understanding the physiologic demands that the surgery will place on the patient, and its relation to their preoperative hemoglobin, age, gender, weight, and underlying medical comorbidities, is essential (**Table 2**).

Table 2
Studies that described the patient-related factors and the risk for blood loss

Author, Year	Number of Arthroplasties	Risk Factor	Blood Loss (Case vs Control)	P Value	LOE
Guerin et al,[6] 2007	162	Age >70 y	850 vs 659 mL	.035	III
Mesa-Ramos et al,[10] 2008	121	Increase age by 1 y	Increase by 0.314 g/dL	<.001	II
Pola et al,[21] 2004	85	Age >75 y	1741 vs 1524 mL	.07	III
Mesa-Ramos et al,[10] 2008	121	Female gender	5.46 vs 4.78 g/dL decrease in Hb	.02	II
Guerin et al,[6] 2007	162	Female gender	988 vs 780 mL (THA) and 780 vs 689 mL (TKA)	<.05	III
Pola et al,[21] 2004	85	Male gender BMI <27 kg/m^2	1797 vs 1528 mL 1639 vs 1531 mL 5.2 vs 4.3 g/dL decrease in Hb	.04 >.05 .005	III III III
Prasad et al,[35] 2007	66	RA	235 vs 216 mL	>.05	III
Pola et al,[21] 2004	85	Hypertension	1707 vs 1474 mL	.02	III
Grosflam et al,[37] 1995	295	ASA >III	NR	<.05	III

Abbreviations: Hb, hemoglobin; LOE, level of evidence; NR, not reported.
Data from Refs.[6,10,21,35,37]

Preoperative Hemoglobin/Anemia

Preoperative anemia has been cited in multiple articles as the strongest and most predictive factor in determining risk for postoperative transfusion (**Table 3**).[6,10–15]

Hatzidakis and colleagues[16] analyzed the incidence of transfusion in relation to preoperative hemoglobin level in 489 consecutive patients who underwent primary lower extremity TJA. They noted that patients who had a hemoglobin level of less than 13 g/dL were 5.6 times more likely to receive a transfusion than those with a hemoglobin level greater than this (*P*<.0001). The investigators noted that patients who had a hemoglobin level between 13 and 15 g/dL were also at an increased risk of transfusion, with the exception of those younger than 65 years of age. However, no patient who had a hemoglobin level greater than 15 g/dL preoperatively required a transfusion. Similarly, Guerin and colleagues[6] prospectively reported on the impact of preoperative hemoglobin on transfusion risk in 162 patients following total hip arthroplasty (THA) or total knee arthroplasty (TKA). The investigators reported that preoperative anemia (hemoglobin <13 g/dL) had a 1.5 times greater risk of receiving an allogeneic blood transfusion compared with those with levels between 13 and 15 g/dL, and a 4 times greater risk than patients with a hemoglobin level greater than 15 g/dL (*P* = .001). More recently, Aderinto and Brenkle[12] evaluated 1016 patients who underwent unilateral THA and found that a hemoglobin level less than 12 g/dL was associated with a 3-fold increase in risk of receiving allogeneic blood postoperatively (*P*<.001).

In the Orthopedic Surgery Transfusion Hemoglobin European Overview (OSTHEO) study, Rosencher and colleagues[17] collected data on 3996 patients undergoing total hip and knee arthroplasty. They reported that patients who had a preoperative hemoglobin level of 8 mg/dL had a 75% and 69% probability of receiving a transfusion for women and men, respectively (*P*<.001). The same study demonstrated that in patients who had similar risk factors, but a preoperative hemoglobin level of 16 g/dL, that the probability of transfusion in men and women reduced to 13% and 7%, respectively (*P*<.001). Extrapolating on their results, Mesa-Ramos and colleagues[10] and Frisch and colleagues[8] found that a mean increase in 1 g/dL in preoperative hemoglobin resulted in a reduced risk for transfusion (odds ratio 0.62), which highlights the importance of preoperative patient optimization.

Preoperative anemia plays an influential role on blood loss and risk of transfusion. Having knowledge of preoperative laboratory studies at least 3 weeks before can allow for adequate preparation and action, if needed.[18]

Age

As the proportion of elderly patients undergoing lower extremity joint arthroplasty grows, one must understand how this may affect blood loss and transfusion risk. Advanced age has been associated with decreased hematopoietic activity, reduced functioning of platelets, and a diminished response from the marrow following acute blood loss.[19] The decreased hematopoietic activity predisposes the elderly to preoperative anemia, which decreases the margin between their baseline hemoglobin and the threshold to transfuse.

Multiple studies have demonstrated a correlation between age and blood loss or risk of transfusion (**Table 4**). In a retrospective analysis of 489 TJA patients, Hatzidakis and colleagues[16] found that patients greater than the age of 65 years had an increased risk of transfusion (relative risk of 2.8). In addition, Browne and colleagues[20] analyzed data collected from the US Nationwide

Table 3
Studies describing the preoperative hemoglobin level and the associated risk of transfusion

Author, Year	Number of Arthroplasties	Risk Factor	Relative Risk for Transfusion	P Value	LOE
Hatzidakis et al,[16] 2000	489	Hb <13 g/dL	5.6	<.0001	IV
Guerin et al,[6] 2007	162	Hb <13 g/dL	1.5	.001	III
Aderinto and Brenkel,[12] 2004	1016	Hb <12 g/dL	3	<.001	III
Rosencher et al,[17] 2003	3996	Hb <8 mg/dL	NR	NR	III
Frisch et al,[8] 2014	1573	Increase Hb by 1 mg/dL	0.62	NR	III

Abbreviations: Hb, hemoglobin; LOE, level of evidence; NR, not reported.
Data from Refs.[6,8,12,16,17]

Table 4
Studies describing patient age and the associated risk of transfusion

Author, Year	Number of Arthroplasties	Risk Factor	Relative Risk for Transfusion	P Value	LOE
Hatzidakis et al,[16] 2000	489	Age >65 y	2.8	NR	IV
Browne et al,[20] 2013	129,901	Age >85 y	2.9	NR	III
Guerin et al,[6] 2007	162	Age >70 y	NR	>.05	III
Mesa-Ramos et al,[10] 2008	121	Increase age by 1 y	NR	>.05	II
Pola et al,[21] 2004	85	Age >75 y	NR	>.05	III

Abbreviations: LOE, level of evidence; NR, not reported.
Data from Refs.[6,10,16,20,21]

Inpatient Sample (NIS) to assess risk factors associated with increased transfusion rates in patients who underwent THA (n = 129,901). They observed that the strongest risk factor for postoperative transfusion was increasing age, with patients greater than 85 years old at the highest risk (odds ratio 2.9).

Other studies have demonstrated that increasing age may be associated with higher rates of blood loss. Guerin and colleagues[6] found that patients greater than 70 years of age who underwent TKA had significantly higher total blood loss (TBL) than those less than 70 years of age (850 vs 659 mL; P = .035). For the patients undergoing THA, there was no significant difference in blood loss between those younger or older than 70 years (P>.05). In addition, the risk of transfusion in either cohort was not found to be associated with age.

A prospective, randomized trial of 121 TKA patients by Mesa-Ramos and colleagues[10] concluded that for every 1-year increase in age, there was an associated increase of 0.314 g/dL in blood loss (P<.001). However, they also noted that there was no association with age and risk of transfusion. In a study by Pola and colleagues[21] evaluating patients who underwent THA (n = 85), they noted that patients older than 75 years of age had more blood loss compared with those who were younger, which trended toward significance (1741 mL vs 1524 mL, respectively; P = .07). In addition, they observed that there was a significant decrease in the postoperative hemoglobin in patients greater than 75 years of age (5.3 mg/dL vs 4.53 mg/dL, respectively; P = .03). However, in regards to postoperative transfusion, they found that older age independently was not a significant risk factor, yet when analyzed concomitantly with gender, hypertension, body mass index (BMI), or preoperative anemia, the risk of transfusion became significantly higher (P = .02).

Elderly patients are at risk of greater blood loss following lower extremity TJA due to malnutrition, poor preoperative hemoglobin, and decreased intrinsic coagulation capabilities. Thus, it is essential to appropriately discuss these risks with the patient and take the appropriate steps to mitigate this factor.

Gender

Several studies have reported that women are at a higher risk for transfusion following lower extremity arthroplasty, which has been hypothesized to be due to a lower preoperative hematocrit and smaller body habitus (**Table 5**).[22] Frisch and colleagues,[8] in a retrospective review of 1573 patients undergoing primary total hip and knee arthroplasty, found an overall transfusion rate of 9.27% for TKA and 26.6% for THA. From their analysis, female patients were found to have a 2.6 times higher risk of receiving a transfusion than men (P = .001). This conclusion was supported by Browne and colleagues,[20] who in 129,901 patients, found that women had a higher likelihood of receiving a transfusion than men after THA (odds ratio 2.1; P<.001). Furthermore, Walsh and colleagues,[23] in evaluating 1035 patients after THA, noted that women were also almost 2 times more likely to receive a blood transfusion (relative risk 1.9; P<.01).

There are studies that reveal no gender-specific differences in transfusion rates, despite differences in blood loss. Mesa-Ramos and colleagues[10] analyzed 121 patients undergoing unilateral TKA and found no significant difference in transfusion rates between men and women (P>.05), although there was a significant difference in blood loss, whereby men were found to lose a mean of 5.46 g/dL and women a mean of 4.78 g/dL (P = .02). Guerin and colleagues[6] prospectively evaluated 162 consecutive patients, and they demonstrated that men had greater blood loss than women in both THA and TKA cohorts (988 vs 780 mL and 780 vs 689 mL, respectively;

Table 5
Studies describing the patient's gender and the associated risk of transfusion

Author, Year	Number of Arthroplasties	Risk Factor	Relative Risk for Transfusion	P Value	LOE
Frisch et al,[8] 2014	1573	Female gender	2.6	.001	III
Browne et al,[20] 2013	129,901	Female gender	2.1	<.001	III
Walsh et al,[23] 2007	1035	Female gender	1.9	<.01	III
Mesa-Ramos et al,[10] 2008	121	Female gender	NR	>.05	II
Guerin et al,[6] 2007	162	Female gender	NR	.47	III
Pola et al,[21] 2004	85	Female gender	NR	.4	III

Abbreviations: LOE, level of evidence; NR, not reported.
Data from Refs.[6,8,10,20,21,23]

$P<.05$). The investigators also noted that male patients had larger decreases in postoperative hemoglobin levels ($P<.05$). However, differences in postoperative transfusion rates were not significant ($P = .47$).

Pola and colleagues[21] found that men had significantly more blood loss after THA than women (1797 vs 1528 mL, respectively; $P = .04$). They also noted no significant differences in transfusion rates between the 2 cohorts (20 vs 30%, respectively; $P = .4$). The investigators concluded that there was difficulty in predicting transfusion rates in patients postoperatively, particularly in nonanemic individuals.

Men may be at risk of greater blood loss, but this does not necessarily translate into a higher risk for transfusion. This disparity may be explained by the fact that men have been shown to have higher circulating hemoglobin levels,[24] and thus a greater reserve before reaching the transfusion threshold. Conclusively, there is still no clear evidence regarding whether there are gender-specific differences in risk for transfusion, and further evaluation is needed.[12]

Weight/Body Mass Index

Recent data have found that approximately one-third of the population in the United States over the age of 20 is obese.[25] Obesity has been linked to a multitude of complications associated with TJA, including infection, early failure, and wound dehiscence.[26–30] Nevertheless, the effects of obesity on blood loss and transfusion rates remain debatable (**Table 6**). Physiologically, increases in weight are known to produce a nonlinear increase in circulating blood volume.[31] However, this should be tempered against the possibility that obesity may make surgery more difficult with associated longer operative times and greater blood loss.

Ahmed and colleagues[32] evaluated the impact of weight on blood loss in patients who underwent TKA (n = 227). The investigators observed that patients who weighed less than 70 kg had an increased rate of transfusion postoperatively compared with those weighing greater than 70 kg (17 vs 8%, respectively; $P<.001$). Similarly, Aderinto and Brenkel[12] prospectively studied

Table 6
Studies describing the patient's weight and the associated risk of transfusion

Author, Year	Number of Arthroplasties	Risk Factor	Relative Risk for Transfusion	P Value	LOE
Ahmed et al,[32] 2012	227	Weight <70 kg	2.1	<.001	III
Aderinto and Brenkel,[12] 2004	1016	Weight <70 kg	2.3	<.001	III
Salido et al,[13] 2002	370	Weight ≤72 kg	NR	.002	III
Walsh et al,[23] 2007	1035	BMI ≥30 kg/m²	0.5	NR	III
Frisch et al,[8] 2014	1573	Increase BMI by 5 kg/m²	0.84	NR	III
Pola et al,[21] 2004	85	BMI >27 kg/m²	NR	.1	III

Abbreviations: LOE, level of evidence; NR, not reported.
Data from Refs.[8,12,13,21,23,32]

1016 patients who underwent a unilateral THA and found that a lower body weight was an independent risk factor for receiving a blood transfusion. Their data showed that patients who weighed less than 70 kg had a 37% transfusion risk compared with 16% in those weighing more than 70 kg ($P<.001$). In addition, Salido and colleagues[13] retrospectively reviewed 296 patients who underwent hip and knee arthroplasties (n = 209 hips, 161 knees), and their results showed that patients who had a mean weight of 72 kg or less were significantly more likely to receive a transfusion compared with those with a mean weight of 76 kg or more ($P = .002$). The investigators concluded that a 1-kg increase in body weight was associated with a 1.05 times reduction in the probability of transfusion.

Several reports have also evaluated the effect of BMI on TBL and rate of transfusions following THA and TKA. Walsh and colleagues[23] reviewed 1035 THA cases to identify predictors of blood transfusion. The investigators found that patients with a BMI of 30 kg/m^2 and greater had a 46% decreased risk of transfusions than those with a BMI less than 30 kg/m^2. In addition, Frisch and colleagues[8] noted that BMI was a significant predictor for transfusion in patients who underwent TKA and THA (n = 949 vs 624, respectively), and they concluded that an increase in BMI of 5 kg/m^2 correlated with a decreased odds ratio of 0.84 for blood transfusion.

Alternatively, Pola and colleagues[21] reported no significant association between BMI, when considered alone, and TBL in 85 patients who underwent primary THA. Their findings indicated that patients with a BMI of less than 27 kg/m^2 and greater than 27 kg/m^2 had a mean blood loss of 1639 and 1531 mL, respectively ($P>.05$). Patients with a BMI less than 27 kg/m^2 had a greater drop in postoperative hemoglobin (5.2 vs 4.3 g/dL, respectively; $P = .005$), but this did not lead to a significant difference in the rate of transfusions between the less than 27 kg/m^2 and greater than 27 kg/m^2 BMI cohorts (37% vs 22%, respectively; $P = .1$).

Low weight may be associated with a higher risk of transfusion, possibly due to a lower circulating blood volume and smaller body habitus.[33] As a result, these patients have a greater likelihood of receiving a transfusion because of a smaller physiologic reserve. However, it is difficult to conclude that patients with higher BMIs are less likely to receive a transfusion, because surgeons need to take into account the difficulty and complicated nature of surgery on these patients.

Comorbidities/American Society of Anesthesiologists Score

As the population continues to age and the demand for joint arthroplasty increases, more patients are presenting with a larger number of medical comorbidities. It is therefore important to understand the effect that these comorbidities have on patient outcomes (**Table 7**).

Patients with a preoperative diagnosis of rheumatoid arthritis (RA) may have a higher risk for transfusion than those with OA; this may be due to a lower preoperative hemoglobin secondary to their commonly found anemia, or possibly due to longer and more difficult surgeries in this patient population.[34] Prasad and colleagues[35] evaluated 66 patients who underwent a primary cemented TKA and found that RA patients had a significantly higher risk of transfusion (up to 3 times as often as OA patients) ($P = .04$). RA patients had significantly lower preoperative hemoglobin levels than those with OA (10.9 vs 12.16 g/dL; $P = .009$), which may be the explanation for the increased transfusion risk. However, the investigators found no significant difference in intraoperative blood loss between both cohorts (216 vs 235 mL in OA

Table 7
Studies describing the patient's comorbidities and the associated risk of transfusion

Author, Year	Number of Arthroplasties	Risk Factor	Relative Risk for Transfusion	P Value	LOE
Prasad et al,[35] 2007	66	RA	3	.04	III
Cushner and Friedman,[34] 1991	112	RA	2.16	<.001	III
Pola et al,[21] 2004	85	Hypertension	NR	>.05	III
Browne et al,[20] 2013	129,901	One or more comorbidities	1.3	NR	III
Ahmed et al,[32] 2012	2281	ASA score ≥III	NR	<.001	III

Abbreviations: LOE, level of evidence; NR, not reported.
  Data from Refs.[20,21,32,34,35]

and RA patients, respectively; $P>.05$). Cushner and Friedman[34] evaluated 112 primary TKA patients and also found no statistical difference in the TBL between OA and RA patients, but there was a significant increase in postoperative transfusions in those with RA (69 vs 32%, respectively; $P<.001$). They also noted lower baseline hematocrit levels in RA patients, likely from anemia of chronic disease.

In addition, Pola and colleagues[21] found that patients with hypertension who underwent THA had significantly higher TBL (1707 vs 1474 [normotensive] mL, respectively; $P = .02$). However, these patients did not have a significantly increased risk of transfusion (38 vs 21%, respectively; $P>.05$). In addition, they noted that when hypertension was combined with female gender, age greater than 75 years, or a BMI less than 27 kg/m^2, the rate of transfusion did reach statistical significance ($P = .02$), alluding to the likelihood that risk for transfusion is multifactorial.

To assess the effect of multiple comorbidities, Browne and colleagues[20] used the Charlson Index scoring system to predict transfusion risk in 129,901 patients from the NIS database. The Charlson Index predicted the 10-year mortality of these patients based on their medical conditions (**Box 1**).[36] Patients with a higher Charlson Index were more likely to receive a transfusion postoperatively (odds ratio 2.2). They also found that patients with one or more comorbidities had a higher risk of transfusion (odds ratio 1.3).

A prospective cohort study by Grosflam and colleagues[37] of 295 consecutive THA found that hypertension was not associated with increased TBL, but the presence of any other comorbidity was. They also reported that an American Society of Anesthesiologists (ASA) score greater than III (severe systemic illnesses that are not incapacitating; **Table 8**) resulted in a significant increase in TBL ($P<.05$). Ahmed and colleagues,[32] in a review of 2281 TKA patients, found a higher risk of transfusions in patients with an ASA score of III or IV versus those with an ASA score of I or II (16% and 40%, respectively, vs 4% and 10%, respectively; $P<.001$). They noted that most patients with ASA scores greater than III were elderly, which as mentioned previously, can be an independent predictor of blood loss. It seems obvious that having patients medically optimized with an ASA score of I or II would lead to the lowest blood loss.

From these studies, it can be surmised that a patient's comorbid state is a significant preoperative predictor of blood loss and may play a role in postoperative transfusion risk. An adequate preoperative assessment and management of coexisting medical conditions is crucial before surgery.

INTRAOPERATIVE FACTORS

Multiple intraoperative factors may play a role in predicting the degree of blood loss and risk of transfusion. These factors include, but are not limited to, the type of surgery performed, the length of operative time, tourniquet use, and the type of anesthesia used (**Table 9**).

Type of Surgery

Whether a patient is undergoing a THA or a TKA (primary or revision) may influence the extent of blood loss due to differences in surgical dissection and operative time. Guerin and colleagues[6] assessed TBL in 162 patients who had a THA or a TKA. They observed that there was a significant difference in blood loss between the 2 cohorts (902 vs 764 mL, respectively; $P = .04$). However, there were no significant differences between THA or TKA patients in postoperative hemoglobin (3.22 vs 3.08 g/dL, respectively; $P>.05$) or transfusion rates (25 vs 23%, respectively; $P>.05$). In contrast, Bierbaum and colleagues[7] prospectively evaluated 9482 patients who underwent THA and TKA and found that a greater proportion of THA patients required blood transfusions than TKA patients (57 vs 39%, respectively).

Hatzidakis and colleagues[16] compared the differences in blood loss and transfusion rates between patients who underwent primary and revision total hip and knee arthroplasties (n = 320 primary, 140 revision). They noted significantly less blood loss during primary compared with revision knee arthroplasty (185 vs 310 mL, respectively; $P = .004$). In addition, patients who had received a primary knee arthroplasty had lower rates of transfusions (6%) compared with those who had revisions or bilateral arthroplasty (28% and 34%, respectively; $P<.05$). In the THA cohort, patients who had a primary had significantly less blood loss than those who had a revision (503 vs 844 mL, respectively; $P<.0001$) as well as lower rates of transfusion (11 vs 33%, respectively; $P<.001$). On the contrary, Rosencher and colleagues,[17] in the OSTHEO study, found no difference in the mean calculated blood loss between primary THA and TKA and revision THA and TKA, respectively (2143 vs 2072 mL and 3060 vs 2634 mL, respectively, $P>.05$).

Although differences in blood loss and transfusion rates between THAs and TKAs may not be clear, it seems that a patient undergoing a revision or bilateral arthroplasty may be at a significantly higher risk for increased blood loss and a transfusion (**Table 10**). Understanding these risks allots time for proper counseling to patients undertaking these procedures and allows for the allocation of blood products, if deemed necessary.

Box 1
Charlson index

Scoring: Comorbidity component (apply 1 point to each unless otherwise noted)

1. Myocardial infarction
2. Congestive heart failure
3. Peripheral vascular disease
4. Cerebrovascular disease
5. Dementia
6. Chronic obstructive pulmonary disease
7. Connective tissue disease
8. Peptic ulcer disease
9. Diabetes mellitus (1 point uncomplicated, 2 points if end-organ damage)
10. Moderate to severe chronic kidney disease (2 points)
11. Hemiplegia (2 points)
12. Leukemia (2 points)
13. Malignant lymphoma (2 points)
14. Solid tumor (2 points, 6 points if metastatic)
15. Liver disease (1 point mild, 3 points if moderate to severe)
16. AIDS (6 points)

Scoring: Age

1. Age less than 40 years: 0 points
2. Age 41 to 50 years: 1 points
3. Age 51 to 60 years: 2 points
4. Age 61 to 70 years: 3 points
5. Age 71 to 80 years: 4 points

Interpretation

1. Calculate Charlson score or index (i)

    a. Add comorbidity score to age score

    b. Total denoted as "i" below

2. Calculate Charlson probability (10-year mortality)

    a. Calculate $Y = e^{(i*0.9)}$

    b. Calculate $Z = 0.983Y$

    c. Where Z is the 10-year survival

From Charlson ME, Pompei P, Ales KL, et al. A new method of classifying prognostic comorbidity in longitudinal studies: development and validation. J Chronic Dis 1987;40(5):377–79; with permission.

Operative Time

Several studies have reported on the relationship between operative time and blood loss (**Table 11**). Hrnack and colleagues[31] retrospectively analyzed 94 primary TKA and 78 primary THA patients and found that increases in operative time were associated with greater intraoperative blood loss. The mean operative times were 133 and 134 minutes for the TKA and THA, respectively. The investigators noted that a 1-minute increase in anesthesia time resulted in 3.2 mL of increased blood loss in patients who underwent TKA and 1.5 mL of blood loss in THA patients ($P<.01$).

Furthermore, Noticewala and colleagues[19] retrospectively reviewed 644 primary unilateral TKA to predict the need for allogeneic transfusion. They reported that large increases in surgical time

Table 8
American Society of Anesthesiologists scores

ASA Score	Description
I	Healthy patient
II	Mild systemic disease (HTN, DM)
III	Severe systemic disease that is not incapacitating
IV	Incapacitating disease that can threaten the patient's life (CHF)
V	Patient expected to live <24 h with or without surgery

Abbreviations: CHF, congestive heart failure; DM, diabetes mellitus; HTN, hypertension.
From American Society of Anesthesiologists. ASA Physical Status Classification System. Available at: http://www.asahq.org/resources/clinical-information/asa-physical-status-classification-system.

significantly increased the likelihood of transfusion ($P<.0001$). In particular, a 30-minute increase in operative time led to a 1.8 times increased likelihood of receiving allogeneic blood. In addition, the mean operative time for patients who had a transfusion versus those who did not was 124 minutes and 109 minutes, respectively ($P = .004$).

Moreover, Salido and colleagues[13] and Frisch and colleagues[8] showed that an increase in operative time was associated with a higher risk of transfusion. In a retrospective review by Salido and colleagues[13] that assessed 370 total hip and knee arthroplasties, the mean surgical time in patients that were transfused was longer than in those who were not (96 vs 87 minutes, respectively; $P = .0001$). In further agreement, Frisch and colleagues[8] extrapolated their data from 1573 patients following total hip and knee arthroplasty and noted that an increase of 40 minutes in operative time resulted in an increase in risk for a transfusion (odds ratio 1.25; $P = .029$). From these studies, it seems that judicious use of time intraoperatively not only will improve productivity but also may decrease blood loss and subsequent transfusions.

Tourniquet Use

The use of pneumatic tourniquets during TKA has been controversial among orthopedic surgeons. Their use has been associated with improved

Table 9
Studies that described the surgical-related factors and the risk for blood loss

Author, Year	Number of Arthroplasties	Risk Factor	Blood Loss	P Value	LOE
Hatzidakis et al,[16] 2000	489	Revision TKA Revision THA	310 vs 185 mL 844 vs 503 mL	.004 <.0001	IV IV
Rosencher et al,[17] 2003	3996	Revision TKA Revision THA	2634 vs 2072 mL 3060 vs 2143 mL	>.05 >.05	III III
Hrnack et al,[31] 2012	172	Increase in anesthesia time by 1 min	3.2 mL (TKA) and 1.5 mL (THA) increase loss	<.01	III
Aglietti et al,[38] 2000	20	No tourniquet	482 vs 350 mL	>.05	II
Vandenbussche et al,[39] 2002	80	No tourniquet	1557 vs 1235 mL	.017	II
Fukuda et al,[40] 2007	48	No tourniquet	1089 vs 691 mL	<.0001	III
Zan et al,[41] 2015	608	Tourniquet release before wound closure	184 mL increase in blood loss	<.0001	II
Stevens et al,[51] 2000	60	Regional anesthesia	166 mL decrease in blood loss	.0006	II
Sculco and Ranawat,[52] 1975	234	Spinal anesthesia	600 mL decrease in blood loss	<.001	III
Guay,[53] 2006	1074	Regional anesthesia	1336 vs 1623 mL	.001	III
Keith,[50] 1977	27	Epidural anesthesia	734 vs 986 mL	>.05	III

Abbreviation: LOE, level of evidence.
Data from Refs.[16,17,31,38–41,50–53]

Table 10
Studies describing the type of surgery the associated risk of transfusion

Author, Year	Number of Arthroplasties	Risk Factor	Relative Risk for Transfusion	P Value	LOE
Guerin et al,[6] 2007	162	THA	NR	>.05	III
Bierbaum et al,[7] 1999	9482	THA	1.46	NR	III
Hatzidakis et al,[16] 2000	489	Revision TKA	5	<.05	IV
		Revision THA	3	<.001	IV

Abbreviations: LOE, level of evidence; NR, not reported.
Data from Refs.[6,7,16]

visualization of the operative field, but the effect on blood loss has not fully been determined.

Aglietti and colleagues[38] found that patients who did not have a tourniquet experienced greater intraoperative blood loss than those who did (482 vs 350 mL, respectively). However, postoperatively, patients in the tourniquet group had increased blood loss, and the investigators concluded that the difference in TBL between both cohorts was not statistically significant (P>.05). One should note that this was only a small study with a total of 20 patients.

Vandenbussche and colleagues[39] prospectively compared 40 TKA patients with tourniquet use at 350 mm Hg to 40 TKA patients without a tourniquet and found a statistically significant higher mean TBL in those without a tourniquet (1557 vs 1235 mL, respectively; P = .0165). However, there was no statistically significant difference in the number of transfusions between the 2 groups (P>.05). In contrast, Jones and colleagues[11] reported a higher transfusion rate for TKA patients (n = 186) with a tourniquet (35 vs 26%, respectively; P<.05).

Fukuda and colleagues[40] evaluated 48 consecutive patients undergoing cemented TKAs and found that intraoperatively patients without a tourniquet had a mean blood loss of 631 mL compared with 228 mL (P<.0001). They also found that TBL was also significantly higher in the tourniquet-less patients (1089 vs 691 mL, respectively; P<.0001).

A meta-analysis of randomized controlled trials was performed by Zan and colleagues[41] evaluating the role of releasing the tourniquet before or after wound closure (n = 608 knees). There was a significantly greater TBL when the tourniquet was released before wound closure than following wound closure (+184 mL; P<.0001). Postoperative blood loss was also evaluated by assessing drain output, and patients with tourniquet release before closure had greater loss (+90 mL; P = .007). Theoretically, releasing the tourniquet before closure would allow for coagulation of any significant bleeding and help to decrease total and postoperative blood loss, but this was not found. The investigators concluded that it may be due in part to the increase in

Table 11
Studies describing the intraoperative variables and the associated risk of transfusion

Author, Year	Number of Arthroplasties	Risk Factor	Relative Risk for Transfusion	P Value	LOE
Noticewala et al,[19] 2012	644	30-min increase in operative time	1.8	NR	III
Frisch et al,[8] 2014	1573	40-min increase in operative time	1.25	.029	III
Vandenbussche et al,[39] 2002	80	No tourniquet	NR	>.05	II
Jones et al,[11] 2004	186	No tourniquet	NR	<.05	III
Guay,[53] 2006	1074	Regional anesthesia	0.5	<.0001	III
Keith,[50] 1977	27	Epidural anesthesia	0.39	NR	III

Abbreviations: LOE, level of evidence; NR, not reported.
Data from Refs.[8,11,19,39,50,53]

fibrinolytic activity that occurs the first time the tourniquet is deflated. They hypothesized that if this first release occurs after the joint capsule and skin are closed and a compressive dressing is in place, the increased fibrinolytic activity can be suppressed from the tamponade effect.[41]

The introduction of a tourniquet for TKA allows for improved visualization of the operative field, improved interdigitation of cement, and the possible benefit of decreased blood loss. However, tourniquet release before wound closure may be associated with a higher risk of bleeding. Furthermore, surgeons need to be aware of the risks associated with tourniquet use, which include skin damage, quadriceps muscle weakness, neuropraxia, vascular injury, or deep vein thrombosis.[42–48] To clarify the effects of tourniquet use, further studies are needed.

Type of Anesthesia

Regional anesthesia has been shown to decrease postoperative nausea, improve postoperative pain control, and decrease the rate of deep vein thrombosis when compared with general anesthesia.[49] It has also been postulated to decrease blood loss as a result of a reduction in sympathetic tone, decreased blood flow to the operative extremity, and lower hydrostatic pressure in the venous system.[50]

In a randomized double-blind trial by Stevens and colleagues,[51] 60 patients undergoing THA were prospectively evaluated to determine if lumbar plexus blockade reduced blood loss when compared with general anesthesia. It was found that intraoperative blood loss was not altered significantly with regional versus general anesthesia (434 vs 538 mL, respectively; $P = .09$), but postoperatively, there was a significantly decreased amount of loss in the lumbar plexus block group (-166 mL, $P = .0006$). However, it was difficult to assess transfusion rates because patients who preoperatively donated blood received the units postoperatively, regardless of hemoglobin levels or symptoms. Sculco and Ranawat[52] also evaluated 234 total hip arthroplasties and compared the use of spinal and general anesthesia. They noted that there was a total reduction in blood loss in patients who received spinal anesthesia (-600 mL; $P<.001$).

In a meta-analysis of 24 studies by Guay,[53] the effect of neuraxial blocks on THA blood loss was reviewed. From these studies, 10 specifically assessed the effect of regional anesthesia versus general anesthesia on blood. Despite no significant difference in intraoperative loss between the 2 groups (789 vs 1055 mL; $P>.05$), TBL was significantly lower in the regional group (1336 vs 1623 mL, respectively; $P = .001$). Patients undergoing regional anesthesia also had a significantly lower rate of blood transfusion postoperatively (19 vs 41%, respectively; $P<.0001$). On the contrary, Keith[50] prospectively assessed 27 patients undergoing THA and found no significant difference in TBL between patients who received epidural or general anesthesia (734 vs 986 mL, respectively; $P>.05$). Although mean intraoperative blood loss for the epidural group was significantly less compared with the general anesthesia group (342 vs 648 mL, respectively; $P<.05$), the epidural group had a greater amount of blood loss postoperatively. However, only 30% of the epidural patients required a blood transfusion compared with 77% of the general anesthesia patients.

The use of regional anesthesia seems to result in lower rates of transfusion, with variable effects on blood loss. However, the authors think that working closely with the anesthesiologist and having discussions with patients about the risks and benefits of regional anesthesia may lead to better management and potentially decrease intraoperative blood loss and lower rates of transfusion postoperatively.

POSTOPERATIVE ANTICOAGULATION

In light of the new American Academy of Orthopedic Surgeons and American College of Chest Physician guidelines, physicians have more autonomy for determining postoperative deep vein thrombosis prophylaxis. Prophylaxis includes the use of mechanical compression devices, such as the use of compression stockings, or the use of pharmacologic agents, which act on the coagulation cascade or platelet aggregation. However, by promoting anticoagulation, these agents consequently increase the bleeding risk. As a result, clinicians face the difficulty of balancing the intended effect and the potential side effects of these prophylactic medications (**Tables 12** and **13**).

A meta-analysis by Freedman and colleagues[54] evaluated studies involving low-molecular-weight heparin, warfarin, aspirin, low-dose heparin, and pneumatic compression. Fifty-two studies demonstrated a higher risk for a minor bleeding event with low-molecular-weight heparin and low-dose heparin compared with a placebo (8.9% and 7.6% vs 2.2%, respectively; $P<.05$). The risk of bleeding with aspirin was similar to that of pneumatic compression devices (1.2 vs 1.1%, respectively; $P>.05$). Turpie and colleagues[55] also performed a meta-analysis of 4 randomized double-blinded studies comparing the effects of fondaparinux and enoxaparin. It was observed

Table 12
Studies that described anticoagulation and the risk for blood loss

Author, Year	Number of Arthroplasties	Risk Factor	Blood Loss	P Value	LOE
Colwell et al,[56] 1999	3011	LMWH prophylaxis	549 vs 554 mL	>.05	I
Warwick et al,[57] 1998	290	LMWH prophylaxis	623 vs 670 mL	>.05	I
Alshryda et al,[3] 2013	161	TXA	129 mL decrease in loss	.002	I
Sukeik et al,[9] 2011	370	TXA	289 mL decrease in loss	<.002	II

Abbreviations: LMWH, low-molecular-weight heparin; LOE, level of evidence; NR, not reported.
   Data from Refs.[3,9,56,57]

that fondaparinux was associated with a higher incidence of major bleeding than enoxaparin (2.7 vs 1.7%, respectively; $P = .008$). It was also noted that most of the bleeding episodes associated with fondaparinux were related to injections commenced at 3 to 9 hours postoperatively.

Colwell and colleagues[56] assessed the effect of enoxaparin and warfarin on postoperative outcomes in 3011 patients who underwent THA. The patients were treated with 30 mg of enoxaparin every 12 hours within 24 hours from the conclusion of surgery, whereas those receiving warfarin received their first dose from 48 hours before surgery until the first 24 hours postoperatively. The mean operative blood loss was 549 mL with enoxaparin and 554 mL while using warfarin ($P>.05$), but there was a significantly higher rate of major bleeding events in the enoxaparin versus the warfarin group (1.2 vs 0.5%, respectively; $P = .055$). It was noted that 14 of the 18 patients who had major bleeding events in the enoxaparin group received their first injection within 0 to 12 hours postoperatively. Furthermore, more patients required transfusion while being treated with enoxaparin versus warfarin (2.8 vs 1.5%, respectively).

Warwick and colleagues[57] prospectively compared the use of low-molecular-weight heparin against foot pumps in a randomized trial of 290 patients following THA. They found no difference in the intraoperative blood loss between the use of heparin and foot pumps (623 vs 670 mL, respectively; $P>.05$). However, in the low-molecular-weight heparin cohort, there was a significantly higher postoperative drain output when compared with the patients with foot pump (578 vs 492 mL, respectively; $P = .014$). Also, the percentage of patients who had wound oozing was significantly higher in the low-molecular-weight heparin group compared with the foot pump group at both 4 and 7 days postoperatively (90 vs 67% and 49 vs 10%, respectively; $P<.001$). However, there was no statistically significant difference in the frequency of transfusions between the 2 groups ($P>.05$). In a study by Walsh and colleagues[23] retrospectively reviewing 1035 patients who underwent THA, the investigators found that patients using low-molecular-weight heparin for deep vein thrombosis prophylaxis required significantly more transfusions compared with patients who used aspirin and a foot pump (relative risk 1.54, $P<.05$). However, there was no significant difference in transfusion rates between the 2 cohorts ($P>.05$).

Although there is a risk of bleeding, the use of anticoagulants remains crucial,[58,59] as it has been reported that approximately 1 of 100 patients following TKA and 1 of 200 following THA will develop a symptomatic venous thromboembolism before hospital discharge.[60] In conclusion, each

Table 13
Studies describing the type of anticoagulation and the associated risk of transfusion

Author, Year	Number of Arthroplasties	Risk Factor	Relative Risk for Transfusion	P Value	LOE
Colwell et al,[56] 1999	3011	LMWH	1.87	NR	I
Warwick et al,[57] 1998	290	LMWH (vs foot pump)	NR	>.05	I
Walsh et al,[23] 2007	1035	LMWH (vs ASA)	1.54	<.05	III

Abbreviations: ASA, acetyl salicylic acid; LMWH, low-molecular-weight heparin; LOE, level of evidence; NR, not reported.
   Data from Refs.[23,56,57]

Table 14
Studies describing the use of tranexamic acid and the associated risk of transfusion

Author, Year	Number of Arthroplasties	Risk Factor	Relative Risk for Transfusion	P Value	LOE
Alshryda et al,[3] 2013	161	TXA	NR	.004	I
Sabatini et al,[2] 2014	45	TXA	NR	<.05	IV
Samujh et al,[61] 2014	113	TXA	0.25	.03	III
Sukeik et al,[9] 2011	370	TXA	NR	<.001	II

Abbreviations: LOE, level of evidence; NR, not reported.
   Data from Refs.[2,3,9,61]

patient should have a tailored postoperative regimen based on their personal risk profile.

TRANEXAMIC ACID IN LOWER EXTREMITY TOTAL JOINT ARTHROPLASTIES

There has been abundant recent literature on the use of TXA to attempt to reduce blood loss in TJA. TXA is a synthetic derivative of lysine that promotes hemostasis by inhibiting the action of plasminogen and therefore exerting an antifibrinolytic effect.[2] However, there have been concerns that using TXA may lead to side effects and a potential increase in thromboembolic risk.

Alshryda and colleagues[3] conducted a double-blind randomized trial on 161 patients who underwent THA. They concluded that the use of intra-articular TXA reduced the risk of blood transfusion by 20% ($P = .004$) and blood loss by 129 mL ($P = .002$). In addition, it was observed that patients who received TXA had a lower cost per surgical admission ($-$458; $P = .05$). Sabatini and colleagues[2] evaluated the use of intravenous TXA on 45 patients who underwent TKA and noted that the transfusion requirement was significantly lower in the TXA group than patients who received a fibrin tissue adhesive ($P<.05$).

In addition, Samujh and colleagues[61,62] reviewed 113 patients who underwent revision TKA and found that patients who received a single intravenous TXA dose of 10 mg per kilogram had fewer transfusions than the control group (5 vs 19%, respectively; $P = .03$). Sukeik and colleagues[9] assessed the effect of TXA on thromboembolic risk in patients who underwent THA and concluded that there were no significant increases in deep vein thrombosis or pulmonary embolism ($P>.05$). However, they did note that the use of TXA reduced TBL ($-$289 mL; $P<.002$) and risk of allogeneic blood transfusion (risk difference -0.2; $P<.001$).

It seems that TXA has beneficial effects on blood loss and transfusion rates (**Table 14**). If TXA becomes widely incorporated in THA and TKA, this may change many of the prior conclusions and minimize the role of various perioperative factors in blood loss.

SUMMARY

Marked blood loss during lower extremity TJA may lead to higher rates of transfusion, which may negatively affect surgical outcomes and yield greater complication rates. It is therefore ideal to identify factors that may increase the likelihood of blood loss, so they can be modified. From this review, it can be concluded that preoperative anemia, older age, multiple comorbidities, increased operative time, and use of postoperative anticoagulation may lead to higher blood loss and transfusion rates, although the influence of other factors remains controversial. Ultimately, it is difficult to implicate individual factors, as prediction of blood loss seems to be multifactorial, and further studies are needed to understand the complex relationships. The use of blood management strategies such as TXA may reduce bleeding in all patients regardless of risk factors and thus minimize the role these factors play in the future, but this is yet to be widely implemented. In the meantime, identifying patient-specific risk factors associated with blood loss will allow clinicians to safely prepare for perioperative adverse events and take proper preoperative measures. Using these predictive factors with a strict postoperative transfusion protocol can lead to a safer and more successful perioperative experience for the patient.

REFERENCES

1. Cherian JJ, Kapadia BH, Issa K, et al. Preoperative blood management strategies for total hip arthroplasty. Surg Technol Int 2013;23:261–6.
2. Sabatini L, Atzori F, Revello S, et al. Intravenous use of tranexamic acid reduces postoperative blood loss in total knee arthroplasty. Arch Orthop Trauma Surg 2014;134(11):1609–14.

3. Alshryda S, Mason J, Sarda P, et al. Topical (intra-articular) tranexamic acid reduces blood loss and transfusion rates following total hip replacement: a randomized controlled trial (TRANX-H). J Bone Joint Surg Am 2013;95(21):1969–74.

4. Ha CW, Noh MJ, Choi KB, et al. Initial phase I safety of retrovirally transduced human chondrocytes expressing transforming growth factor-beta-1 in degenerative arthritis patients. Cytotherapy 2012;14(2):247–56.

5. Klein HG. How safe is blood, really? Biologicals 2010;38(1):100–4.

6. Guerin S, Collins C, Kapoor H, et al. Blood transfusion requirement prediction in patients undergoing primary total hip and knee arthroplasty. Transfus Med 2007;17(1):37–43.

7. Bierbaum BE, Callaghan JJ, Galante JO, et al. An analysis of blood management in patients having a total hip or knee arthroplasty. J Bone Joint Surg Am 1999;81(1):2–10.

8. Frisch NB, Wessell NM, Charters MA, et al. Predictors and complications of blood transfusion in total hip and knee arthroplasty. J Arthroplasty 2014;29(9 Suppl):189–92.

9. Sukeik M, Alshryda S, Haddad FS, et al. Systematic review and meta-analysis of the use of tranexamic acid in total hip replacement. J Bone Joint Surg Br 2011;93(1):39–46.

10. Mesa-Ramos F, Mesa-Ramos M, Maquieira-Canosa C, et al. Predictors for blood transfusion following total knee arthroplasty: a prospective randomised study. Acta Orthop Belg 2008;74(1):83–9.

11. Jones HW, Savage L, White C, et al. Postoperative autologous blood salvage drains–are they useful in primary uncemented hip and knee arthroplasty? A prospective study of 186 cases. Acta Orthop Belg 2004;70(5):466–73.

12. Aderinto J, Brenkel IJ. Pre-operative predictors of the requirement for blood transfusion following total hip replacement. J Bone Joint Surg Br 2004;86(7):970–3.

13. Salido JA, Marin LA, Gomez LA, et al. Preoperative hemoglobin levels and the need for transfusion after prosthetic hip and knee surgery: analysis of predictive factors. J Bone Joint Surg Am 2002;84-A(2):216–20.

14. Keating EM, Meding JB, Faris PM, et al. Predictors of transfusion risk in elective knee surgery. Clin Orthop Relat Res 1998;(357):50–9.

15. Clarke AM, Dorman T, Bell MJ. Blood loss and transfusion requirements in total joint arthroplasty. Ann R Coll Surg Engl 1992;74(5):360–3.

16. Hatzidakis AM, Mendlick RM, McKillip T, et al. Preoperative autologous donation for total joint arthroplasty. An analysis of risk factors for allogenic transfusion. J Bone Joint Surg Am 2000;82(1):89–100.

17. Rosencher N, Kerkkamp HE, Macheras G, et al. Orthopedic Surgery Transfusion Hemoglobin European Overview (OSTHEO) study: blood management in elective knee and hip arthroplasty in Europe. Transfusion 2003;43(4):459–69.

18. Levine BR, Haughom B, Strong B, et al. Blood management strategies for total knee arthroplasty. J Am Acad Orthop Surg 2014;22(6):361–71.

19. Noticewala MS, Nyce JD, Wang W, et al. Predicting need for allogeneic transfusion after total knee arthroplasty. J Arthroplasty 2012;27(6):961–7.

20. Browne JA, Adib F, Brown TE, et al. Transfusion rates are increasing following total hip arthroplasty: risk factors and outcomes. J Arthroplasty 2013;28(8 Suppl):34–7.

21. Pola E, Papaleo P, Santoliquido A, et al. Clinical factors associated with an increased risk of perioperative blood transfusion in nonanemic patients undergoing total hip arthroplasty. J Bone Joint Surg Am 2004;86-A(1):57–61.

22. Scott BH, Seifert FC, Glass PS, et al. Blood use in patients undergoing coronary artery bypass surgery: impact of cardiopulmonary bypass pump, hematocrit, gender, age, and body weight. Anesth Analg 2003;97(4):958–63 [table of contents].

23. Walsh M, Preston C, Bong M, et al. Relative risk factors for requirement of blood transfusion after total hip arthroplasty. J Arthroplasty 2007;22(8):1162–7.

24. Tong E, Murphy WG, Kinsella A, et al. Capillary and venous haemoglobin levels in blood donors: a 42-month study of 36,258 paired samples. Vox Sang 2010;98(4):547–53.

25. Ogden CL, Carroll MD, Kit BK, et al. Prevalence of childhood and adult obesity in the United States, 2011–2012. JAMA 2014;311(8):806–14.

26. Namba RS, Paxton L, Fithian DC, et al. Obesity and perioperative morbidity in total hip and total knee arthroplasty patients. J Arthroplasty 2005;20(7 Suppl 3):46–50.

27. Amin AK, Clayton RA, Patton JT, et al. Total knee replacement in morbidly obese patients. Results of a prospective, matched study. J Bone Joint Surg Br 2006;88(10):1321–6.

28. Patel VP, Walsh M, Sehgal B, et al. Factors associated with prolonged wound drainage after primary total hip and knee arthroplasty. J Bone Joint Surg Am 2007;89(1):33–8.

29. Peersman G, Laskin R, Davis J, et al. Infection in total knee replacement: a retrospective review of 6489 total knee replacements. Clin Orthop Relat Res 2001;(392):15–23.

30. Winiarsky R, Barth P, Lotke P. Total knee arthroplasty in morbidly obese patients. J Bone Joint Surg Am 1998;80(12):1770–4.

31. Hrnack SA, Skeen N, Xu T, et al. Correlation of body mass index and blood loss during total knee and total hip arthroplasty. Am J Orthop 2012;41(10):467–71.

32. Ahmed I, Chan JK, Jenkins P, et al. Estimating the transfusion risk following total knee arthroplasty. Orthopedics 2012;35(10):e1465–71.

33. Walsh TS, Palmer J, Watson D, et al. Multicentre cohort study of red blood cell use for revision hip arthroplasty and factors associated with greater risk of allogeneic blood transfusion. Br J Anaesth 2012; 108(1):63–71.

34. Cushner FD, Friedman RJ. Blood loss in total knee arthroplasty. Clin Orthop Relat Res 1991;(269):98–101.

35. Prasad N, Padmanabhan V, Mullaji A. Blood loss in total knee arthroplasty: an analysis of risk factors. Int Orthop 2007;31(1):39–44.

36. Charlson ME, Pompei P, Ales KL, et al. A new method of classifying prognostic comorbidity in longitudinal studies: development and validation. J Chronic Dis 1987;40(5):373–83.

37. Grosflam JM, Wright EA, Cleary PD, et al. Predictors of blood loss during total hip replacement surgery. Arthritis Care Res 1995;8(3):167–73.

38. Aglietti P, Baldini A, Vena LM, et al. Effect of tourniquet use on activation of coagulation in total knee replacement. Clin Orthop Relat Res 2000;(371): 169–77.

39. Vandenbussche E, Duranthon LD, Couturier M, et al. The effect of tourniquet use in total knee arthroplasty. Int Orthop 2002;26(5):306–9.

40. Fukuda A, Hasegawa M, Kato K, et al. Effect of tourniquet application on deep vein thrombosis after total knee arthroplasty. Arch Orthop Trauma Surg 2007;127(8):671–5.

41. Zan PF, Yang Y, Fu D, et al. Releasing of tourniquet before wound closure or not in total knee arthroplasty: a meta-analysis of randomized controlled trials. J Arthroplasty 2015;30(1):31–7.

42. Din R, Geddes T. Skin protection beneath the tourniquet. A prospective randomized trial. ANZ J Surg 2004;74(9):721–2.

43. Abdel-Salam A, Eyres KS. Effects of tourniquet during total knee arthroplasty. A prospective randomised study. J Bone Joint Surg Br 1995;77(2):250–3.

44. Irvine GB, Chan RN. Arterial calcification and tourniquets. Lancet 1986;2(8517):1217.

45. Silver R, de la Garza J, Rang M, et al. Limb swelling after release of a tourniquet. Clin Orthop Relat Res 1986;(206):86–9.

46. Newman RJ. Metabolic effects of tourniquet ischaemia studied by nuclear magnetic resonance spectroscopy. J Bone Joint Surg Br 1984;66(3): 434–40.

47. O'Leary AM, Veall G, Butler P, et al. Acute pulmonary oedema after tourniquet release. Can J Anaesth 1990;37(7):826–7.

48. Gielen M. Cardiac arrest after tourniquet release. Can J Anaesth 1991;38(4 Pt 1):541.

49. Hu S, Zhang ZY, Hua YQ, et al. A comparison of regional and general anaesthesia for total replacement of the hip or knee: a meta-analysis. J Bone Joint Surg Br 2009;91(7):935–42.

50. Keith I. Anaesthesia and blood loss in total hip replacement. Anaesthesia 1977;32(5):444–50.

51. Stevens RD, Van Gessel E, Flory N, et al. Lumbar plexus block reduces pain and blood loss associated with total hip arthroplasty. Anesthesiology 2000;93(1):115–21.

52. Sculco TP, Ranawat C. The use of spinal anesthesia for total hip-replacement arthroplasty. J Bone Joint Surg Am 1975;57(2):173–7.

53. Guay J. The effect of neuraxial blocks on surgical blood loss and blood transfusion requirements: a meta-analysis. J Clin Anesth 2006;18(2):124–8.

54. Freedman KB, Brookenthal KR, Fitzgerald RH Jr, et al. A meta-analysis of thromboembolic prophylaxis following elective total hip arthroplasty. J Bone Joint Surg Am 2000;82-A(7):929–38.

55. Turpie AG, Bauer KA, Eriksson BI, et al. Fondaparinux vs enoxaparin for the prevention of venous thromboembolism in major orthopedic surgery: a meta-analysis of 4 randomized double-blind studies. Arch Intern Med 2002;162(16):1833–40.

56. Colwell CW Jr, Collis DK, Paulson R, et al. Comparison of enoxaparin and warfarin for the prevention of venous thromboembolic disease after total hip arthroplasty. Evaluation during hospitalization and three months after discharge. J Bone Joint Surg Am 1999;81(7):932–40.

57. Warwick D, Harrison J, Glew D, et al. Comparison of the use of a foot pump with the use of low-molecular-weight heparin for the prevention of deep-vein thrombosis after total hip replacement. A prospective, randomized trial. J Bone Joint Surg Am 1998; 80(8):1158–66.

58. Surin VV, Sundholm K, Backman L. Infection after total hip replacement. With special reference to a discharge from the wound. J Bone Joint Surg Br 1983;65(4):412–8.

59. Saleh K, Olson M, Resig S, et al. Predictors of wound infection in hip and knee joint replacement: results from a 20 year surveillance program. J Orthop Res 2002;20(3):506–15.

60. Januel JM, Chen G, Ruffieux C, et al. Symptomatic in-hospital deep vein thrombosis and pulmonary embolism following hip and knee arthroplasty among patients receiving recommended prophylaxis: a systematic review. JAMA 2012;307(3): 294–303.

61. Samujh C, Falls TD, Wessel R, et al. Decreased blood transfusion following revision total knee arthroplasty using tranexamic acid. J Arthroplasty 2014; 29(9 Suppl):182–5.

62. Larocque BJ, Gilbert K, Brien WF. A point score system for predicting the likelihood of blood transfusion after hip or knee arthroplasty. Transfusion 1997; 37(5):463–7.

Iliopsoas Irritation as Presentation of Head-Neck Corrosion After Total Hip Arthroplasty: A Case Series

Laura Matsen Ko, MD[a], Jacob J. Coleman, BS[b,*],
Venessa Stas, MD[a], Paul J. Duwelius, MD[a]

KEYWORDS

- Total hip arthroplasty • Corrosion • Metallosis • Complication • Iliopsoas • Pseudotumor

KEY POINTS

- Corrosion of modular components at the femoral neck remains a complication of total hip arthroplasty.
- The authors have found the iliopsoas sign (pain on resisted flexion of the hip) to be suggestive of femoral component corrosion.
- The operative reports were reviewed, and corrosion was documented at the head-neck junction in all cases. After the revisions, all iliopsoas tendonitis symptoms resolved.
- Based on the authors' experience and the recent literature, they recommend that the iliopsoas sign or presentation of a sterile iliopsoas abscess in a previously well-functioning total hip arthroplasty be concern for corrosion of the femoral component of the total hip.

INTRODUCTION

Total hip arthroplasty (THA) is generally a highly successful operation.[1] However, occasionally patients do return with pain in the hip without an obvious cause, such as dislocation, fracture, wear, or infection. In evaluating the painful total hip, it is helpful to use the history and the physical examination to focus on the workup.[2]

Modularity at the head-neck junction of the femoral component has been accepted as an option for adjusting the femoral component geometry since the late 1980s. There were initial concerns about fretting and crevice corrosion at the taper junctions, and these were reduced by design improvements. Nevertheless, corrosion from the femoral component remains a complication of

THA. Recently Rush University published a case series of 10 patients demonstrating that there can be an adverse local tissue reaction after THA caused by corrosion at the head-neck taper. This corrosion is correlated with the unique laboratory finding of serum cobalt levels being elevated more than serum chromium levels.[3,4]

The authors have found the iliopsoas sign (pain on resisted flexion of the hip) to be suggestive of the presence of femoral component corrosion. This physical examination test was originally described for the detection of appendicitis or iliopsoas abscess.[5] The authors think the relationship of iliopsoas irritation and intraarticular corrosion may be caused by the close relationship of the iliopsoas and the joint capsule. In most hips, the joint capsule and the iliopsoas sheath are

a Orthopedic + Fracture Specialists, Providence St. Vincent Medical Center, 11782 Southwest Barnes Road #300, Portland, OR 97225, USA; b Providence Health & Services, Orthopedic Institute, 5251 Northeast Glisan Street, Building A, Suite 326, Portland, OR 97213, USA
* Corresponding author.
E-mail address: jacob.coleman@providence.org

Orthop Clin N Am 46 (2015) 461–468
http://dx.doi.org/10.1016/j.ocl.2015.06.009
0030-5898/15/$ – see front matter © 2015 Elsevier Inc. All rights reserved.

physically separated by the substantial ligaments of the hip: the iliofemoral, pubofemoral, and ischiofemoral ligaments.[6] Occasionally there is a communication in a native hip between the hip capsule and the iliopsoas.[7] After a THA, there is iatrogenic damage to the joint capsule that may lead to communication between the iliopsoas and the joint capsule.

The authors present a case series to demonstrate the relationship of a positive iliopsoas sign and/or iliopsoas sterile abscess to the presence of clinically important head-neck corrosion.

MATERIAL AND METHODS

From a retrospective review of the authors' records from May 29, 2012 to April 23, 2014, they identified 8 hips having revision arthroplasty for a concern of corrosion, with corrosion identified at the revision procedure. The authors' suspected patients with corrosion preoperatively as having elevated cobalt over chromium levels, MRI findings of a pseudotumor, and iliopsoas symptoms. Iliopsoas symptoms were defined as examination findings of severe groin pain with resistance of hip flexion. Some patients exhibited a sterile psoas abscess that required either aspiration or drainage. Intraoperatively, corrosion was defined as a finding of black debris between the trunnion and the femoral head and identifiable metallosis debris in the soft tissue.

Mechanical causes of iliopsoas tendonitis, such as an oversized or inadequately anteverted cup, were excluded. None of the patients had a metal-on-metal bearing. All patients had a larger femoral metal head (32 mm, 36 mm, or 40 mm) on Ultra-high-molecular-weight polyethylene (UHMWPE). Six of the original implants were M/L Taper prostheses with Kinectiv modular neck technology (Zimmer, Warsaw, In, USA); one was a VerSys

beaded full-coat prosthesis (Zimmer, Warsaw, In, USA); one patient had his or her primary THA placed in Thailand with unrecognizable implants. Each case had (1) acceptable radiographs, at least anteroposterior (AP) pelvis, AP hip, and lateral hip of the primary THA, including cup position, stem position, and lack of implant loosening; (2) elevation of both cobalt and chromium levels, with the cobalt levels being more elevated than their chromium levels; (3) a negative workup for infection, including erythrocyte sedimentation rate, C-reactive protein, and hip aspiration; and (4) a metal suppression MRI demonstrating a soft tissue reaction.

For these patients, the authors reviewed the intraoperative findings, histology, clinical symptoms, and radiographs. They were particularly interested in the presence of pain on resisted hip flexion, a positive psoas sign, or the presence of an iliopsoas sterile abscess.

RESULTS

The demographics and preoperative data for these patients are described in **Table 1**. These patients represented 8 of the 120 revision hip arthroplasties (7%) performed at the authors' institution from May 29, 2012 to April 23, 2014. The study group consisted of 3 women and 5 men with an average age of 65 years (range 57–71 years) at the time of revision. The average body mass index (BMI) was 27 (range 20–33). The preoperative cobalt levels ranged from 4.3 to 13.5 μg/mL. The average time between the primary THA and revision surgery was 5 ± 2 years (see **Table 1**). Data about the revision surgery are found in **Table 2**. All patients had a femoral head made of cobalt chromium; 7 of the 8 patients had a titanium stem. Patient 6 had a full-coat cobalt chrome stem. In 6 of the 8 patients,

Table 1
Demographic and preoperative data

Patient Number	Age at Second Surgery (y)	Time Between Primary/Revision (y)	Sex	BMI	Preop Cr Levels (μg/mL)	Preop Co Levels (μg/mL)
1	69	5.0	M	27	1.0	6.0
2	57	3.0	F	30	2.3	6.3
3	77	4.5	M	28	—	—
4	71	9.5	M	25	2.3	12.1
5	68	4.3	M	30	4.0	13.5
6	59	6.0	F	24	2.7	4.3
7	60	4.7	M	33	<1.0	4.7
8	61	3.8	F	20	0.2	4.4

Abbreviations: BMI, body mass index; Co, cobalt; Cr, chromium; F, female; M, male; Preop, preoperative.

Table 2
Revision surgery data

Patient Number	Positive Iliopsoas Sign	Complication After Revision	Extent of Revision	Head Size	Stem Type Before Revision	Approach	Iliopsoas Drain
1	Yes	Yes	Stem/cup (all)	32, −4	Kinectiv	Posterior	Yes
2	Yes	No	Stem/cup (all)	40	Kinectiv	Posterior	No
3	—	No	Modular neck/head/liner	40	Kinectiv	Posterior	No
4	No	No	Stem/cup	—	—[a]	Posterior	No
5	Yes	Yes	Stem/head/liner	40	Kinectiv	Posterior	Yes
6	—	No	Stem/cup (all)	32, +7	Beaded	Posterior	Yes
7	Yes	No	Cup/head/liner	40, −4	Kinectiv	2-Incision posterior	No
8	Yes	No	Modular neck/head/liner	36	Kinectiv	Posterior	No

[a] Specifics unknown; primary THA done abroad.

the femoral component was modular with titanium stem and neck components. Five of the 8 patients had a positive iliopsoas sign before revision. One patient had a negative iliopsoas sign, and the iliopsoas sign was not documented in 2 of the patients. Three of the 8 patients had their iliopsoas drained before revision because of effusions visualized on MRI within the iliopsoas (see **Table 2**). Prerevision radiographs were read as normal on all patients.

The operative reports were reviewed, and corrosion was documented as being found at the head-neck junction in all patients. In cases of modularity, the authors saw corrosion at the head-neck junction and not at the neck-stem junction (**Fig. 1**). Intraoperative gross pathology findings were similar to the senior author's experience with aseptic lymphocyte-dominated vasculitis-associated lesion (ALVAL) responses found during

revision of metal-on-metal THA (**Fig. 2**). Intraoperative pathology findings were similar with the findings described by Cooper and colleagues[3]: necrotic tissue and all the cultures were read as negative (**Figs. 3–7**).

In 4 of the 8 patients (50%), the stem and cup were explanted followed by a complete revision of both the femoral as well as the acetabular prostheses. In 2 of the 8 patients (25%), there was a revision of the neck, head, and acetabular liner. In one patient, there was a revision of the stem in addition to an exchange of the liner. In the final patient, there was a revision of the cup in addition to exchange of the head (see **Table 2**).

Patient 4 (**Figs. 8–10**) sustained an anterior hip dislocation around 1.5 weeks postoperatively, which was not diagnosed until the 6-week postoperative visit (**Fig. 11**). The dislocation could not be reduced without an open surgical revision

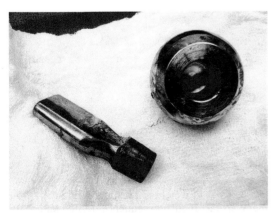

Fig. 1. Intraoperative images from patient 8. Corrosion was noted at the head-neck taper but not at the neck-stem taper.

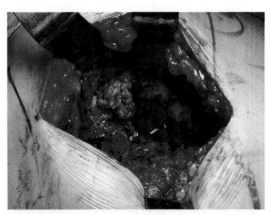

Fig. 2. Extensive soft tissue destruction noted in patient 3, similar to ALVAL findings seen with revision of metal-on-metal THA.

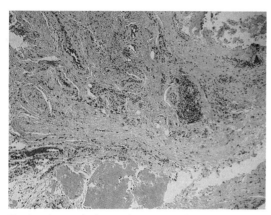

Fig. 3. Histopathology of patient 7 showing a mixed lymphocytic and plasmacytic infiltrate. Cultures were negative (hematoxylin-eosin, original magnification ×100).

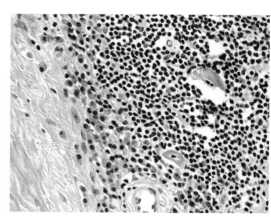

Fig. 6. Histopathology of patient 8 showing primarily a lymphocytic infiltrate with associated macrophages. Rare plasma cells present. Cultures were negative (hematoxylin-eosin, original magnification ×100).

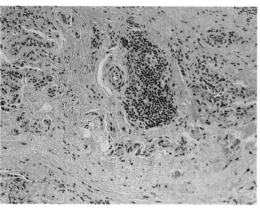

Fig. 4. Histopathology of patient 7 showing a mixed lymphocytic and plasmacytic infiltrate. Cultures were negative (hematoxylin-eosin, original magnification ×200).

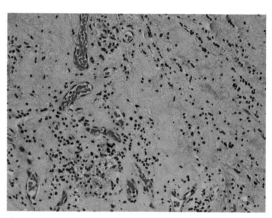

Fig. 7. Histopathology of patient 8 showing primarily a lymphocytic infiltrate with associated macrophages. Rare plasma cells present. Cultures were negative (hematoxylin-eosin, original magnification ×200).

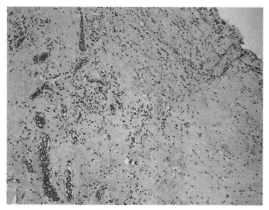

Fig. 5. Histopathology of patient 7 showing a mixed lymphocytic and plasmacytic infiltrate. Cultures were negative (hematoxylin-eosin, original magnification ×400).

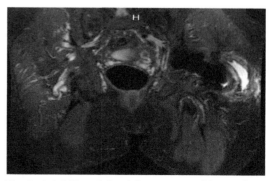

Fig. 8. Axial T1 weighted fat suppressed image from metal artifact reduction sequence (MARS) MRI of the hips demonstrate a total hip replacement on the left with pseudotumor formation surrounding the prosthesis at the level of the greater trochanter.

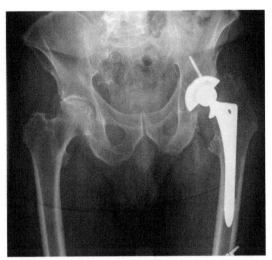

Fig. 9. Patient 4 is a 71-year-old man with a BMI of 25. Before revision, the cobalt level was 12.1 μg/mL and the chromium level was 2.3 μg/mL. Primary THA was done abroad, and implant records were not available. A total of 9.5 years transpired between primary THA and revision. Preoperative images.

that included a surgical relocation and placement of a constrained liner. Patient 1 had urinary retention 4 days after the operation and required a Foley catheter. No other complications were

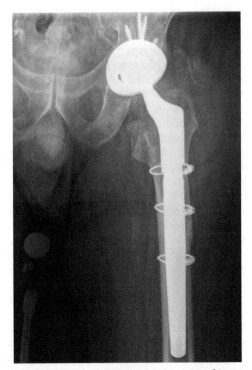

Fig. 10. Patient 4 postoperative images, after complete revision of stem and cup.

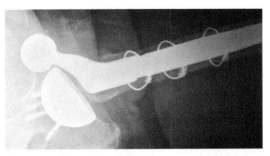

Fig. 11. Patient 4 postoperative complication (anterior hip dislocation), which required surgical reduction and placement of a constrained liner. He has not had further complications.

noted in the postoperative period. Seven of the 8 patients though their symptoms and strength subjectively improved after their revision operation.

In patient 1, the delay in diagnosis was greater than 11 months. This patient did very well for his first 2 years after his primary total hip when he began having symptoms located in his groin. His inflammatory markers were within normal limits. A computed tomography scan demonstrated a fluid collection, and sterile fluid was drained from his iliopsoas. When his symptoms did not improve, tissue was obtained percutaneously, which demonstrated necrotic tissues. He then had a drain placed in the iliopsoas sterile abscess. The patient was explored by general surgery via an anterior approach, and the pathology findings were negative for infection. Postoperatively, the patient had developed a femoral neuropathy and was unable to fire his quadriceps. He was explored a week later in a combined procedure with a neurosurgery, vascular surgery, and the initial orthopedic surgeon. Intraoperatively, no nerve action was found in the quadriceps. A large mass with metal-appearing material was noted. The patient's stem was revised; postoperatively, the symptoms of pain nearly completely resolved at the 6-week and 1-year follow up. The patient continues to have femoral nerve palsy.

Patient 8 presented to the authors' clinic with severe unremitting pain of her right hip 3.5 years postoperatively (**Fig. 12**). Unfortunately, because of a change in her insurance, she had been to another surgical clinic where she had undergone debridement and repair of her gluteus medius 6 months before her representation and almost 3 years after her original operation (**Fig. 13**). On her presentation to the authors, her sedimentation rate and C-reactive protein levels were found to be normal. Synovial fluid was then analyzed for infection and was also found to be negative. Her

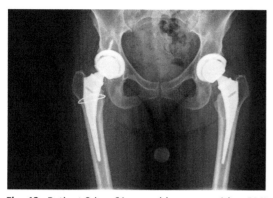

Fig. 12. Patient 8 is a 61-year-old woman with a BMI of 20. Prerevision cobalt level was 4.4 µg/mL, and the chromium level 0.2 µg/mL. Symptomatic on right side. Preoperative images demonstrate that she is status post primary bilateral THAs. Right side required cable because of concern of intraoperative calcar compromise.

blood cobalt and chromium levels were obtained and found to be elevated. An MRI scan showed a mass extending from her hip capsule into her iliopsoas (see **Fig. 8**). In her functional examination, she presented with weakness and pain with flexion. She underwent a revision of her modular neck, revision of the ceramic femoral head with a titanium inner femoral sleeve, and acetabular liner (**Fig. 14**). The pathology findings are demonstrated in **Figs. 6** and **7**. At her 6-week follow-up, she was nearly pain free, including no pain with resisted hip flexion; her gluteal strength was returning.

After the revisions, all of the symptoms of iliopsoas tendonitis resolved at a minimum of 6 months and a mean 1.2 years of follow-up.

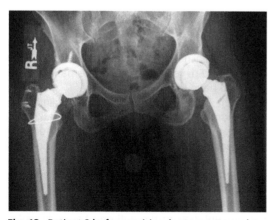

Fig. 13. Patient 8 before revision (note suture anchors present as treatment of misdiagnosed gluteal tear at outside hospital); 3.8 years between primary and revision.

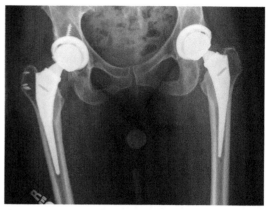

Fig. 14. Patient 8 after revision: revision of modular neck, head, and acetabular liner. Cable was removed because of interval healing and integrity of calcar.

DISCUSSION

Although it is accepted that corrosion may occur at the head-neck taper,[8,9] the specific signs and symptoms associated with corrosion have not been identified. Although a positive iliopsoas sign seems to be sensitive to the presence of corrosion, it is not specific to this condition. Anterior groin pain after a THA may also be associated with anterior iliopsoas impingement caused by excessive acetabular version,[10] recurrent hematomas,[11] acetabular loosening, stress fracture, iliopsoas tendonitis,[12] appendicitis, iliopsoas abscess, lumbosacral radiculopathy, inguinal hernia, gynecologic pathology, undescended testes, and femoral artery aneurysm.[13,14]

The reported series from Rush[3] lead the senior surgeon to obtain metal ion levels and be suspicious for corrosion. The MRI findings were suggestive of an ALVAL response on MRI with metal artifact reduction software (MARS). Because this was not a metal-on-metal hip, the conclusion was reached that corrosion may be the culprit.[4,15–17] Given that 2 of the authors' 8 patients had a cobalt ion level less than 4.5, the authors agree with Griffin's[4] recent article that they should use a cobalt level of 4.5 as the trigger for obtaining an MRI. Additionally if patients are symptomatic with a positive iliopsoas sign and there is a concern for corrosion, MRI should be obtained if cobalt levels are less than 4.5. Of note, 4 of the retrieved femoral heads were size 40. Larger femoral heads cause more corrosion, perhaps because of the greater torque.[18]

The authors think the iliopsoas symptoms are likely related to the close proximity, and possible communication, of the iliopsoas and the hip capsule. The iliopsoas bursa is located near the most vulnerable portion of the anterior capsule of the hip[6,19] (**Fig. 15**). Therefore, a defect in the anterior capsule, such as from an anterior acetabular retractor, may lead to communication between the bursa and the hip joint. Additionally, even if the bursa is not disrupted during surgery, it is possible that the capsule is stretched from prior degenerative joint disease and inflammatory wear interarticularly; with the overproduction of synovial fluid, the capsule ruptures.[6,7,19]

One study has demonstrated a communication between the bursa and the hip joints in patients with iliopsoas bursitis. MRI demonstrated a communication between the hip capsule and iliopsoas bursae in all 18 patients who had iliopsoas bursitis.[6] Another study suggested that 15% of healthy adults have a communication between iliopsoas and the hip capsule.[7]

Nearly all of the total hip arthroplasties in place in North America have a modular metal-on-metal articulation at the head-neck junction. Some of the total hip arthroplasties have additional metal on metal articulations, such as metal on metal (MOM) hips and modular hips. The prevalence of modular stems in this series may be related to the high frequency with which this prosthesis was used in the authors' practice during this time period. The authors no longer routinely use modular stems because they found no clinical

benefit in improving the head center compared with a nonmodular stem and because of the additional concerns about corrosion with an extra modular junction.[20] All stems except one from Thailand were from the same manufacturer, but this was not surprising given that the senior author uses only Zimmer stems.

The authors' group agrees with the Rush group that exchange to a titanium sleeve ceramic implant is the preferred treatment at this time. Obviously more complex revisions are required in the face of component malposition or severe corrosion of the femoral neck. In situations of severe corrosion of the neck stem, revision should be considered.

Strengths of this study include a single series done at one center. The high incidence of iliopsoas findings in this series and the initial delay in diagnosis were the compelling reasons for the authors to share their experience. Another strength of this study is the awareness that anatomically deformed hips and surgical corrections, such as THA, may cause disruptions in the capsule, thereby causing a communication between the iliopsoas bursae and hip capsule.

Limitations of this study are the small numbers involved and the fact that it is a retrospective case series. Another potential weakness of this study is that there maybe silent cases of minor corrosion and that these cases may be underreported. The authors realize that the iliopsoas sign may also be positive in cases of infection, loosening of the components, or any process which causes joint inflammation. None of these diagnoses were seen in the authors' series. However, the authors think that the high incidence of iliopsoas findings in this small series warrants clinical identification.

Certainly the incidence of the diagnosis of corrosion will increase along with the number of total hips in the general population. Clinical awareness of iliopsoas findings in patients with THA and pain of unexplained cause deserves a workup described in this article and by the group at Rush.[3]

SUMMARY

Based on the authors' experience and the recent literature, they recommend that the iliopsoas sign or presentation of a sterile iliopsoas abscess in a previously well-functioning THA be concern for corrosion of the femoral component of the total hip. Patients presenting with this sign after a THA merit further evaluation for the possibility of corrosion. Diagnostic workup includes obtaining serum cobalt and chrome levels to look for corrosion, C-reactive protein and sedimentation rate to rule out infection, a metal-suppression MRI to evaluate

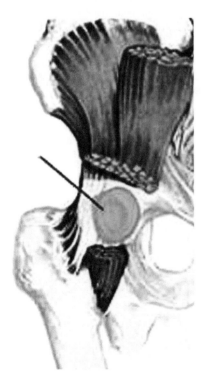

Fig. 15. The hip capsule and iliopsoas are adjacent anatomic structures. The *black line* is pointing to the iliopsoas bursa.

for iliopsoas involvement, ALVAL, or other soft tissue involvement.[3] Early surgical intervention is warranted in the face of elevated cobalt over chrome levels and especially with positive findings on MRI with MARS.

The authors present their series with physical findings that may aid the orthopedic surgeon in a prompt diagnosis that can prevent further soft tissue injury.

REFERENCES

1. Callaghan JJ, Albright JC, Goetz DD, et al. Charnley total hip arthroplasty with cement. J Bone Joint Surg Am 2000;82-A:487–97.
2. Bozic KJ, Rubash HE. The painful total hip replacement. Clin Orthop Relat Res 2004;420:18–25.
3. Cooper J, Della Valle CJ, Berger RA, et al. Corrosion at the head-neck taper as a cause for adverse local tissue reactions after total hip arthroplasty. J Bone Joint Surg Am 2012;94-A:1–7.
4. Griffin WL. Metal ion levels: how can they help us? J Arthroplasty 2014;29(4):659–60.
5. Wagner JM, McKinney WP, Carpenter J. Does this patient have appendicitis? JAMA 1996;276(19):1589–94.
6. Zembrzuska H, Papadopoulos PJ, Gilliland WR, et al. Iliopsoas bursitis. Available at: http://www.rheumatologynetwork.com/articles/iliopsoas-bursitis#sthash.6ncWhma0.dpuf. Accessed April 6, 2014.
7. Wunderbaldinger P, Bremer C, Schellenberger E, et al. Imaging features of iliopsoas bursitis. Eur Radiol 2002;12:409–15.
8. Collier JP, Surprenant VA, Jensen RE, et al. Corrosion at the interface of cobalt-alloy heads on titanium-alloy stems. Clin Orthop Relat Res 1991;271:305–12.
9. Cook SD, Barrack RL, Baffes GC, et al. Wear and corrosion of modular interfaces in total hip replacements. Clin Orthop Relat Res 1994;298:80–8.
10. Lachiewicz PF, Kauk JR. Anterior iliopsoas impingement and tendinitis after total hip arthroplasty. J Am Acad Orthop Surg 2009;17(6):337–44.
11. Bartelt RB, Sierra RJ. Recurrent hematomas within the iliopsoas muscle caused by impingement after total hip arthroplasty. J Arthroplasty 2011;26(4):665.
12. Henderson RA, Lachiewicz PF. Groin pain after replacement of the hip: etiology, evaluation and treatment. J Bone Joint Surg Br 2012;94(2):145–51.
13. Kozlov DB, Sonin AH. Iliopsoas bursitis: diagnosis by MRI. J Comput Assist Tomogr 1998;22:625–8.
14. Parziale JR, O'Donnell CJ, Sandman DN. Iliopsoas bursitis. Am J Phys Med Rehabil 2009;88:690–1.
15. Kwon YM. Cross sectional imaging in evaluation of soft tissue reactions secondary to metal debris. J Arthroplasty 2014;29(4):653–6.
16. Lombardi AV. Case studies in management of THA failure secondary to taper corrosion, modular junctions and metal-on-metal bearings. J Arthroplasty 2014;29(4):663–7.
17. Engh CA, MacDonald SJ, Sritulanondha S, et al. Metal ion levels after metal-on-metal total hip arthroplasty: a five-year, prospective randomized trial. J Bone Joint Surg Am 2014;96(6):448–55.
18. Dyrkacz R, Brandt JM, Olanrewaju AO, et al. The influence of head size on corrosion and fretting behavior at the head-neck interface of artificial hip joints. J Arthroplasty 2013;28(6):1036–40.
19. Toohey AK, LaSalle TL, Martinez S, et al. Iliopsoas bursitis: clinical features, radiographic findings, and disease associations. Semin Arthritis Rheum 1990;20:41–7.
20. Duwelius PJ, Burkart B, Carnahan C, et al. Modular versus nonmodular neck femoral implants in primary total hip arthroplasty: which is better? Clin Orthop Relat Res 2014;472(4):1240–5.

Liposomal Bupivacaine
A Comparative Study of More Than 1000 Total Joint Arthroplasty Cases

John W. Barrington, MD[a], Oluseun Olugbode, MS[b],
Scott Lovald, PhD, MBA[c],*, Kevin Ong, PhD[d],
Heather Watson, PhD[c], Roger H. Emerson Jr, MD[b]

KEYWORDS

- Liposomal bupivacaine • Knee arthroplasty • Hip arthroplasty • Pain control • Analgesia

KEY POINTS

- Pain after total joint arthroplasty (TJA) can be severe and difficult to control. A single-dose local analgesic has been introduced that delivers bupivacaine in a liposomal time-release platform.
- The study included 2248 consecutive hip and knee arthroplasty cases, in half of which (Pre) the subjects were treated using a well-established multimodal analgesia, including periarticular injection (PAI).
- In a matching number of procedures the PAI was substituted for a liposomal bupivacaine injection technique (Post).
- Visual analog scale pain scores were significantly lower for patients treated with liposomal bupivacaine for both hip (1.67 vs 2.30; $P<.0001$) and knee (2.21 vs 2.52; $P<.0001$) procedures.
- We found improvement in pain relief in a large series of patients who had TJA after the introduction of a liposomal bupivacaine as part of an established multimodal protocol.

INTRODUCTION

More than 1.1 million total joint arthroplasties (TJAs) are performed annually in the United States[1] and are widely considered highly successful in terms of improving the quality of life of patients with osteoarthritis.[2] Despite its success, pain after TJA can be severe and difficult to control.[3] Clinical studies and hospital record analysis have shown that severe postoperative pain can be associated with an increased risk of complications, including rehabilitation delay,[4] prolonged return to normal functioning,[5,6] progression to persistent pain states,[7,8] prolonged hospital stay,[9] and increased readmission rate,[10] all of which can lead to increased cost of care.[11–14]

Many complications after TJA may be associated with the pain management strategies. Opioid analgesics, including intravenous patient controlled and oral, have been a standard modality for postoperative pain management, but are associated with the risk of nausea, pruritus, vomiting, respiratory depression, prolonged ileus, and cognitive dysfunction.[15–17] Regional pain control techniques, such as femoral nerve blockade, may limit exposure to opioid related adverse events (ORAE), but may cause quadriceps weakness, neuropathy, and postoperative falls.[18,19] Periarticular injection (PAI) has been shown in case series and randomized controlled trials to decrease pain, increase function, and reduce ORAEs after TJA.[20–22] PAI has also been suggested to

Funding: Support for statistical analysis and associated article preparation was provided by Pacira, Inc.
[a] Plano Orthopedic Sports Medicine & Spine Center, 5228 W Plano Pkwy, Plano, TX 75093, USA; [b] Texas Center for Joint Replacement, 6020 West Parker Road, Suite 470, Plano, TX 75093, USA; [c] Exponent, Inc, 149 Commonwealth Drive, Menlo Park, CA 94025, USA; [d] Exponent, Inc, 3440 Market Street, Suite 600, Philadelphia, PA 19104, USA
* Corresponding author.
E-mail address: slovald@exponent.com

be cheaper and easier to perform than other regional modalities, such as femoral neck blocks.[3]

A single-dose local analgesic has recently been introduced that delivers bupivacaine in a liposomal time-release platform. To date, there is still little clinical evidence concerning the effect of the time-release mechanism on patient-reported pain among differing PAI modalities. This comparative study compared a large sample of procedures using a novel extended-release liposomal bupivacaine during PAI, to a control group of procedures previously conducted using PAI without liposomal bupivacaine, using pain control as the primary outcome measure. Because of the time-release mechanism incorporated in liposomal bupivacaine, we hypothesized that this group would have demonstrably lower visual analog scale (VAS) pain scores for the immediate postoperative period.

MATERIALS AND METHODS

In the period between December 2011 and October 2012, 1124 consecutive hip and knee arthroplasty procedures were performed using a well-established multimodal analgesia (including PAI with Marcaine, with or without ketorolac, and morphine) and therapy protocols (the Pre group). This sample included all procedures representative of a traditional hip and knee arthroplasty practice, including primary and revision hip and knee procedures, and unicompartmental knee arthroplasty procedures. Four surgeons in a dedicated arthroplasty practice provided cases for this study.

In the period that immediately followed (October 2012 to August 2013), a matching number of 1124 consecutive hip and knee arthroplasty procedures were performed with similar therapy protocols, but substituting the established PAI for an US Food and Drug Administration (FDA)–approved liposomal bupivacaine surgical site soft tissue injection (PAI) technique (EXPAREL, Pacira Pharmaceuticals, Parsippany, NJ) as part of their multimodal analgesia protocol (the Post group). The procedures covered during this period also represented the complete hip/knee arthroplasty practice and were performed by the same 4 surgeons. The sample size was chosen to maximize the number of patients who could be compared in a 1:1 fashion with a commensurate sample of patients receiving liposomal bupivacaine. Because more than 1000 patients were recruited for each group, this study has more than 90% power at an alpha level of 0.05 to detect an effect size of 0.20 in the average VAS pain score based on post-hoc power calculations.

The primary outcome measures were the average VAS pain score for each patient and the percentage of VAS pain scores during hospitalization that were 0, which is a result of patients answering that they had no pain. The average pain score was aggregated for each patient for the entire stay as well as for each individual day of stay. VAS pain data were collected by nursing personnel, who were blinded to the surgical analgesia treatment protocol, at every instance in which they had contact with the patient, which resulted in an average of 9 VAS scores taken for each day of hospital stay for each patient. The collection of VAS pain scores was implemented through a robust prospective data gathering system that is the result of a custom effort at the study site that occurred before the initiation of the current study protocol. VAS data and other relevant medical parameters are collected routinely on every case that passes through the study center.

Secondary outcome measures were analyzed for a subset of the patient sample (2000 patients) and included an analysis of the rate of mortality, infection, hemorrhage/hematoma, falls, deep venous thrombosis, major cardiopulmonary events (including pulmonary embolus), autologous transfusion, readmission, and missed therapy caused by nausea/vomiting. For this subgroup, which was selected based on direct data from hospital records, patient satisfaction and cost were also compared between groups. Overall patient-reported satisfaction was measured blind to the surgeon and hospital via the Press Ganey survey. The cost analysis included a comparison of total direct hospital costs for all supplies and pharmaceuticals for each treatment group, as reported by hospital administration. All patient information was deidentified, and this is an institutional review board–approved study via exemption. Statistical analysis was performed with SAS software (SAS Institute Inc, Cary, NC) version 9.4, comparing demographics, pain scores, complications, length of stay (LOS), and patient satisfaction. The study sample size was large enough that 2-sample Student t-tests were implemented to test for differences in the means between Pre and Post groups for age, body mass index (BMI), and LOS even though the variables were not normally distribution. For categorical variables, including gender, χ^2 tests were used. Differences in pain scores were tested using 2-sample t-tests to compare differences between group means. Furthermore, regression analyses were implemented to investigate associations between patient demographics, surgery, or treatment group with average pain scores overall and by day. Variables in the regression analysis included race, ethnicity, BMI, gender, hip/knee, LOS, surgeon, Pre/Post, and patient age at surgery. Satisfaction scores and complications were compared between groups via a 2-sample *t*-test. For all tests, statistical significance was adjusted for multiple comparisons ($P = .00179: 0.05/28$).

RESULTS

The distribution of procedures was comparable between the Pre and Post groups, with the percentage of patients in the Post group for each procedure as follows: primary knee (48%), revision knee (45%), unicompartmental knee (56%), bilateral knee (46%), primary hip (50%), revision hip (47%), and bilateral hip (50%) **(Fig. 1)**. There were no differences in age, BMI, and gender breakdown between groups, aside from patients in the Post group for hip being slightly older (65.8 years vs 63.1 years; $P = .0002$) **(Table 1)**.

VAS pain scores were significantly lower for patients in the Post group for hip (1.67 vs 2.30; $P<.0001$), knee (2.21 vs 2.52; $P<.0001$), and all procedures combined (1.98 vs 2.43; $P<.0001$) **(Fig. 2)**. There was also a significantly higher percentage of patients in the Post group who reported having no pain for hip (57.3% vs 43.4%; $P<.0001$) and knee (47.2% vs 42.1%; $P<.0001$) procedures. Regression analysis also showed the Post group to have significantly lower VAS pain scores by 0.39 ($P<.0001$), after controlling for available demographic and surgical factors. Regression analysis also showed the Post group to have higher pain scores by 0.15 on the day of surgery but to have lower pain scores from days 1 to 4, ranging 0.62 to 0.96 points lower ($P<.0001$) **(Fig. 3)**.

The effect on VAS pain scores varied by surgeon ($P<.001$). The largest improvement in the Post group pain scores was for surgeon 1 (2.5–1.7; $P<.0001$) and surgeon 4 (2.1–1.6; $P<.0001$), who operated on most of the patients (68%). The remaining 2 surgeons who operated on 32% of the patients observed no significant differences.

There were few significant differences in complications between the Pre and Post groups, though 2 differences are notable **(Table 2)**. Both falls (10 Pre vs 2 Post; $P = .0207$) and autologous transfusion (73 vs 32; $P<.0001$) were less common in the Post group, although after adjusting for multiple comparisons the reduction in falls was not statistically significant. Seven of 10 falls occurred in patients with a femoral nerve catheter, in spite of using knee immobilizers and physical therapy blocking techniques in these patients.

There were trends for improvement in LOS, patient satisfaction, and associated costs for the Post group (see **Table 2**; **Table 3**). LOS decreased from 2.69 days to 2.40 days in the Post group for knee procedures ($P<.001$). Overall patient-reported satisfaction as measured by Press Ganey improved in the Post group from 96.7% to 98.3% ($P = .0221$), although this finding was not significant after adjusting for multiple comparisons. For the sample collected, the hospital's overall direct cost for all supplies and pharmaceuticals was decreased on average by $1246 per patient (see **Table 3**).

DISCUSSION

There was significant improvement in pain relief in a large series of patients with TJA after the introduction of a liposomal bupivacaine as part of an already well-established multimodal protocol. There was improved pain relief for both hip and knee procedures, as measured by both mean VAS pain scores and the percentage of patients who reported no pain. For the treatment group, 57% of hip patients and 47% of knee patients reported zero pain at some point during their acute

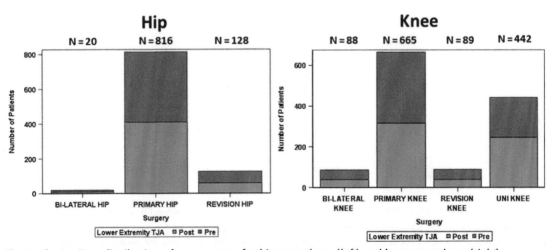

Fig. 1. The Pre/Post distribution of surgery type for hip procedures (*left*) and knee procedures (*right*).

Table 1
Difference in age, BMI, and gender (percentage male) between Pre and Post patients for the hip and knee groups using χ^2 and t-tests

	Hip			Knee		
	Pre (Range)	Post (Range)	P Value	Pre (Range)	Post (Range)	P Value
Age (y)	63.1 (19.0–95.0)	65.8 (32.0–96.0)	P<.001[a]	66.7 (36.0–93.0)	66.7 (38.0–97.0)	P = .890
BMI	29.3 (18.0–49.7)	29.0 (16.5–53.6)	P = .470	31.2 (18.2–55.3)	31.3 (16.6–58.5)	P = .765
Gender (% male)	43.5	42.8	P = .838	41.3	42.5	P = .685

[a] Statistically significant.

hospitalization. With more than 1000 patients in each group, the power of this study is more than 90% to detect an effect size of at least 0.20.

Pain control has a critical role in patient prognosis after large joint arthroplasty, primarily in its role to encourage earlier ambulation and initiation of physiotherapy.[23] Aggressive pain control improves patient compliance with rehabilitation immediately after surgery.[18] In contrast, poorly controlled pain can lead to delayed or diminished ambulation, anxiety, delays in recovery of normal function and lifestyle, poor sleep, urinary retention, and reduced quality of life,[24] as well as increased cost of care.[25–27] Aside from slower rehabilitation, adverse outcomes associated with poorly controlled pain include delayed wound healing, increased risk of pulmonary morbidity (including pneumonia) and thrombosis, increased mortality risk, and hypertension.[24] The elimination of

analgesic gaps,[28–30] preemptive procedure/site-specific analgesia, and elimination of cognitive/age/cultural barriers[31–33] may be the mechanisms whereby many of the patients in this study experienced improved pain control.

The primary difference in the Post group was the administration of a liposomal bupivacaine as part of the analgesic protocol. Liposomal bupivacaine is a 72-hour local anesthetic formulation that was FDA-approved in 2013 for surgical site soft tissue injection. This formulation uses a novel delivery system to combine the well-established benefits of bupivacaine with time-release delivery and prolonged duration of effect. Efficacy and safety of liposomal bupivacaine have been established in more than 21 clinical trials, including 10 double-blind, randomized controlled trials that collectively involved 823 patients undergoing a range of surgical procedures, including total knee

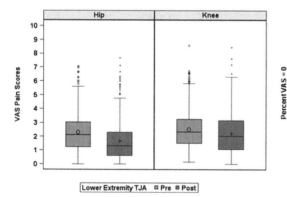

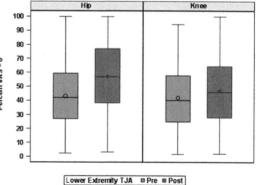

Fig. 2. Average total VAS pain scores (*left*) and the percentage of patients with a VAS pain score of 0 (*right*) are shown for hip and knee procedures. [a] Statistical significance after adjusting for multiple comparisons. Avg, average; CI, confidence interval.

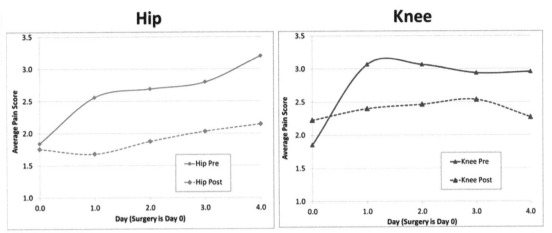

Fig. 3. Average VAS pain scores for hip and knee procedures for the Pre and Post groups for each day up to 4 days after the surgery.

arthroplasty.[20,34–42] Importantly, this study describes a surgical soft tissue injection, not an intra-articular infusion.[43] Regional techniques such as liposomal bupivacaine act as a substitute for traditional methods of pain control, primarily patient-controlled morphine or other opioids. By reducing narcotic consumption, there is a great potential to reduce nausea and vomiting, the hospital LOS, improve patient satisfaction, and increase physical therapy participation.[18] In a pooled study of 37,031 patients, those who experienced an ORAE had a 55% longer LOS, 47% higher costs of care, 36% increased risk of

30-day readmission, and 3.4 times higher risk of inpatient mortality compared with patients who did not experience an ORAE.[9]

Both falls (10 Pre vs 2 Post; $P = .0207$) and autologous transfusion (73 vs 32; $P<.0001$) were less common in the Post group, although after adjusting for multiple comparisons the reduction in falls was not statistically significant. Most of the falls (7 out of 10) occurred in patients with a femoral nerve catheter. Prolonged quadriceps weakness remains a concern with femoral nerve block use.[18,23,44,45] It is estimated that motor block complications, including falls, fractures, and neurologic dysfunction, are

Table 2
Secondary outcomes for Pre and Post groups, including complications, LOS, and overall satisfaction

Complication	Pre	Post	P Value
Mortality	0	0	$P = 1$
Infection (%)	0.40	0.50	$P = .738$
Hemorrhage/hematoma (%)	0.20	0.20	$P = 1$
Missed PT b/o nausea (%)	0.90	0.50	$P = .284$
Falls (%)	1.00	0.20	$P = .021$
Deep vein thrombosis (%)	0.70	0.60	$P = .781$
PE (%)	0.50	0.90	$P = .284$
Major cardiopulmonary event (%)	0.60	0.30	$P = .317$
PE/CV event (%)	1.10	1.20	$P = .834$
Autologous transfusion (%)	7.30	3.20	$P<.0001^a$
Readmission (%)	2.20	2.60	$P = .559$
LOS, hip (days)	2.98	3.02	$P = .784$
LOS, knee (days)	2.69	2.40	$P<.0001^a$
Press Ganey overall satisfaction (%)	96.70	98.30	$P = .022$

Abbreviations: b/o, because of; CV, cardiovascular; PE, pulmonary embolism; PT, physical therapy.
  [a] Indicates statistical significance after adjusting for multiple comparisons.

Table 3
Aggregate cost data for supplies and pharmaceuticals for a subset of patients in the Pre and Post groups

Cost	Pre	Post	Change
Cost of Supplies ($)	11,900,847	10,394,427	1,506,420
Cost of Pharmaceuticals ($)	371,506	631,813	−260,307
Total Change			1,246,113

observed in about 2% of patients.[23] Sharma and colleagues[18] described a cohort of 709 patients with total knee arthroplasty who underwent femoral nerve blocks, and they reported 12 (1.6%) falls, 5 (0.7%) cases of femoral neuritis, and 3 (0.4%) reoperations secondary to falls.

For the current study, no other complications were statistically different between the 2 groups. Specifically, use of liposomal bupivacaine did not predispose patients to increased infection, hemorrhage, hematoma, or adverse cardiopulmonary events.

LOS was decreased in the Post group for knee procedures, despite there being no attempted change in an already well-established rehabilitation protocol. Nuelle and Mann[46] described how, using the same traditional TJA procedure, accelerated rehabilitation protocols allow patients to achieve goals for discharge earlier. Cognizant of this potential bias, this study made no change to rehabilitation protocols. This study occurred in a practice and hospital model that already had in place an established total joint institute, including preoperative education,[24] patient-focused care initiatives,[47] multimodal analgesia regimens,[48,49] and postoperative rehabilitation pathways. Thus, the results of this study point to the difference in local soft tissue analgesia regimen: patients' pain experience and satisfaction drove their ability to return home, which was the discharge disposition for 85% of patients in both cohorts. Along with a reduction in pain scores and a reduced LOS for knee procedures, patient satisfaction trended toward increasing in the Post group, despite having already been very high at 96.7% for the baseline Pre group. Although this is a small improvement in a sample with a high baseline satisfaction, this can also be considered as a nearly 50% reduction in dissatisfied patients from 3.3% to 1.7%. Local and regional patient satisfaction surveys, including information sent to the Hospital Consumer Assessment of Healthcare Providers and Systems (HCAHPS), are major factors in the daily operations and future direction of hospital initiatives.[50]

In addition, the hospital saw cost savings after the introduction of liposomal bupivacaine. The cost reductions were found in spite of pharmacy cost increases of $260 per patient, because the hospital saved more than $1.5 million on supply costs, predominantly by eliminating femoral nerve catheters, patient-controlled analgesia pumps, and knee immobilizers. Although the cost analysis relied on costs for only supplies and pharmaceuticals but did not consider costs from other sources (eg, facility, professional services), these results indicate that there is a potential for reducing hospital supply costs in transitioning toward local infiltration analgesia. Furthermore, more difficult-to-measure cost savings, such as LOS decreases, satisfaction improvement scores, and subsequent referral increases, were not factored in this analysis, and may lead to additional economic benefit to the hospital. Hospital perspective is important: the quality and safety of pain management provided at a hospital, and by its providers, have become key performance markers. Patients' self-reported pain scores are commonly used as a factor in ranking health care facilities (and rankings can be viewed online by patients and the public),[51] and selection of one facility rather than a nearby competitor may be influenced by published rankings or superiority in providing pain management. An era is beginning in which reimbursement rates from government and private payers will depend on pain management and other performance markers.[52,53]

This retrospective comparative study, comparing the first 1124 cases using a novel extended-release liposomal bupivacaine with a 1124 patient control group, showed improved overall mean VAS pain scores, an increased number of pain-free patients, decreased LOS, trends toward decreased falls, and decreased overall cost. Strengths of the study include the definition of specific primary and secondary outcome measures, a well-powered comparative study, and a global stakeholder perspective on arthroplasty surgery, including patient-reported satisfaction scores, payer-directed focus on minimizing complications, and hospital-required and systems-required diligence in controlling costs. Although classified as a retrospective study, the data were collected as part of a prospective data gathering system, improving the consistency and completeness of relevant study data relative to a traditional retrospective chart review. Further, the high frequency of VAS score time points reduces the risk for inaccuracy caused by sampling errors. In a conscious effort to analyze the treatment effect across a typical mix of cases within a TJA practice, primary and revision hip and knee procedures were aggregated to analyze the effect of transitioning the pain control regimen throughout the practice case mix. Assessing clinically meaningful differences in VAS scores will be more appropriate in follow-on studies targeted to specific procedures. Limitations of this study include the lack of a standardizing technique between surgeons, the gradual and sporadic introduction of other medications during the study period (eg, tranexamic acid contributing to decreased transfusion), and the nonrandomized design of the study. Although a historical control is used, this control sample was treated immediately before the treatment group, thus minimizing any differences in the patient samples that may be affected by time. An ongoing multicenter randomized controlled trial is underway, which is focused on standardizing the anesthesia and injection protocol.

ACKNOWLEDGMENTS

The authors thank Richard D. Reitman, MD, and John M. Hillyard, MD, who contributed excellent care to the patients in this study, and Marque Broussard, RN, for his assistance in data collection.

REFERENCES

1. Hall MJ, DeFrances CJ, Williams SN, et al. National Hospital Discharge Survey: 2007 summary. Natl Health Stat Report 2010;(29):1–20, 24.

2. Ethgen O, Bruyere O, Richy F, et al. Health-related quality of life in total hip and total knee arthroplasty. A qualitative and systematic review of the literature. J Bone Joint Surg Am 2004;86A(5):963–74.

3. Affas F, Nygards EB, Stiller CO, et al. Pain control after total knee arthroplasty: a randomized trial comparing local infiltration anesthesia and continuous femoral block. Acta Orthop 2011;82(4):441–7.

4. Morrison RS, Magaziner J, McLaughlin MA, et al. The impact of post-operative pain on outcomes following hip fracture. Pain 2003;103(3):303–11.

5. Dihle A, Helseth S, Kongsgaard UE, et al. Using the American Pain Society's patient outcome questionnaire to evaluate the quality of postoperative pain management in a sample of Norwegian patients. J Pain 2006;7(4):272–80.

6. Dihle A, Helseth S, Paul SM, et al. The exploration of the establishment of cutpoints to categorize the severity of acute postoperative pain. Clin J pain 2006;22(7):617–24.

7. Kehlet H, Jensen TS, Woolf CJ. Persistent postsurgical pain: risk factors and prevention. Lancet 2006;367(9522):1618–25.

8. Perkins FM, Kehlet H. Chronic pain as an outcome of surgery. A review of predictive factors. Anesthesiology 2000;93(4):1123–33.

9. Kessler ER, Shah M, Gruschkus SK, et al. Cost and quality implications of opioid-based postsurgical pain control using administrative claims data from a large health system: opioid-related adverse events and their impact on clinical and economic outcomes. Pharmacotherapy 2013;33(4):383–91.

10. Coley KC, Williams BA, DaPos SV, et al. Retrospective evaluation of unanticipated admissions and readmissions after same day surgery and associated costs. J Clin Anesth 2002;14(5):349–53.

11. Azim SA, Sangster R, Curcio C, et al. Characterization of patients with difficult-to-treat acute pain following total knee arthroplasty using multi-modal analgesia. Open Pain J 2013;6:1–6.

12. Pogatzki-Zahn EM, Schnabel A, Zahn PK. Room for improvement: unmet needs in postoperative pain management. Expert Rev Neurother 2012;12(5): 587–600.

13. Holzer P. Opioid receptors in the gastrointestinal tract. Regul Pept 2009;155(1–3):11–7.

14. Oderda GM, Evans RS, Lloyd J, et al. Cost of opioid-related adverse drug events in surgical patients. J Pain Symptom Manage 2003;25(3):276–83.

15. Wheeler M, Oderda GM, Ashburn MA, et al. Adverse events associated with postoperative opioid analgesia: a systematic review. J Pain 2002;3(3):159–80.

16. Oderda GM, Said Q, Evans RS, et al. Opioid-related adverse drug events in surgical hospitalizations: impact on costs and length of stay. Ann Pharmacother 2007;41(3):400–6.

17. Cepeda MS, Farrar JT, Baumgarten M, et al. Side effects of opioids during short-term administration: effect of age, gender, and race. Clin Pharmacol Ther 2003;74(2):102–12.

18. Sharma S, Iorio R, Specht LM, et al. Complications of femoral nerve block for total knee arthroplasty. Clin Orthop Relat Res 2010;468(1):135–40.

19. Beaupre LA, Johnston DB, Dieleman S, et al. Impact of a preemptive multimodal analgesia plus femoral nerve blockade protocol on rehabilitation, hospital length of stay, and postoperative analgesia after primary total knee arthroplasty: a controlled clinical pilot study. ScientificWorldJournal 2012;2012:273821.

20. Kerr DR, Kohan L. Local infiltration analgesia: a technique for the control of acute postoperative pain following knee and hip surgery: a case study of 325 patients. Acta Orthop 2008;79(2):174–83.

21. Parvataneni HK, Shah VP, Howard H, et al. Controlling pain after total hip and knee arthroplasty using a multimodal protocol with local periarticular injections: a prospective randomized study. J Arthroplasty 2007;22(6 Suppl 2):33–8.

22. Busch CA, Shore BJ, Bhandari R, et al. Efficacy of periarticular multimodal drug injection in total knee arthroplasty. A randomized trial. J Bone Joint Surg Am 2006;88(5):959–63.

23. Paul JE, Arya A, Hurlburt L, et al. Femoral nerve block improves analgesia outcomes after total knee arthroplasty: a meta-analysis of randomized controlled trials. Anesthesiology 2010;113(5):1144–62.

24. Practice guidelines for acute pain management in the perioperative setting: an updated report by the American Society of Anesthesiologists Task Force on Acute Pain Management. Anesthesiology 2012; 116(2):248–73.

25. Kehlet H. Surgical stress: the role of pain and analgesia. Br J Anaesth 1989;63(2):189–95.

26. Pavlin DJ, Chen C, Penaloza DA, et al. A survey of pain and other symptoms that affect the recovery process after discharge from an ambulatory surgery unit. J Clin Anesth 2004;16(3):200–6.

27. Wu CL, Naqibuddin M, Rowlingson AJ, et al. The effect of pain on health-related quality of life in the immediate postoperative period. Anesth Analg 2003; 97(4):1078–85 [table of contents].

28. Carr DB, Reines HD, Schaffer J, et al. The impact of technology on the analgesic gap and quality of acute pain management. Reg Anesth Pain Med 2005;30(3):286–91.

29. Ng A, Hall F, Atkinson A, et al. Bridging the analgesic gap. Acute Pain 2000;3(4):1–6.

30. Chen PP, Chui PT, Ma M, et al. A prospective survey of patients after cessation of patient-controlled analgesia. Anesth Analg 2001;92(1):224–7.

31. Green CR, Anderson KO, Baker TA, et al. The unequal burden of pain: confronting racial and ethnic disparities in pain. Pain Med 2003;4(3):277–94.

32. Atherton MJ, Feeg VD, el-Adham AF. Race, ethnicity, and insurance as determinants of epidural use: analysis of a national sample survey. Nurs Econ 2004;22(1):6–13, 13.

33. Joshi GP, Kehlet H. Procedure-specific pain management: the road to improve postsurgical pain management? Anesthesiology 2013;118(4):780–2.

34. Davidson EM, Barenholz Y, Cohen R, et al. High-dose bupivacaine remotely loaded into multivesicular liposomes demonstrates slow drug release without systemic toxic plasma concentrations after subcutaneous administration in humans. Anesth Analg 2010;110(4):1018–23.

35. Bergese SD, Ramamoorthy S, Patou G, et al. Efficacy profile of liposome bupivacaine, a novel formulation of bupivacaine for postsurgical analgesia. J Pain Res 2012;5:107–16.

36. Dasta J, Ramamoorthy S, Patou G, et al. Bupivacaine liposome injectable suspension compared with bupivacaine HCl for the reduction of opioid burden in the postsurgical setting. Curr Med Res Opin 2012;28(10):1609–15.

37. Golf M, Daniels SE, Onel E. A phase 3, randomized, placebo-controlled trial of DepoFoam® bupivacaine (extended-release bupivacaine local analgesic) in bunionectomy. Adv Ther 2011;28(9):776–88.

38. Cohen SM. Extended pain relief trial utilizing infiltration of Exparel(®), a long-acting multivesicular liposome formulation of bupivacaine: a phase IV health economic trial in adult patients undergoing open colectomy. J Pain Res 2012;5:567–72.

39. Marcet JE, Nfonsam VN, Larach S. An extended pain relief trial utilizing the infiltration of a long-acting Multivesicular liposome formulation of bupivacaine, EXPAREL (IMPROVE): a Phase IV health economic trial in adult patients undergoing ileostomy reversal. J Pain Res 2013;6:549–55.

40. Vogel JD. Liposome bupivacaine (EXPAREL®) for extended pain relief in patients undergoing ileostomy reversal at a single institution with a fast-track discharge protocol: an IMPROVE Phase IV health economics trial. J Pain Res 2013;6:605–10.

41. Haas E, Onel E, Miller H, et al. A double-blind, randomized, active-controlled study for post-hemorrhoidectomy pain management with liposome bupivacaine, a novel local analgesic formulation. Am Surg 2012;78(5):574–81.

42. Bergese SD, Onel E, Morren M, et al. Bupivacaine extended-release liposome injection exhibits a favorable cardiac safety profile. Reg Anesth Pain Med 2012;37(2):145–51.

43. Syed HM, Green L, Bianski B, et al. Bupivacaine and triamcinolone may be toxic to human chondrocytes: a pilot study. Clin Orthop Relat Res 2011;469(10):2941–7.

44. Richman JM, Liu SS, Courpas G, et al. Does continuous peripheral nerve block provide superior pain control to opioids? A meta-analysis. Anesth Analg 2006;102(1):248–57.

45. Capdevila X, Barthelet Y, Biboulet P, et al. Effects of perioperative analgesic technique on the surgical outcome and duration of rehabilitation after major knee surgery. Anesthesiology 1999;91(1):8–15.

46. Nuelle DG, Mann K. Minimal incision protocols for anesthesia, pain management, and physical therapy with standard incisions in hip and knee arthroplasties: the effect on early outcomes. J Arthroplasty 2007;22(1):20–5.

47. Committee on Advancing Pain Research, Care, and Education. Relieving pain in America: a blueprint for transforming prevention, care, education, and research. Washington, DC: Institute of Medicine of the National Academies. 2011.

48. Southworth S, Peters J, Rock A, et al. A multicenter, randomized, double-blind, placebo-controlled trial

of intravenous ibuprofen 400 and 800 mg every 6 hours in the management of postoperative pain. Clin Ther 2009;31(9):1922–35.

49. Sinatra RS, Jahr JS, Reynolds LW, et al. Efficacy and safety of single and repeated administration of 1 gram intravenous acetaminophen injection (paracetamol) for pain management after major orthopedic surgery. Anesthesiology 2005;102(4):822–31.

50. US Department of Health and Human Services CfMaM. HCAHPS: Patients' Perspectives of Care Survey. Avialable online at: http://www.cms.gov/Medicare/Quality-Initiatives-Patient-Assessment-instruments/Hospital QualityInits/HospitalHCAHPS.html.

51. Report UW. US World Report rankings of pain management at major hospitals in the United States. Available online at: http://health.usnews.com/health-news/best-hospitals/articles/2009/10/20/which-best-hospitals-are-best-and-worst-at-pain-management.

52. Lansky D, Nwachukwu BU, Bozic KJ. Using financial incentives to improve value in orthopaedics. Clin Orthop Relat Res 2012;470(4):1027–37.

53. So JP, Wright JG. The use of three strategies to improve quality of care at a national level. Clin Orthop Relat Res 2012;470(4):1006–16.

Trauma

Preface

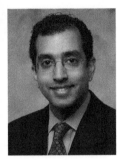

Saqib Rehman, MD
Editor

The current issue of *Orthopedic Clinics of North America* has three review articles in the field of orthopedic trauma. In the first article, Dr Lachman and coauthors review the management of traumatic knee dislocations. These are injuries frequently occurring in trauma patients and are often treated at trauma centers. Consequently, surgeons who manage orthopedic trauma are often faced with these complex injury patterns, which often require timely surgical treatment. It is my hope that this article will help those surgeons who see these injuries infrequently but are tasked with managing them.

In our second article, Dr Yarboro and colleagues review practical applications of local antibiotics in orthopedic trauma. Antibiotic cements, both absorbable and nonabsorbable, are useful for dead space management as well as for treatment of acute and chronic infection. Dr Yarboro's article reviews the basic science as well as the clinical uses of local antibiotic therapy.

In our last article, Dr Iorio and colleagues review the techniques and hazards of percutaneous sacroiliac screw fixation of the posterior pelvic ring. This treatment has become a familiar tool for the orthopedic trauma surgeon but is not without its risks. Newer imaging modalities such as intraoperative CT scans, 3D imaging, and computed navigation potentially can make these procedures safer, but basic principles to stay out of trouble are reviewed here.

I hope you will enjoy this issue of the *Orthopedic Clinics of North America*, particularly the section on orthopedic trauma.

Saqib Rehman, MD
Department of Orthopaedic Surgery
Temple University Hospital
3401 North Broad Street
Philadelphia, PA 19140, USA

E-mail address:
Saqib.rehman@tuhs.temple.edu

Orthop Clin N Am 46 (2015) xvii
http://dx.doi.org/10.1016/j.ocl.2015.07.002
0030-5898/15/$ – see front matter © 2015 Published by Elsevier Inc.

Traumatic Knee Dislocations
Evaluation, Management, and Surgical Treatment

James R. Lachman, MD[a,*], Saqib Rehman, MD[a],
Paul S. Pipitone, DO[b]

KEYWORDS

- Knee dislocation • Multi-ligament knee injury • Multi-ligament reconstruction knee • Knee reduction

KEY POINTS

- Knee dislocation is a relatively uncommon but often missed diagnosis leading to significant morbidity.
- Serial examination of a suspected knee dislocation is essential in the prevention of missed arterial injury. Routine arteriography is not recommended.
- Augmenting primary repair of the medial and lateral ligamentous structures with graft reconstruction can be beneficial, particularly with posteromedial or posterolateral corner disruptions. Cruciate graft longevity is compromised if collateral structures are not restored.
- Currently, angiography (routine or computed tomographic angiography/magnetic resonance angiography) is recommended for patients demonstrating insufficient perfusion or any asymmetry in physical examination. Universal angiography is not recommended.
- Clinicians must be aware of the existence of an irreducible knee dislocation. Use caution during reduction and cognizant of signs (dimple sign, excessive force required for reduction, joint asymmetry after reduction attempt). The cases should undergo open reduction in the operating room.

INTRODUCTION

Incidences of knee dislocations have historically been reported as less than 0.02% of all musculoskeletal injuries.[1,2] This number is most likely an underestimate caused by spontaneous reductions and missed diagnosis.[1,3] Knee dislocations have, in recent years, become increasingly recognized because of the advances in imaging modalities and a better understanding of the dynamic nature of knee stability through 3 major ligamentous structures and the joint capsule.[4,5] Radiographic evidence of frank dislocation is not always available, and the clinician must be aware of other clues of a dislocation that may have spontaneously reduced in the field. Most knee dislocations are the result of high-energy mechanisms, and careful history and physical examination in a systematic approach will aid in identifying patients at risk for this injury.

CAUSE
Mechanism

The available literature on knee dislocations includes several retrospective studies with very few patients owing to the relatively rare nature of the injury. Incidence in males out number females

[a] Department of Orthopaedic Surgery and Sports Medicine, Temple University Hospital, 3509 North Broad Street #5, Philadelphia, PA 19140, USA; [b] Department of Orthopaedic Surgery, Nassau University Medical Center, East Meadow, NY 11554, USA
* Corresponding author.
E-mail address: james.lachman2@tuhs.temple.edu

Orthop Clin N Am 46 (2015) 479–493
http://dx.doi.org/10.1016/j.ocl.2015.06.004
0030-5898/15/$ – see front matter © 2015 Elsevier Inc. All rights reserved.

almost 2.5:1.0; these injuries usually result from a high-energy mechanism, the most common being motor vehicle collision (up to 50% of reported cases).[6,7] The other 2 most common mechanisms include sports injuries (up to 33%) and simple falls (up to 12%).[8] Patients in the high-energy group are often polytrauma patients with associated fractures and ipsilateral joint dislocations.[9,10] A fourth subset, designated ultralow energy, has been recently described and some patterns elucidated.[8]

Classification

As with all traumatic injuries, the first description of a knee dislocation includes whether the injury is closed versus open and the time from injury to presentation. It is important for the examiner to determine if the dislocation is partial (subluxed), spontaneously reduced, or complete.[3] The classification systems used in the past for knee dislocations are summarized in **Table 1**. Kennedy described knee dislocations based on the direction of tibial translation relative to a stationary femur (**Fig. 1**). This system enables effective communication if the knee remains dislocated. The major limitation with this system is the variability in injured ligaments when only accounting for the dislocation direction.[15] McCoy and colleagues[11] and Shelbourne[12] created classification systems, and each used the energy of the injury mechanism. High-, low-, and ultralow energy mechanisms were described; higher-energy injuries have a higher incidence of vascular injury. Taking a thorough history is always important with these injuries. Palmer[13] classified knee dislocations based on the time since the injury, defining

the 3-week mark as an important date. Before 3 weeks, the joint capsule has not healed and surgical intervention for ligament repair was not advised. Boisgard and colleagues[14] created a classification system that included all bicruciate ligament injuries but also included knees that did not dislocate (see **Table 1**).

Schenk developed a classification system that is based on the anatomic structures injured. This system was modified by Wascher and then Yu and is now the most widely used and accepted classification available. It accounts for injured ligaments, vascular or neurologic injury, and also whether an associated fracture is present. Schenk's classification is strictly for knee dislocations and does not include knees with bicruciate injuries that did not dislocate (**Table 2**).

Schenk's classification was later modified to include 3 letter designations. Dislocations with an associated fracture were designated V, those with associated arterial injury designated C, and those with associated nerve injury designated N (**Table 3**).[15]

EVALUATION
Acute Assessment

Cases of suspected knee dislocation in the acute setting are often the result of high-energy mechanisms. Initial evaluation includes the primary survey according to the Advanced Trauma and Life Support protocol before the secondary survey, which includes prompt but careful evaluation of the neurologic and vascular status of the affected limb.

The diagnosis is relatively straightforward in patients with an unreduced knee dislocation (**Fig. 2**). Proceeding in a stepwise pattern is

Table 1				
Historical knee dislocation classification systems				
Author, Date	Basis of Classification	Types	Drawbacks	Utility
Kennedy,[10] 1963	Direction of tibial dislocation as related to femur	1. Anterior 2. Posterior 3. Medial 4. Lateral 5. Rotatory	Difficult to identify direction of dislocation in spontaneously reduced knees	Limited: direction of dislocation not reliable predictor of injured structures
McCoy et al,[11] 1987; S helbourne,[12] 1991	Energy imparted at time of injury	1. High 2. Low 3. Ultralow	Requires detailed history and patients who are not obtunded	Higher-energy mechanisms associated with increased incidence of vascular and soft tissue compromise
Palmer,[13] 2007; Boisgard et al,[14] 2009	Period of time from injury to management	Acute vs chronic	3 wk is the division point between acute and chronic	Management recommendations based on injury acuity

Data from Refs.[10–14]

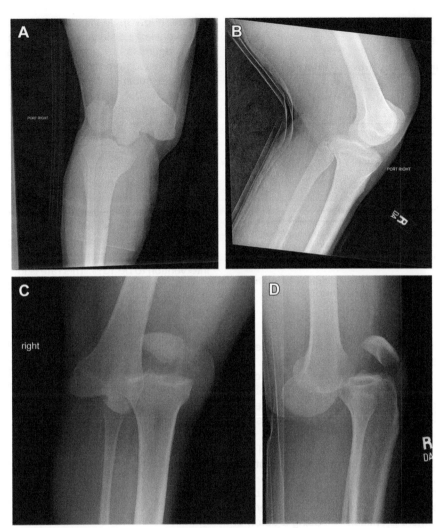

Fig. 1. (*A–D*) (*A, B*) Anteroposterior (AP) and lateral radiographs of knee before reduction attempt demonstrating frank joint incongruity and medial dislocation. (*B, C*) AP and lateral radiographs of knee before reduction attempt demonstrating frank joint incongruity and posterolateral knee dislocation.

recommended. In patients with a spontaneously reduced knee dislocation, identifying those at risk for vascular or soft tissue compromise is much more difficult. Subtle signs of bruising or swelling surrounding the knee may suggest capsular disruption. It is for this reason that significant hemarthrosis is often not present.

The incidence of open knee dislocations varies between sources from 15% to more than 35%.[16,17] As with all open injuries, the complication rates increase; long-term outcomes and satisfaction rates are poor.[17]

Vascular Examination

The incidence of vascular injury in knee dislocations ranges in the literature from less than 5% up to 65%, depending on the mechanisms of

injury. A review of larger numbers of patients shows the overall incidence is 20%.[4] Historically, high-energy mechanisms resulting in a hyperextension moment were thought to be more likely to cause vascular compromise. A more recent review of available literature did not demonstrate an association between direction of dislocation and vascular insult.[18,19] The popliteal artery has anatomic features that put it at risk during any high-energy mechanism. It has a fibrous tethering on either side of the knee, proximally at the adductor hiatus and distally at the soleus arch. It lays in close proximity to the posterior knee joint capsule and is protected by a very thin layer of fat. Leg compartment syndrome is a known complication. The anatomic proximity of the trifurcation of the popliteal artery to the knee attributes to this risk.

Table 2 Schenk classification		
Grade	Injured Structures	Intact Structures
I	Single cruciate + collateral	ACL + collateral PCL + collateral
II	ACL/PCL	Collaterals
III M	ACL/PCL/MCL/ LCL + PLC	LCL + PLC
III L	ACL/PCL/LCL + PLC	MCL
IV	ACL/PCL/MCL/ LCL + PLC	—
V	Fracture dislocation	

Abbreviations: ACL, anterior cruciate ligament; LCL, lateral collateral ligament; MCL, medial collateral ligament; PCL, posterior cruciate ligament; PLC, posterolateral corner.
Adapted from Schenk R. Classification of knee dislocations. Oper Tech Sports Med 2003;11(3):193–8; with permission.

Establishing a well-perfused limb is essential in all cases of suspected knee dislocation. The mechanisms for doing so, however, are controversial. A standard examination includes palpating dorsalis pedis and posterior tibial pulses bilaterally and assessing for any asymmetry. Vasospasm is common with tension injuries on arteries, and this can be a pitfall for thorough evaluation. There is literature to suggest that, in the absence of any asymmetry, further assessment is not necessary.[20,21] Other investigators think obtaining bilateral ankle-brachial-indices (ABI) evaluations in the initial assessment is critical.[22,23] Using a cutoff of less than 0.9, the sensitivity of ABI in detecting vascular injury requiring surgical intervention approaches 100%.[23]

The concept of a routine angiogram for all suspected knee dislocations has been the focus of numerous studies and the center of significant

Table 3 Moore classification	
	Fracture-Dislocation of the Knee
I	Split fractures through medial or lateral plateau
II	Complete fractures separating entire medial or lateral plateau
III	Rim avulsion fracture
IV	Rim compression fracture
V	4-Part fractures

From Moore TM. Fracture dislocation of the knee. Clin Orthop Relat Res 1981;(156):128–40; with permission.

debate (**Fig. 3**). Multiple investigators contend that every knee dislocation should undergo angiogram regardless of physical examination.[10,24–26] These investigators indicate that vascular injuries are often subintimal, and physical examination can often be unreliable. Other investigators contend that angiography should be reserved for those that have signs of inadequate circulation in the effected extremity.[18–22,27] Currently, angiography (routine computed tomographic angiography [CTA] or magnetic resonance angiography [MRA]) is recommended for patients demonstrating insufficient perfusion or any asymmetry in physical examination, though practice varies between institutions and clinicians.

One of the largest available studies cites an incidence of popliteal artery injury requiring surgical intervention to be 13%. This rate is lower than previously reported, and the study recommends a more judicious use of angiography. The study failed to identify any commonalities among the patients sustaining vascular injury.[28]

Green and Allen[24] described the importance of timely identification of vascular injury. Of the patients who were identified with vascular compromise, those treated surgically within 8 hours had a significantly lower amputation rate (11%) than those treated after 8 hours (86%).[24]

Neurologic Examination

The physical examination should include a detailed neurologic examination including sensation in the tibial, deep peroneal, and superficial peroneal distributions to light touch, pinprick, and temperature if available. Motor examination including the flexor and extensor hallucis longus, tibialis anterior, and gastrocnemius is important to establish the baseline function.

The incidence of nerve injury associated with knee dislocation ranges from 4.5% to 40.0%.[7,9,18,29] Most commonly, the common peroneal is the injured nerve, though isolated tibial nerve palsy has been reported.[30] The nerve is at risk for injury as well, similar to the artery, due to its anatomic constraints both proximally and distally (**Fig. 4**). The fibular neck tethers the nerve proximally, and the fibrous arches of the intermuscular septum form the distal tether. Kadiyala and colleagues[31] demonstrated the precarious blood supply of the common peroneal nerve caused by its lack of intraneural vessels in the region of the fibular neck. Of those that do have neurologic deficit, the recovery is unpredictable. In one series, 21% had full neurologic recovery and 29% only partial recovery. The remaining 50% had no useful motor recovery.[32]

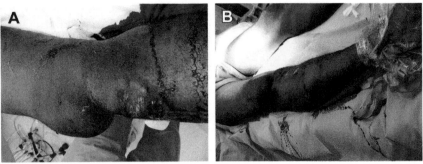

Fig. 2. (*A*, *B*) These clinical photographs depict a gross deformity secondary to knee dislocation (which is also an open injury in this case).

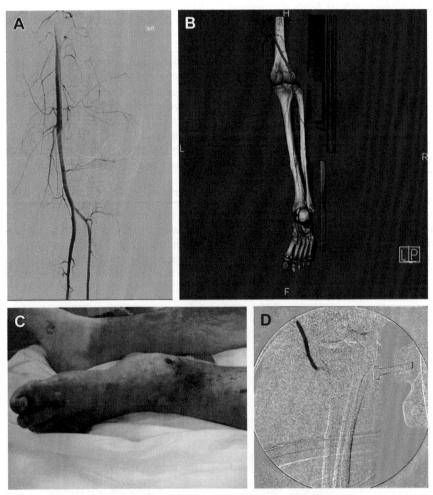

Fig. 3. (*A*) Routine angiogram showing normal 3-vessel runoff after passing through popliteal hiatus. (*B*) Here is demonstrated a normal computed tomographic angiography reconstruction after knee dislocation. The arterial reconstruction is continuous from femoral artery through the trifurcation of the popliteal artery distal to the knee. (*C*) This clinical photograph shows a patient after a knee dislocation with an asymmetric vascular examination. A cold, mottled foot that appears pale in comparison with the uninjured leg is a clear sign evaluation with angiogram emergently in the operating room is essential. (*D*) This image is a routine angiogram demonstrating disruption at the distal popliteal artery with extravasation of contrast in a patient with a knee dislocation.

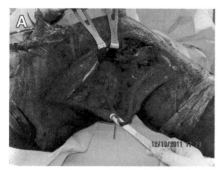
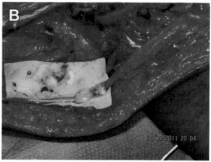

Fig. 4. (*A, B*) Here is an intraoperative photograph showing near-complete disruption of the common peroneal nerve at the popliteal hiatus after knee dislocation. The common peroneal nerve is located at the end of the forceps.

Contrary to intuition, the reported incidence of nerve injury in ultralow-energy knee dislocations is higher (44.4%) than the incidence in the higher-energy trauma patients. These patients are often obese; though the operative times are longer and the procedures more difficult, knee range of motion in those operated on was significantly better (average 91.4°) than those treated nonoperatively (average 53.6°).[8]

RADIOGRAPHIC EVALUATION
Immediate

After confirmation of limb perfusion and before physical examination of ligamentous integrity, standard views of the knee are obtained immediately after reduction. This timing enables the clinician to confirm adequate reduction, evaluate for any fracture, and assess overall knee alignment that may suggest a grossly unstable knee.

Associated fracture has a reported incidence ranging from 10% to 20%.[3] These fractures are often in locations where the injured ligaments originate or insert. Fibular head (arcuate fracture), tibial spine, and lateral tibial condyle (Segond fracture) avulsions are common (**Fig. 5**). These fractures are often treated by ligament reconstruction but occasionally, if the fragment is large enough, involve internal fixation of the fracture fragments.[3] Routine anteroposterior, oblique, and lateral views of the knee along with full-length tibia and full-length femur films, including the joint above and the joint below, should be obtained.

Secondary

After the limb is reduced, vascular injury is ruled out and grossly unstable knees are stabilized; advanced imaging is appropriate. Computed tomography (CT), MRI, or both may be appropriate. CT is used to better understand the personality of

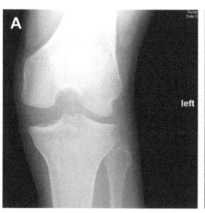
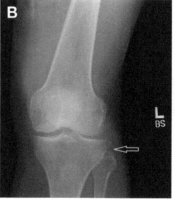
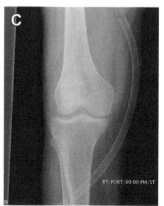

Fig. 5. Subtle signs of knee dislocation. (*A*) Here is an anteroposterior radiograph of the knee demonstrating medial joint space widening, which can often be the only finding suggestive of more severe injury. (*B*) Anteroposterior (AP) radiograph of the knee depicting the classic arcuate fragment (*arrow*). This is an avulsion of the fibular head, which suggests a lateral ligament complex injury. (*C*) AP radiograph of knee dislocation with Segond fracture. Notice the small avulsion off of lateral tibia, which is often a subtle sign of a more severe injury and occurs in high association with ACL rupture.

any fracture, whereas MRI can elucidate soft tissue and ligament injuries not appreciated on physical examination. Both aid in operative planning.

EXAMINATION OF KNEE STABILITY

Examination of ligamentous integrity is often limited secondary to patient discomfort, and some of the more specific diagnostic tests require patient cooperation impossible in these circumstances. Clues to ligament injury in a spontaneously reduced knee dislocation are any asymmetry in the joint space, minor subluxations in any direction, and Segond fractures. One should attempt examination, however; intra-articular injection of lidocaine after aspiration of any hemarthrosis can aid in patient comfort (**Fig. 6**). The Lachman test and anterior drawer (anterior cruciate ligament [ACL] rupture) (**Fig. 7**), varus/valgus stressing (medial collateral ligament [MCL]/lateral collateral ligament [LCL] compromise) (**Fig. 8**), and posterior sag (posterior cruciate ligament [PCL] disruption) (**Fig. 9**) are the most reliable maneuvers in the acute setting.[33] The pivot shift, dial test, reverse pivot shift, and weight-bearing examinations are impractical at the bedside but can aid in the diagnosis while under anesthesia.

The most common ligament injury pattern for knee dislocations is both cruciates and the medial ligament complex.[6,7] The posterolateral corner (PLC) is second to the medial ligament complex in frequency of injury. Rarely (>11%) are all 4 major stabilizers injured at the same time.[18,34] Multiple case reports demonstrate less common injury patterns when one cruciate or both cruciates remain intact after a knee dislocation.[35–37] The clinician must not assume every knee dislocation is the same. In addition, reports of tendon injury (patella, popliteus, and biceps femoris) are present; but the incidence is unclear.[3]

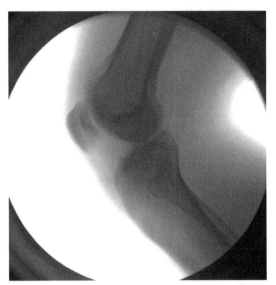

Fig. 7. Here is a fluoroscopic intraoperative image during examination under anesthesia demonstrating anterior translation of the tibial during anterior drawer testing.

Reduction Technique

After a rapid evaluation of neurovascular status (not including ABIs at this point), it is essential to reduce a dislocated knee as soon as possible. Reports of skin necrosis caused by delayed reduction are numerous.[38,39] Often, after palpation of the surface anatomy, gentle in-line traction attempting to bring the knee into extension is enough to reduce a dislocated knee. It is important that no manual pressure be used to aid in any direction, especially in the popliteal fossa, to avoid iatrogenic neurovascular injury.

Occasionally, the knee will not completely reduce or not reduce at all. Clarke[40] first described what is now known as the dimple

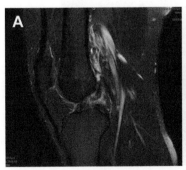
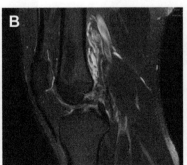
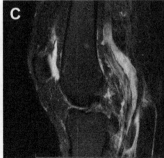

Fig. 6. (A) Sagittal MRI depicting ACL attenuation and midsubstance PCL rupture with associated periarticular edema. (B) Another example of a sagittal MRI demonstrating midsubstance tear of the ACL and a femoral-sided tear of the PCL. (C) This image is a sagittal MRI of knee demonstrating PCL injury.

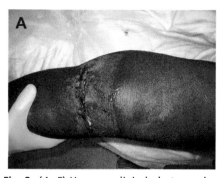
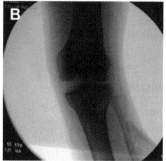
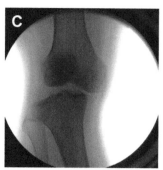

Fig. 8. (*A, B*) Here are clinical photographs demonstrating the valgus stress examination with widening of the medial joint space clinically and under fluoroscopy. (*C*) Another fluoroscopic intraoperative image of the same knee under varus stress testing. Notice the widening of the lateral joint space.

sign in 1942. When the knee is gently brought into extension, a worsening skin dimple between the medial femoral condyle and the medial tibial plateau can be a sign that closed reduction will be unsuccessful. The skin dimple is a sign that the medial femoral condyle has buttonholed through the medial joint capsule and the MCL has become entrapped and is being pulled into the joint with the gentle traction. Multiple case reports cite this as an irreducible knee dislocation and recommend open reduction in the operating room (**Fig. 10**).[39,40]

Once the knee is reduced, repeat neurologic and vascular examination (this time with the more time-consuming ABIs) are done immediately. With any vascular compromise or asymmetry in ABIs whereby the affected leg is less than 0.9, surgical exploration is warranted. With a more equivocal examination, MRA, CTA, or traditional angiography are performed. If patients have a normal neurologic and vascular examination, then the clinician may proceed with further radiographs and ligamentous evaluation.

TREATMENT
Nonoperative Versus Operative Treatment

Kennedy[10] in 1963 and Taylor and colleagues[41] in 1972 suggested that patients with knee dislocations, without arterial injury, treated nonoperatively have better outcomes than those who underwent reconstruction.[10,41] Multiple investigators have shown in more recent studies that ligament injuries left untreated go on to worse functional outcomes and satisfaction scores than those undergoing reconstruction.[6,29,42]

Management of knee dislocations is a topic of hot debate. Direct ligament repair versus ligament reconstruction, use of autograft versus allograft tissue for reconstruction, arthroscopic versus open treatment, and timing of treatment are all areas of controversy in the available literature.

Early Treatment

Arterial injuries
Arterial injuries require immediate exploration and vascular surgery consultation. To aid in any

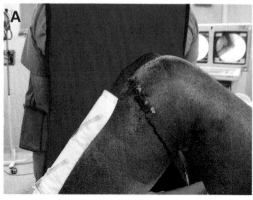
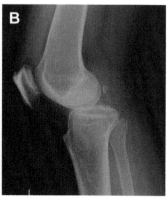

Fig. 9. (*A*) Here is a clinical photograph depicting the posterior sag sign, which indicates PCL compromise. (*B*). Here is a lateral radiograph showing posterior subluxation of the tibia on the femur suggesting injury to the PCL, which corresponds to the sag sign on clinical examination.

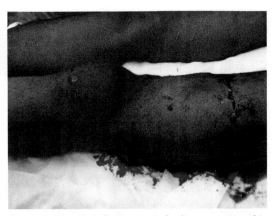

Fig. 10. This clinical photograph demonstrates skin dimpling. Not to be confused with the dimple sign, which represents incarceration MCL in the joint preventing complete reduction, often the joint capsule can become entrapped in the joint preventing complete reduction.

shunt or bypass grafting, it is not uncommon for the vascular team to request knee-spanning external fixation. Reexamination is an important mechanism to prevent a missed arterial injury. An evolving ischemia, changing pulse examination, or change in ABI measurements can all be detected if routine reexamination is part of standard treatment. Prophylactic 4-compartment fasciotomies have also been recommended by numerous investigators after revascularization **(Fig. 11)**.[2,6,11,19]

Ligament injuries

Determination of ligamentous injury in the emergency room will govern the next step in the

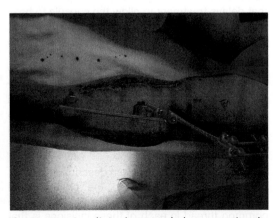

Fig. 11. Here is a clinic photograph demonstrating delayed reconstruction after a multi-ligamentous knee injury. The reconstruction was delayed secondary to arterial injury requiring bypass and 4-compartment fasciotomy.

treatment algorithm. If the postreduction knee is grossly unstable, a temporizing knee-spanning external fixator may be placed to provide stability and allow soft tissues to calm down. If the knee is not grossly unstable, placement into a knee immobilizer is recommended instead of circumferential splinting or casting, which increase the chance of compartment syndrome secondary to limited material compliance.[29,34] Serial examination may reveal increasing swelling and progressing compartment syndrome, which require 4-compartment fasciotomy.

SURGICAL TECHNIQUE
Acute Surgical Intervention

If the surgeon chooses to perform acute ligament reconstruction (earlier than 3 weeks), it should be done as an open procedure because of the capsular disruption precluding arthroscopic assistance.[4] Typically, the involved structure will dictate the surgical approaches necessary. If the PLC is involved, a lateral curvilinear incision is used. This incision also exposes the LCL. Access to the cruciates and MCL can be gained through a midline skin incision with medial para-patellar arthrotomy **(Fig. 12)**. For the posteromedial corner, a posteromedial approach should be performed for a more direct exposure. Imaging should help guide preoperative planning, particularly with identifying the location of the collateral ligament injuries. For instance, if an LCL injury is proximal, the correct windows in the iliotibial band must be entered to find the injury. Midsubstance tears of the MCL and LCL may require additional allograft reconstruction to augment the primary repair while bony avulsions may be reattached to their anatomic origins using standard osteosynthesis methods.[43]

The efficacy of cruciate ligament reconstruction has been well described, and it seems even necessary with avulsions of the tibial spine.[44] The principles of proper graft selection stay true in reconstruction of multi-ligamentous knee injuries after dislocation, although allograft, rather than autograft, is typically used in reconstruction of these injuries.[45,46]

Sequence of Ligament Reconstruction

Cruciate ligament reconstruction typically precedes PLC reconstruction.[47] The sequence of reconstruction is integral to restoring anatomic congruence of the joint. The PCL is reconstructed first to prevent tightening the ACL graft that may force permanent posterior sag of the tibia on the femur. Fixing the PCL graft helps reduce the tibia into its native anatomic position.[1] Next, the ACL

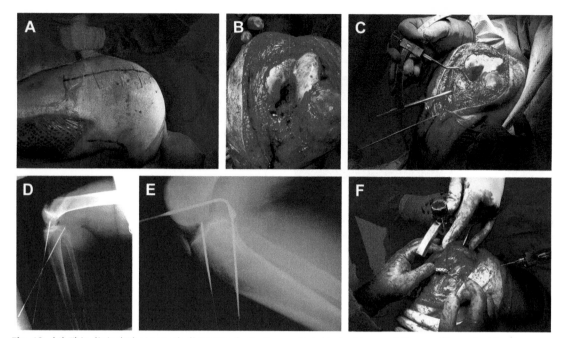

Fig. 12. (*A*) This clinical photograph illustrates both the medial skin incision and the curvilinear incision to access the posterolateral corner. (*B*) Here is an intraoperative photograph illustrating the medial para-patellar open technique for multiple ligament reconstructions. The remnant ACL and PCL have been debrided in preparation for drilling tunnels and graft passage. (*C*) Here is an intraoperative photograph showing placement of tibial tunnels for both ACL and PCL graft passage. (*D*) This fluoroscopic intraoperative lateral image of the knee shows positioning of the tibial-sided tunnels for ACL and PCL graft placement. It is important to spread these tunnels apart in order not to compromise passage of either graft and ensure adequate bone on all sides of both tunnel. (*E*) This fluoroscopic intraoperative lateral image of the knee demonstrates a tool used to prevent posterior migration of the PCL guidewire while drilling the tunnel. Any advancement of this guidewire risks penetration into the popliteal hiatus and damage to the popliteal artery. (*F*) Here is an intraoperative photograph demonstrating femoral-sided tunnel drilling for PCL placement.

graft can be tensioned safely without risking posterior subluxation. Following cruciate reconstruction, attention can then be given to collateral repair versus reconstruction. Finally, PLC reconstruction is appropriate (see **Fig. 12**B–F). When performing both cruciate and collateral ligament repair/reconstruction in surgery, the authors prefer to fix both cruciate grafts to their femoral tunnels and to have the collateral ligaments exposed before fixing the PCL tibial tunnel and proceeding as discussed earlier.

Posterolateral Corner and Lateral Collateral Ligament Injury Treatment

Some investigators argue that acute reconstruction of the PLC is necessary and provides for better outcomes than delayed reconstruction (**Fig. 13**).[6,48–52] Three weeks is cited as the time frame within which outcomes are improved.[49,53–55] Arthroscopic assistance has become routine practice during PLC reconstruction to aid in the diagnosis of cruciate and meniscal pathology as well

as to evaluate the popliteus and lateral compartment structures. This is not the case in patients with multi-ligamentous knee injuries, however. Use of arthroscopy requires an intact joint capsule that delays treatment to allow the capsule to heal. In the acute setting, arthroscopy is not only difficult but can also lead to compartment syndrome caused by fluid extravasation secondary to the significant capsular injury. Some surgeons will delay surgical intervention for 10 to 14 days to allow for quadriceps function to improve, a decrease in soft tissue swelling and ecchymosis, and healing of the joint capsule, whereas others think waiting impairs visualization and makes injury identification more difficult.[1]

Multiple incisions have been described that provide adequate exposure to the posterolateral structures of the knee (see **Fig. 12**A).[48,56] The common thread in each of these incisions is that dissection is carried down through the injured structures while protecting the peroneal nerve, which is in close proximity. Evaluation of the iliotibial tract superficially, biceps femoris and LCL at

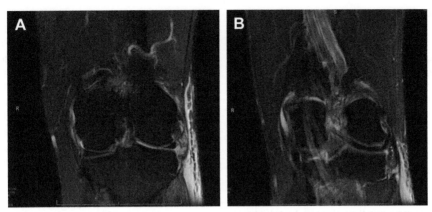

Fig. 13. (A, B) These coronal MRI slices of knee demonstrate disruption of the posterolateral ligament complex including LCL midsubstance tear.

the next layer, and finally the popliteal muscle and tendon and the popliteofibular ligament as one dissects from superficial to deep allows for systematic evaluation as each structure is exposed.[56] Injury severity will dictate whether direct repair is possible or if reconstruction (allograft or autograft) is necessary.[53,56]

Tears of the LCL often occur with PLC injuries. Midsubstance tears can often be primarily repaired in the acute setting. The need to use allograft or autograft material supplementation after direct LCL repair is controversial.[7,57,58] In the multi-ligamentous injured knee with PLC compromise, reconstructing the popliteofibular ligament is necessary as well as restoring the LCL. Failure to recognize and treat this injury in the setting of a reconstructed PCL graft can result in significantly increased graft stresses and possibly jeopardize the cruciate reconstruction.[59] The authors prefer to perform simultaneous allograft lateral reconstructions to augment primary repair, except in cases of large distal bony avulsion injuries **(Fig. 14)**.

The Muller procedure (popliteal bypass procedure), Larson technique, 2- and 3-tail PCL reconstruction, LaPrade technique, and biceps femoris LCL reconstruction have all been proposed as options for reconstruction after PCL injury is sustained.[60] Both the fibular-based (Larson technique) and transtibial double bundle technique have been described and are the most commonly used.[57,58] The fibular-based technique, first described by Fanelli and Larson,[61] involves using a hamstring graft passed through a tunnel in the fibular head. The limb leaving the anterior fibular head is crossed in a figure-of-eight pattern with the limb leaving the posterior fibular head and fixed to the lateral femur. This construct recreates the stability provided by the LCL and the popliteofibular ligament while only using one graft.[61] The transtibial double bundle technique involves using a split Achilles tendon allograft fixed at its midpoint to the isometric point of the lateral femoral condyle. The anterior limb is anchored to the fibular head to reconstruct the LCL while the posterior limb is fixed distally through the

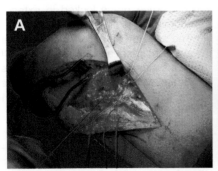
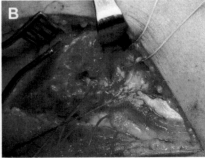

Fig. 14. (A, B) These intraoperative photographs demonstrate direct repair of the LCL with allograft augmentation and reconstruction of the popliteofibular ligament. The krachow suture is in the biceps femoris and iliotibial band, and the sutures adjacent to the Army/Navy retractor are in the lateral femoral condyle at the origin of the LCL. The vessel loop is around the common peroneal nerve.

posterior tibial to reconstruct the popliteofibular ligament.[60]

Posteromedial Corner and Medial Collateral Ligament Injury Treatment

Hughston and Eilers[62] first described the role of the posterior oblique ligament in 1973, and Müller[63] further elucidated the function in 1983. Before these descriptions, injuries to the medial side of the knee were treated nonoperatively and assumed to be MCL related (**Fig. 15**). The semimembranosus, through a broad 5-expansion insertion, also adds dynamic stability, which was underappreciated until that time.[63] Instability on the medial side in the multi-ligament injured knee often requires more than just activity modification and bracing and may warrant surgical treatment when more than just the collateral is involved. This point is especially true in knees where there is concomitant ACL instability. The longevity of the graft in a reconstructed ACL is compromised when there is posteromedial corner (PMC) instability.[64]

In addition to direct repair of the MCL when possible, supplementation with allograft is routinely done. This supplementation is not only to augment the MCL repair but also to recreate the contribution of the semimembranosus and posterior oblique ligaments to dynamic stability. A common technique for PMC reconstruction involved using a semitendinosus autograft. The semitendinosus is harvested from its musculotendinous junction while maintaining its insertion at the pes anserinus. The tendon is then looped into a drill hole in the medial femoral condyle at the insertion site for the MCL. Effort is place on this drill hole at the isometric point so as not to vary the tension placed on the graft at any point during controlled knee flexion. The free end of the graft is then passed from posterior to anterior in a drill hole in the medial tibial condyle and anchored there.[65] The authors' preference is to use a 2-tailed allograft fixed with an interference screw in the femur with one tail passing posterior to the semimembranosus and then meeting the other limb at the tibial insertion of the MCL where both limbs are fixed using a screw and spiked washer (**Fig. 16**).[66]

Multiple techniques for reconstruction of the MCL have been described, which use separate grafts for the MCL and posterior oblique ligament (double bundle techniques) originating from the same point on the medial femoral condyle described earlier. Borden and colleagues[67] described a technique using a tibialis anterior allograft to reconstruct both ligaments with different tibial insertion sites. Marx first described a similar technique using an Achilles allograft. The principles of graft selection apply to any ligament reconstruction decision.

Delayed Surgical Intervention

The use of arthroscopy in a standard fashion can be used in those cases of knee dislocation whereby reconstruction occurs in a delayed time frame. In these cases, direct repair of the collaterals is no longer possible and reconstruction with autograft or allograft is necessary.[12,50–52]

Methods for Protection of Repair Postoperatively

Standard protocols for repair protection in the immediate postoperative period include knee immobilization in extension for the first 4 to 6 weeks in a hinged knee brace locked in extension or knee immobilizer.

The use of a hinged, ringed external fixator has been described and shown to be effective in a resent series. Graft failure was decreased in those patients whose reconstructions were protected using a hinged ring external fixator without any differences in knee range of motion.[68]

Postoperative Complications

Reports of complications from surgical intervention for knee dislocations are plentiful. Complications ranging from injury to nerves and vessels, tourniquet problems, wound problems, compartment syndrome, complex regional pain syndrome,

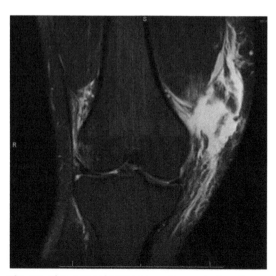

Fig. 15. This coronal MRI image demonstrates disruption of the posteromedial ligament complex. MCL rupture and significant extracapsular edema is visible in the image.

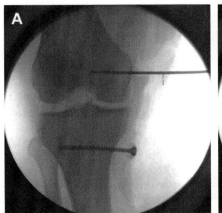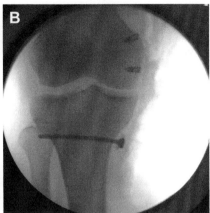

Fig. 16. (*A*, *B*) These fluoroscopic intraoperative radiographs demonstrate femoral tunnel (*marked with pin identifying isometric point*) and screw with spiked washer for PMC reconstruction.

knee stiffness, persistent laxity, osteonecrosis, posttraumatic osteoarthritis, and deep vein thrombosis have all been reported.[2,69]

Physical Therapy

Residual knee stiffness is the most common long-term complication following multi-ligamentous knee injury reconstruction.[29] ACL reconstruction has been associated with loss of extension, and PCL reconstruction has been associated with loss of flexion. Structured physical therapy protocols are essential in obtaining and maintaining a satisfactory result. Emphasis is placed on gaining full terminal extension symmetric with the noninjured knee only in those cases without PLC reconstruction. Emphasis of passive knee extension is limited to 0°, whereas passive knee flexion is limited to less than 90° during the first 6 weeks.[69] Avoidance of knee flexion, specifically hamstring contraction, is avoided to prevent posterior tibial translation after a PCL reconstruction. Avoidance of open-chain exercises is typically advised after cruciate reconstruction.

Outcomes

Knee dislocations are catastrophic injuries that demand emergent evaluation and often require a multidisciplinary approach. Long-term outcome studies are relatively scarce secondary to the variability in any given study population and the wide variety of injury patterns between knee dislocations. Multiple controversies exist with regard to outcomes using various treatment methods (early vs late intervention, graft selection, repair vs reconstruction of medial and lateral structures, rehabilitation regimens).

Levy and colleagues conducted a systematic review that supports early operative intervention

(defined as within 3 weeks) compared with delayed intervention, whereas another study demonstrated no differences between groups treated before and 2 weeks after injury.[34,70,71]

Higher-energy injuries were shown to have inferior outcomes to lower-energy mechanisms in one prospective study, whereas lower-energy injuries were correlated with an increased incidence of neurologic injuries in another study.[8,11,34]

The incidence of posttraumatic osteoarthritis has been reported as high as 87%.[70] One common trend in recent literature is that functional outcomes improve with surgical intervention, but the magnitude of improvement varies depending on the source.[2,20,29,34,72,73]

Careful clinical evaluation is essential when knee dislocation is suspected. Ruling out vascular compromise is the first priority with any initial examination. Although significant improvements have occurred with surgical technique, graft quality, and rehabilitation protocols, return to "normal knee function" remains uncommon.[73]

REFERENCES

1. Peskun CJ, Whelan DB, Fanelli GC, et al. Diagnosis and management of knee dislocations. Physician Sports Med 2010;38(4):101–11.
2. Hegyes MS, Richardson MW, Miller MD. Knee dislocation: complications of non-operative and operative management. Clin Sports Med 2000;19(3): 519–43.
3. Harner CD, Harner CD. The multiple ligament injured knee. Clin Sports Med 1999;18(1):241–62.
4. Keating JF. Acute knee ligament injuries and knee dislocation. European Surgical Orthopaedics and Traumatology 2014;2949–71.

5. Veltri DM, Maynard MJ. The role of cruciate and postero-lateral ligaments in stability of the knee. Am J Sports Med 1995;23:436–43.

6. Harner CD, Waltrip RL, Bennett CH, et al. Surgical management of knee dislocations. J Bone Joint Surg 2004;86-A:262–73.

7. Liow RY, McNicholas MJ, Keating JF, et al. Ligament repair and reconstruction in traumatic dislocation of the knee. J Bone Joint Surg Br 2003; 85(6):845–51.

8. Vaidya R, Roth M, Nanavati D, et al. Knee dislocation from minor trauma in morbidly obese patients. Orthopaedic J Sports Med 2013;1(4).

9. Twaddle BC, Bidwell TA, Chapman JR. Knee dislocations: where are the lesions? A prospective evaluation of surgical findings in 63 cases. J Orthop Trauma 2003;17(3):198–202.

10. Kennedy JC. Complete dislocation of the knee joint. J Bone Joint Surg 1963;45A:889–904.

11. McCoy GF, Hannon DG, Barr RJ, et al. Vascular injuries associated with low velocity dislocations of the knee. J Bone Joint Surg Br 1987;69(2):285–7.

12. Shelbourne KD. Low-velocity knee dislocation. Orthop Rev 1991;20(11):995–1004.

13. Palmer I. On the injuries to ligaments of the knee joint: a clinical study. 1938. Acta Chir Scand 2007; 454:17–22.

14. Boisgard S, Versier G, Descamps S, et al. Bicruciate ligament lesions and dislocation of the knee: mechanisms and classification. Orthop Traumatol Surg Res 2009;95(8):627–31.

15. Schenk R. Classification of knee dislocations. Oper Tech Sports Med 2003;11(3):193–8.

16. King JJ, Cerynik DL, Blair JA. Surgical outcomes after traumatic open knee dislocations. Knee Surg Sports Traumatol Arthrosc 2009;17(9):1027–32.

17. Wright DG, Covey DC, Born CT, et al. Open dislocation of the knee. J Orthop Trauma 1995;9(2):135–40.

18. Wascher DC, Dvirnak PC, DeCoster TA. Knee dislocation: initial assessment and implications for treatment. J Orthop Trauma 1997;11(7):525–9.

19. Wascher DC. High velocity knee dislocation with vascular injury: treatment principles. Clin Sports Med 2000;19:457–77.

20. Hollis JD, Daley BJ. 10-year review of knee dislocations; is angiography always necessary. J Trauma 2005;59(3):672–5.

21. Klineberg EO, Crites BM, Flinn WR, et al. The role of arteriography in assessing popliteal artery injury in knee dislocations. J Trauma 2004;56(4):786–90.

22. Applebaum R, Yellin AE, Weaver FA. Role of routine angiography in blunt lower extremity trauma. Am J Surg 1990;160:221–5.

23. Mills WJ, Barei DP, McNair P. The value of ankle brachial index for diagnosing arterial injury after knee dislocation: a prospective study. J Trauma 2004;56(6):1261–5.

24. Green NE, Allen BL. Vascular injuries associated with dislocation of the knee. J Bone Joint Surg Am 1977;59:236–9.

25. Gable DR, Allen JW, Richardson JD. Blunt popliteal artery injury: is physical exam alone enough for evaluation. J Trauma 1997;43:541–4.

26. McCutchan JD, Gillham NR. Injury to the popliteal artery associated with dislocation of the knee: palpable distal pulses do not negate the requirement for arteriography. Injury 1989;20:307–10.

27. Miranda FE, Dennis JW, Veldenz HC, et al. Confirmation of the safety and accuracy of physical examination in the evaluation of knee dislocation for injury of the popliteal artery: a prospective study. J Trauma 2002;52(2):247–51.

28. Natsuhara KM, Yeranosian MG, Cohen JR, et al. What is the frequency of vascular injury after knee dislocation. Clin Orthop Relat Res 2014;472(9): 2615–20.

29. Sisto DJ, Warren RF. Complete knee dislocation. A follow-up of operative treatment. Clin Orthop 1985; 198:94–101.

30. Frassica FJ, Sim FH, Staeheli JW, et al. Dislocation of the knee. Clin Orthop Relat Res 1991;263:200–5.

31. Kadiyala RK, Ramirez A, Taylor AE, et al. The blood supply of the common peroneal nerve in the popliteal fossa,. J Bone Joint Surg Br 2005; 87(3):337–42.

32. Niall DM, Nutton RW, Keating JF. Palsy of the common peroneal nerve after traumatic dislocation of the knee. J Bone Joint Surg Br 2005;87(5):664–7.

33. Swenson TM. Physical diagnosis of the multiple-ligament-injured knee. Clin Sports Med 2000;19: 415–23.

34. Engebretsen L, Risberg MA, Robertson B, et al. Outcome after knee dislocations; a 2-9 years follow-up of 85 consecutive patients. Knee Surg Sports Traumatol Arthrosc 2009;17(9):1013–26.

35. Bellabarba C, Bush-Joseph CA, Bach BR Jr. Knee dislocation without anterior cruciate ligament disruption. A report of three cases. Am J Knee Surg 1996; 9(4):167–70.

36. Flowers A, Copley LA. High energy knee dislocation without anterior cruciate ligament disruption in a skeletally immature adolescent. Arthroscopy 2003; 19(7):782–6.

37. Bratt HD, Newman AP. Complete dislocation of the knee without disruption of both cruciate ligaments. J Trauma 1993;34(3):383–9.

38. Hill JA, Rana NA. Complications of posterolateral dislocation of the knee: case report and literature review. Clin Orthop 1981;154:212–5.

39. Wand JS. A physical sign denoting irreducibility of a dislocated knee. J Bone Joint Surg Br 1989;71-B:862.

40. Clarke HO. Dislocation of the knee-joint with capsular interposition. Proc Roy Soc Med 1942; 35:759.

41. Taylor AR, Arden GP, Rainey HA. Traumatic disloca-tion of the knee joint: a report of 43 cases with spe-cial reference to conservative management. J Bone Joint Surg 1972;54B:96–102.

42. Almakinders LC, Dedmond BT. Outcomes of opera-tively treated knee dislocations. Clin Sports Med 2000;19(3):503–18.

43. Shelbourne KD, Haro MS, Gray T. Knee dislocation with lateral side injury. Results of an en-masse surgi-cal repair technique of the lateral side. Am J Sports Med 2007;35(7):1105–16.

44. Aderinto J, Walmsley P, Keating JF. Fractures of the tibial spine: epidemiology and outcome. Knee 2008; 15(3):164–7.

45. Shelton WR, Fagan Autografts BC. Commonly used in anterior cruciate ligament reconstruction. J Am Acad Orthop Surg 2011;19:259–64.

46. West RV, Harner Graft CD. Selection in anterior cru-ciate ligament reconstruction. J Am Acad Orthop Surg 2005;13:197–207.

47. Levy BA, Dajani KA, Morgan JA, et al. Repair versus reconstruction of the fibular collateral ligament and posterolateral corner in the multi-ligament-injured knee. Am J Sports Med 2010;38(4):804–9.

48. Hughston JC, Jacobson KE. Chronic posterolateral instability of the knee. J Bone Joint Surg Am 1985; 67:351–9.

49. Krukhaug Y, Molster A, Rodt A, et al. Lateral liga-ment injuries of the knee. Knee Surg Sports Trauma-tol Arthrosc 1998;6:21–5.

50. Fanelli GC, Edson CJ. Arthroscopically assisted combined anterior and posterior cruciate ligament reconstruction in the multiple ligament injured knee: 2- to 10-year follow-up. Arthroscopy 2002;18:703–14.

51. Fanelli GC, Feldmann DD. Management of com-bined ACL/PCL/posterolateral complex injuries of the knee. Oper Tech Sports Med 1999;7:143–9.

52. Hughston JC, Andrews JR, Cross MJ, et al. Classifi-cation of knee ligament instabilities. Part II. The lateral compartment. J Bone Joint Surg Am 1976; 58-A:173–9.

53. Jacobson KE. Technical pitfalls of collateral ligament surgery. Clin Sports Med 1999;18:847–82.

54. LaPrade RF, Hamilton CD, Engebretsen L. Treatment of acute and chronic combined anterior cruciate lig-ament and posterolateral knee injuries. Sports Med Arthrosc Rev 1997;5:91–9.

55. LaPrade RF. Arthroscopic evaluation of the lateral compartment of knees with grade 3 posterolateral knee complex injuries. Am J Sports Med 1997;25: 596–602.

56. Veltri DM, Warren RF. Operative treatment of posterolateral instability of the knee. Clin Sports Med 1994;13:615–27.

57. Bin SI, Nam TS. Surgical outcome of 2-stage management of multiple knee ligament injuries after knee dislocation. Arthroscopy 2007;23(10): 1066–72.

58. Medvecky MJ, Zazulak BT, Hewett TE. A multidisciplinary approach to the evaluation, recon-struction and rehabilitation of the multi-ligament injured athlete. Sports Med 2007;37(2):169–87.

59. Harner CD, Vogrin TM, Höher J, et al. Biomechanical analysis of a posterior cruciate ligament reconstruc-tion: deficiency of the posterolateral structures as a cause of graft failure. Am J Sports Med 2000; 28(1):32–9.

60. Miller M. In: Wiesel SW, editor. Operative techniques: sports knee surgery. Lippincott and Williams; 2008.

61. Fanelli GC, Larson RV. Practical management of posterolateral instability of the knee. Arthroscopy 2002;18:1–8.

62. Hughston JC, Eilers AF. The role of the posterior ob-lique ligament in repairs of acute medial (collateral) ligament tears of the knee. J Bone Joint Surg 1973; 55A:923–40.

63. Müller W. The knee: form, function, and ligament reconstruction. Berlin: Springer–Verlag; 1983.

64. Sims WF, Jacobson KE. The posteromedial corner of the knee; medial-sided injury patterns revisited. Am J Sports Med 2004;32(2):337–45.

65. Lind M, Jakobsen BW, Lund B, et al. Anatomical reconstruction of the medial collateral ligament and posteromedial corner of the knee in patients with chronic medial collateral ligament instability. Am J Sports Med 2009;37(6):1116–22.

66. Stannard JP, Black BS, Azbell C, et al. Posterome-dial corner injury in knee dislocations. J Knee Surg 2012;25(5):429–34.

67. Borden PS, Kantaras AT, Caborn DN. Medial collat-eral ligament reconstruction with allograft using a double-bundle technique. Arthroscopy 2002;18:E19.

68. Stannard JP, Nuelle CW, McGwin G, et al. Hinged external fixators in treatment of knee dislocations: a prospective randomized study. J Bone Joint Surg 2014;96(3):184–91.

69. Manske RC, Hosseinzadeh P, Giangarra CE. Multi-ple ligament knee injury; complications. N Am Jour Sports Phys Ther 2008;3(4):226–33.

70. Marx RG, Hetsroni I. Surgical technique: medial collateral ligament reconstruction using Achilles allo-graft for combined knee ligament injury. Clin Orthop Relat Res 2012;470(3):798–805.

71. Levy BA, Dajani KA, Whelan DB, et al. Decision making in the multi-ligament-injured knee: an evidence-based systematic review. Arthroscopy 2008;25:430–8.

72. Merrill KD. Knee dislocations with vascular injuries. Orthop Clin North Am 1994;25:707–13.

73. Dedmond BT, Almekinders LC. Operative versus non-operative treatment of knee dislocations: a meta-analysis. Am J Knee Surg 2001;14(1):33–8.

Applications of Local Antibiotics in Orthopedic Trauma

Jourdan M. Cancienne, MD, M. Tyrrell Burrus, MD,
David B. Weiss, MD, Seth R. Yarboro, MD*

KEYWORDS

• Infection • Trauma • Local • Antibiotics • Bead • Prophylaxis

KEY POINTS

- Local antibiotics have the advantage of high local concentrations (thus efficacy at the surgical site), and low systemic concentrations (less risk of systemic side effects).
- Local antibiotics have been proven effective for infection prophylaxis and treatment of established infection, and are typically used in concert with systemic antibiotics.
- Multiple delivery systems are available for antibiotic delivery, with each having unique properties that may be advantageous.
- Antibiotic delivery from PMMA is highly variable and depends upon: surface area (bead size), antibiotic used, number of antibiotics, mixing technique, time since implantation, Fluid characteristics around the beads, and others.
- Aqueous antibiotic solution injected locally after wound closure is a simple delivery method that has demonstrated positive results in animal and clinical models.

INTRODUCTION

Local antibiotic use began more than 100 years ago with Joseph Lister, who pioneered safe, antiseptic surgery. Before Lister's innovations, as many as 80% of all operations were complicated by infection. He was the first to apply local antiseptics, including carbolic acid, to surgical wounds to treat open fractures.[1] This led to further use of local antiseptics by Fleming during World War I, and in 1939 with Jensen instilling sulfanilamide crystals as local antibiotic in open fractures for infection prevention.[2,3] Despite significant advances in the use of prophylactic antibiotics and perioperative protocols, orthopedic surgical site infections still remain a significant source of morbidity and mortality and result in a substantial financial burden to the health care system. Surgical site infections are the second most common cause of nosocomial infections in extra-abdominal surgeries, with an incidence of 2% to 5%,[4,5] and approximately 5% of orthopedic internal fixation implants becoming infected. The rate of infection following internal fixation of closed fractures is generally much lower than that of open fractures, with open fractures approaching 30%. Despite the higher infection rate seen in the treatment of particular fractures compared with arthroplasty, there is much less literature available on the prophylactic use of local antibiotics for infection prevention in open and closed fracture treatment.[6–8]

Local antibiotics provide high local concentrations with lower systemic levels than parenterally administered antibiotics. The delivery of local antibiotics can both supplement and sometimes obviate the need for systemic antibiotics. In certain instances, the target area of treatment may be avascular, preventing systemic antibiotics from reaching the targeted site. In these scenarios, local

Division of Orthopaedic Trauma, Department of Orthopaedic Surgery, University of Virginia Health System, PO Box 800159, Charlottesville, VA 22908-0159, USA
* Corresponding author.
E-mail address: SRY2J@virginia.edu

Orthop Clin N Am 46 (2015) 495–510
http://dx.doi.org/10.1016/j.ocl.2015.06.010
0030-5898/15/$ – see front matter © 2015 Elsevier Inc. All rights reserved.

orthopedic.theclinics.com

antibiotics may serve as the only effective option in treating the infection. Perhaps the main advantage of local antibiotic therapy is the ability of an antibiotic to reach a high local concentration while simultaneously having a low or undetectable systemic concentration, thereby avoiding certain negative side effects, such as nephrotoxicity and ototoxicity and decreasing the chances of developing pathogenic resistance.[9–11] At this high level of local concentration, many bacteria that might otherwise be normally resistant to an antibiotic fall within its spectrum of activity.[12]

In addition to infection prophylaxis, local antibiotics may have a role for treatment of established infections. This antibiotic therapy is typically coupled with surgical debridement when necessary,[13] which includes wide excision of infected and devascularized tissues, curettage of abscesses and sequestra, restoration of soft tissue coverage, and removal of all foreign bodies.[14] Although these techniques help to eradicate infection, they also contribute to the formation of dead space. Various antibiotic carriers can help fill and manage this potential space caused by bone or soft tissue defects, preventing subsequent development of infection (**Table 1**).

One potential negative implication of a high local concentration of antibiotics is cytotoxicity, which could inhibit new bone formation and delay fracture union at high enough levels.[15–17] We will review commonly used carriers and methods for local antibiotic administration, their indications, and recent clinical trials evaluating the success of these methods.

Biofilm

One aspect of treating infection involves isolating the pathogen from the infected tissue or bone and determining the sensitivity of that pathogen to different antimicrobial agents. This goal is most readily accomplished when treating the unicellular, planktonic bacteria that are present in an infected wound bed. Conversely, biofilms interfere with this strategy. A biofilm is an extracellular matrix produced by bacteria that offers protection and provides an organizing scaffold to facilitate metabolic activity and communication between the bacteria within the matrix (**Fig. 1**).[18] In a biofilm, bacteria may tolerate antibiotic concentrations up to 1000-fold greater than the same bacteria in planktonic form.[19] Biofilm bacteria are not as mobile or virulent within the body as their unicellular phenotypes; however, they are much more protected from host immunity and systemic antibiotics and thus more difficult to eradicate.

Once established, the biofilm can provide a continual source of bacteria that can detach as planktonic cells or biofilm fragments that can then travel to and infect other sites or cause a systemic infection.[20] Even though they are less virulent, biofilms cause damage by invoking a host inflammatory response that generates adjacent tissue destruction, manifesting clinically as pain and implant loosening.[20] Biofilms, and the bacteria that comprise them, have the ability to attach to orthopedic implants through their unique surface structures.[21] The most common biofilm-producing organisms found in orthopedic infections are

Table 1
The author's preferred concentrations for local antibiotic carriers

	Recommended Mixture	Trade Examples	Other Considerations
PMMA	2 g vancomycin and 2.4 g tobramycin in 40 g PMMA cement	Palacos (Zimmer, Warsaw, IN), Simplex (Stryker, Kalamazoo, MI), SmartSet (DePuy, West Chester, PA)	May take longer to set up and may require additional monomer when additional antibiotics are added
Calcium sulfate	1 g vancomycin and 1.2 g tobramycin in 10 mL packet of calcium sulfate	Osteoset (Wright Medical, Memphis, TN), Stimulan (Biocomposites, Wilmington, NC)	FDA approved as a bone void filler, antibiotic delivery is off-label use; adding tobramycin powder only after mixing $CaSO_4$ will help it set up
Aqueous solution	80 mg tobramycin in 40 mL solution	Available as generic tobramycin, prepared in the OR	Inject into wound AFTER wound closure; if a drain is in place, clamp drain while injecting solution

Abbreviations: PMMA, polymethylmethacrylate; OR, operating room.

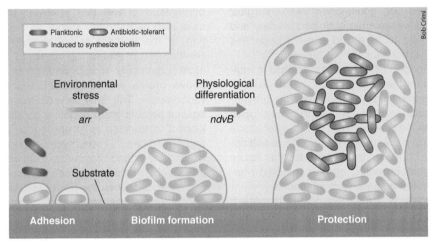

Fig. 1. Planktonic bacteria (*blue*) assemble onto an acceptable substrate, such as an orthopedic implant, to form a biofilm (*green*). A subpopulation within the biofilm (*purple*) develops a tolerance to certain antibiotics, and can withstand much higher concentrations than normally seen with the more singular, unicellular planktonic bacteria. These bacteria are more protected from systemic antibiotics, however are less virulent to the body. arr, CDG phosphodiesterase found within *P aeruginosa* responsible for biofilm defense response when exposed to subinhibitory concentrations of aminoglycosides; ndvB, a gene product that contributes to the protection of the biofilm. (*From* O'Toole GA, Stewart PS. Biofilms strike back. Nat Biotechnol 2005;23(11):1378–9; with permission.)

Staphylococcus aureus, coagulase-negative staphylococci, beta-hemolytic streptococci, and aerobic gram-negative rods, such as *Pseudomonas aeruginosa*.[20,22]

Unfortunately, failure to isolate an organism from an implant-related infection is not uncommon. Although the planktonic bacteria can be isolated and grown with traditional culture techniques, identifying bacteria from biofilms is often unsuccessful.[23] Sonication of explanted implants has been shown to improve the sensitivity of intraoperative cultures.[24] Even with accurate intraoperative cultures, established infections often require formal irrigation and debridement for infection eradication or suppression, depending on the acuity of the infection. In these situations, the ability to eradicate the infection depends on removal of biofilm at the infection site, often through extensive resection and formation of potential space.

Recent research has focused on the prevention of biofilm formation via modification of implants to alter the surfaces, inhibiting bacteria adhesion. One example using this strategy has been the coating of voice prostheses with silicone rubber.[25] Although this has been successful in the field of otolaryngology, these materials may interfere with osseointegration of orthopedic implants, limiting its applicability. Other strategies have focused on covalently linking antibiotics to the implant surface.[26,27] Translational research has shown this technique to be effective in inhibiting *S aureus* implant colonization while still supporting bone healing in a large animal model.[27] However,

there is concern that this novel technique may encourage and even stimulate bacteria to develop resistance. Regardless of the implant, all medical devices are susceptible to biofilm colonization and infection. Strategies for the treatment and prevention of biofilm formation must be considered to reduce the morbidity and cost of orthopedic implant infections.

Delivery Systems

The ideal local antibiotic delivery system has yet to be formulated, but would produce a high local antibiotic level at the target site and concurrently allow a safe systemic level. The elution rates, factors that influence elution rates, and the interaction between the environment and the material would need to be defined. The material would be easily handled and manipulated, removed if nonabsorbable, and nonimmunogenic and inexpensive. For an absorbable material, it would need break down in a relatively short time, such that it did not act as a foreign body once the antibiotic was eluted. In the past 2 decades several different local antibiotic delivery carriers have been used. These can largely be divided into 2 groups based on the biodegradability of the delivery vehicle.

Polymethylmethacrylate

Antibiotic-loaded bone cement may be considered the current gold standard for local antibiotic delivery in orthopedic surgery.[28] Antibiotic-loaded polymethylmethacrylate (PMMA) cement beads are the most popular nonbiodegradable modality used in conjunction with surgical debridement and systemic antibiotic therapy and have been used to treat and prevent bone and soft tissue infections for almost 30 years.[29,30]

Antibiotic-loaded PMMA can be applied in multiple settings for the treatment and prophylaxis of infection. Common indications include the prevention of infection in total joint arthroplasty, open fractures, and the management of potential space (dead space) in patients with large bone or soft tissue deficits.[29] It also can be used to treat acute and chronic osteomyelitis, chronic infected nonunions, and periprosthetic joint infections.

Contraindications are largely limited to patient hypersensitivity or allergy to specific antibiotics as well as the presence of resistant organisms such as *Enterococcus*.[31] The presence of the beads themselves is an attractive surface for slime-producing organisms, such as *Enterococcus*, and this slime barrier decreases the efficacy of the antibiotic.[31,32] The theoretic advantages of antibiotic beads include a high local concentration with low systemic levels, occupation of potential space following surgical debridement, low immunogenic response, and a high surface area of the bead allowing for a rapid release of the antibiotic.[11,29]

The surgical technique involves mixing the antibiotic powder with the powdered cement polymer and then adding the methylmethacrylate liquid monomer. The cement is then inserted into a bead mold or beads can be formed by hand. They are then typically connected with either 26-gauge wire or nonabsorbable heavy suture. The author's preferred technique is to use a 0 Prolene suture and pass the suture through the beads as they are hardening, thus making the beads easier to place and later retrieve at the time of removal.

Regarding the mechanical effect of antibiotic on the PMMA, biomechanical testing performed on Smart Set GHV (DePuy Orthopedics Inc, Warsaw, IN) and CMW 1 (CMW Laboratories Ltd, Devon, United Kingdom) to determine if their structural properties was compromised with the addition of antibiotics (linezolid, gentamycin, vancomycin, linezolid plus vancomycin, linezolid plus gentamicin).[33] With up to 2 g antibiotic per 40 g PMMA packet (5% weight/weight), there was no reduction in the axial compression strength of each brand of cement. However, 4.5 g or greater of antibiotic powder has been shown to weaken PMMA.[34] One method to maintain or increase the mechanical strength of the cement is to vacuum-mix the batch, which will reduce porosity and thus increase strength.[35]

The antibiotic used must be water soluble, available in powder form, be chemically stable, and have a broad antibacterial spectrum with a low percentage of resistant species. The antibiotic must also be thermally stable, as the polymerization of the cement is an exothermic reaction creating temperatures up to 60 to 80°C.[36] The most commonly mixed antibiotics that fit the above profile are gentamicin, tobramycin, and vancomycin. The aminoglycosides are effective against aerobic gram-negative bacilli and staphylococci in addition to streptococci, enterococci, and anaerobes.[37] Tobramycin is more commonly used in the United States due to its wide availability as a pharmaceutical-grade power. Vancomycin can be added when the risk of resistant staphylococcal organisms is present. Vancomycin has been shown to be heat resistant and is readily available in powder form, with effective elution properties.[38]

Although elution is ultimately governed by the difference in the concentration of antibiotic in the cement and its surrounding environment, other factors affecting elution include the type and viscosity of PMMA, the type and concentration of the antibiotic, and the structural characteristics of the beads.[36,39] Increasing the surface area–to-volume ratio (ie, smaller beads) increases the elution of antibiotics.[17] The type of antibiotic also affects elution, with tobramycin able to elute antibiotics longer and sustain concentrations above the minimum inhibitory concentration for longer periods of time than vancomycin at the same dose.[40] Moreover, elution of antibiotics from PMMA beads has been extensively studied and remains a debated issue that is not completely understood.[41–47] In general, there is a biphasic release pattern that occurs with an initial rapid release of approximately 5% to 7% of the total amount of antibiotic released within the first 24 hours, followed by a sustained secondary elution of antibiotic that steadily decreases over weeks or months.[11,48] In fact, elution has been reported up to 5 years after PMMA bead implantation.[49] Ultimately, multiple factors contribute to the elution profile of an antibiotic from PMMA beads, making it quite difficult to standardize the system for consistent antibiotic delivery.

Antibiotic-loaded PMMA beads also can be administered in an antibiotic bead pouch (**Fig. 2**).[50–52] With this technique, antibiotic-loaded beads are placed into a bony or soft tissue defect, and the wound is not closed, but is covered with an occlusive dressing, such as Ioban (3M, St. Paul, MN) (**Figs. 3** and **4**). Negative-pressure wound therapy (NPWT) may be used in conjunction, although this is at the surgeon's discretion and has produced somewhat conflicting results in recent studies.[53] Although Stinner and colleagues[53] showed decreased efficacy of bead

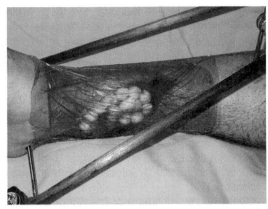

Fig. 2. Lower extremity wound managed with an antibiotic bead pouch sealed with Ioban dressing until definitive wound closure obtained. (*From* Zalavras CG, Marcus RE, Levin LS, et al. Management of open fractures and subsequent complications. J Bone Joint Surg Am 2007;89(4):889; with permission.)

pouch used with NPWT, Warner and colleagues[54] found that for extremity blast injuries, compared with a Vacuum-Assisted Closure Therapy system (KCI Inc, San Antonio, TX), a bead pouch resulted in less late methicillin-resistant *Staphylococcus aureus* infections, although more unanticipated returns to the operating room for wound problems,

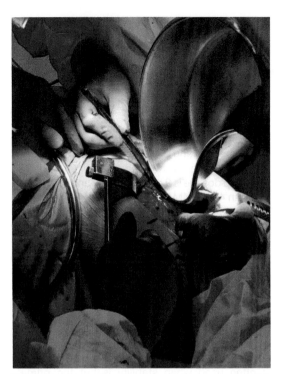

Fig. 4. Bead insertion into the surgical wound, in this scenario an infected hip.

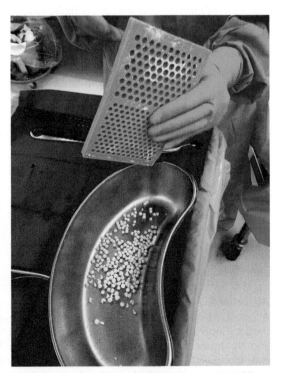

Fig. 3. Once beads have set, they are removed from the tray and collected into a metal basin in preparation for insertion into the surgical site.

and the bead pouch group required more surgeries overall until closure of the wounds.

Several animal and clinical studies have been conducted that have supported the beneficial role of PMMA beads in the prevention of infection following bone contamination.[39,51,52,55–58] Fitzgerald and colleagues[56] demonstrated a 90% prevention rate in the development of osteomyelitis following contamination with *S aureus* after insertion of gentamicin-loaded cement, whereas Chen and colleagues[55] reported a significant reduction in the bacterial count of *S aureus* after the insertion of tobramycin-loaded beads in a rabbit model.[56] In one of the largest clinical trials, Ostermann and colleagues[58] compared the addition of an antibiotic bead pouch versus systemic antibiotics alone in preventing infection in 1085 open fractures. The group reported infection rates of 3.7% in those treated with the antibiotic bead pouch in addition to systemic antibiotics, compared with 12% in those treated with systemic antibiotics alone. Furthermore, several animal and clinical studies have investigated the potential therapeutic applications of PMMA beads in the treatment of osteomyelitis.[49,59–62] A randomized controlled study by Calhoun and colleagues[62] suggested that long-term systemic antibiotic therapy following debridement and reconstructive surgery for infected nonunions can be substituted by local antibiotic therapy in the form of PMMA beads. Patzakis and colleagues[61] further corroborated the effectiveness of PMMA beads after demonstrating a 100% union rate in patients with chronic osteomyelitis and bony defects who underwent debridement, systemic antibiotics, and bead placement.

Several different doses of antibiotics in PMMA have been reported in the orthopedic literature. Most arthroplasty studies report a range of 1 to 2 g of vancomycin and 2.4 to 3.6 g of tobramycin.[63–65] Although there is no consensus, the author's preferred dosage is 2 g vancomycin and 2.4 g tobramycin in 40 g PMMA cement.

Intramedullary nails made from antibiotic-loaded PMMA cement may be used for antibiotic delivery in long-bone infections.[66,67] Two approaches are commonly used, each having its advantage. A nail composed of PMMA can be fabricated with a 40-French chest tube, which has an 11-mm inner diameter. A 16-gauge or 18-gauge Luque wire is commonly placed in the middle of the nail to allow removal if it breaks. The advantage of this technique is maximal antibiotic delivery, as there is more cement present, and it is often used when stability is not the primary objective. The other technique involves coating a titanium nail (either pediatric nail or standard 9-mm tibia nail) with antibiotic-loaded PMMA cement. This may be either formed by hand, or injected into a chest tube around the nail. If done by hand, the interlock screw holes may be preserved. This technique allows some antibiotic to be delivered to the target site, but its primary advantage is stability. For either technique, removal of the chest tube surrounding the antibiotic nail is facilitated by cooling the nail in a water bath and coating the inside of the chest tube with mineral oil before filling with cement.[68]

One additional application of antibiotic-loaded PMMA cement is the Masquelet technique, which is a 2-stage strategy for the reconstruction of segmental diaphyseal defects.[69,70] Developed in 1986, the technique takes advantage of induced membranes to reconstruct the defects with nonvascularized bone autograft.[69] The first stage includes standard debridement, and insertion of PMMA antibiotic-loaded cement spacer into the defect, and closure or coverage of soft tissue. The second stage occurs 6 to 8 weeks later after definitive healing of the soft tissue envelope has occurred. The spacer is taken out with careful attention paid to not disrupt the membrane that has been induced by the cement. This cavity now surrounded by the membrane is packed with cancellous bone autograft that can be combined with demineralized bone matrix to fill the void. The technique relies on the theory that the

biological membrane induced by the PMMA cement has a protective and positive effect on the cancellous autograft.[69,70] A recent retrospective study reported on 84 posttraumatic diaphyseal long-bone reconstructions using the technique over a 20-year period.[71] The series was composed of largely open fractures (89%) of which union was obtained in 90% at a mean of 14 months after the first stage of the reconstruction. The investigators report that the technique provides a successful way to manage segmental defects and control infection before bone reconstruction.

Controversies concerning PMMA beads and other forms of nonbiodegradable local antibiotic therapy include length of implantation and the need for removal. Prolonged implantation may lead to the development of drug-resistant bacteria. Despite killing glycocalyx-forming bacteria during the elution phase, bacteria can persist and adhere to the retained PMMA beads, now acting as foreign bodies, and may survive on their surface after release of antibiotic has fallen below therapeutic levels.[72] This adherence might provide an environment for recurrence and resistance, as has been seen in the wounds of patients that have been treated with gentamicin-loaded acrylic cement beads in the past.[73] One center has reported an increase in the prevalence of resistant bacteria with the introduction of antibiotic-loaded bone cement.[74] PMMA itself has been associated with decreased immune function and response, which might further impair the eradication of any remaining infection.[75] In response to these concerns over prolonged implantation, bead removal within 4 to 6 weeks from implantation has been recommended because the beads progressively become incorporated within callus and entrapped in fibrous tissue, which likely reduces elution and can complicate retrieval.[76]

In summary, PMMA beads have proven to be an effective nonbiodegradable option for local antibiotic therapy for prevention and treatment of infections in open fractures and osteomyelitis. For maximal effectiveness, the author recommends that the beads be used as an adjunct in the care of infection and not as a substitute for debridement.

Absorbable options

Although PMMA may be considered the gold standard for local antibiotic delivery for the prevention and treatment of orthopedic infection, concerns over the use of PMMA has led to the investigation of alternate biodegradable materials as delivery vehicles. Concerns include variable release properties of PMMA and retained PMMA acting as a foreign body after antibiotic release falls below therapeutic levels, creating a surface for reinfection and bacterial resistance.[72,77] In contrast, a biodegradable implant with a faster, complete, release of antibiotic would theoretically decrease the risk of recurrence of infection and generation of resistance. Furthermore, biodegradable implants obviate the need for a second surgery for removal. An osteoconductive, bioabsorbable bone substitute that is clinically as effective as PMMA in infection eradication has several clinical advantages.[78] Biodegradable antibiotic delivery vehicles can be broadly grouped into 4 different categories: bone graft, bone graft substitutes or extenders, natural polymers, and synthetic polymers.[79]

Bone Graft

Bone autograft and allograft, combined with antibiotics, have been used clinically for more than 2 decades as a delivery vehicle to treat infection.[79] The concept was developed in 1984 and centered on using a material that was already required for the reconstruction at the time of a secondary surgery to remove the antibiotic-laden cement. The morselized bone incorporates during bone regeneration and remodeling, allowing the recruitment of host defenses to protect the now vascularized bone graft and zone of previous infection.[79] Antibiotics are added as a powder to the morselized bone autograft or allograft or the graft can be soaked in an antibiotic solution.[69] The antibiotic is absorbed directly to the bone surface, and release is known to occur through first-order kinetics.[69] In vitro and in vivo studies in a rabbit model demonstrated first-order kinetics for release of tobramycin and vancomycin over a period of 3 weeks with levels exceeding usual bactericidal concentrations.[80] In a clinical study, tobramycin and vancomycin levels were studied in 26 patients with antibiotic morselized cancellous bone grafts greater than 20 mL. Data demonstrated continued release for at least 3 weeks, safe serum levels, and drain fluid levels 10 to 100 times the reported effective levels of both vancomycin and tobramycin.[80] At minimum 2-year follow-up, the investigators reported no evidence of active infection in any patient.

Antibiotic-loaded autologous cancellous bone grafting also has shown positive results. Chan and colleagues[81] in 1998 combined iliac cancellous bone grafts with piperacillin and/or vancomycin and implanted the mixture at the site of similar infected osseous defects. All fractures in the 36 study patients went on to union within 4 to 5 months with the only complications reported as skin rashes. In a more recent study by the same group, Chan and colleagues[82] evaluated 96 patients for infected tibial nonunions treated with local antibiotic bead therapy and staged antibiotic-loaded versus pure autogenous bone graft. In the antibiotic-loaded group, the infection-eradication rate was 95% at more than 4 years' follow-up with a 100% union rate versus 82% eradication and 98% union rate in the pure autogenous group. A more recent study by Khoo and colleagues[83] reported no early infections after the insertion of antibiotic-loaded iontophoresed segmental allografts for various orthopedic limb salvage surgeries with a mean follow-up of 51 months. More studies are needed to evaluate the local antibiotic concentration level and the effect this has on eventual bone graft incorporation and bone healing. In one study comparing bone healing with autogenous cancellous bone grafting with and without admixed tobramycin, there was no effect in bone healing with large concentrations of local tobramycin.[63] Given the differences in bone and antibiotics used in addition to loading method and dosing, firm conclusions cannot be drawn from the literature at this time and more clinical comparative studies are needed to guide future use.

Bone Graft Substitutes or Extenders

Bone graft substitutes, such as calcium sulfate, calcium phosphate, hydroxyapatite, and tricalcium phosphate, have gained interest because they are osteoconductive and are compatible with and can promote the regeneration of bone during the time of material degradation. They are also desirable because they avoid the risk of transmitting disease pathogens associated with the use of allograft. Many of these products have Food and Drug Administration–approved treatment indications for bone void filler and are readily available in most operating rooms. However, they all show a rapid release of the antibiotic at a relatively uncontrolled rate.[79]

Of the bone graft substitutes, calcium sulfate is used most commonly in the clinical setting as an antibiotic delivery vehicle.[12] It is commercially available and was first used as bone defect filler in 1982.[84] Its advantages as bone void filler include its steady and gradual resorption, osteoconductive properties, lack of immunogenic side effects, and consistent clinical record.[85–88] Blaha[89] further demonstrated that calcium sulfate supports the infiltration of new blood vessels and osteogenic cells, and prevents ingrowth of soft tissue. Water-soluble antibiotics can be incorporated into the crystalline structure rather easily, although as mentioned previously, the antibiotic in this form is often eluted at an uncontrolled rate.[90] Tobramycin, which is generally effective against the most common species responsible for osteomyelitis, can be incorporated to produce an extremely high local concentration as the pellets are resorbed.[85,87] The most appropriate antibiotic dosage regimen remains unclear; however, common formulations used clinically have ranged from approximately 1 g vancomycin and/or 1.2 g tobramycin or gentamicin per 25 g calcium sulfate.[37,91,92] Even in infections when certain organisms are not sensitive to tobramycin at levels obtainable with systemic therapy, the high local concentrations released by the calcium sulfate pellets may be effective at eradicating the infection.[93,94]

Several human and animal studies have demonstrated the safety and efficacy of antibiotic-loaded calcium sulfate beads with infection-eradication rates of more than 90% (**Fig. 5**).[78,95,96] In a recent prospective randomized clinical trial, McKee and colleagues[97] compared tobramycin-loaded calcium sulfate pellets with PMMA and demonstrated similar infection-eradication rates and new bone growth with the clinical benefit of requiring fewer subsequent procedures. A recent in vitro study reported that calcium sulfate as an antibiotic carrier is at least equivalent, and potentially superior to

PMMA, in inhibiting bacterial growth in liquid and agar cultures.[98] There is building evidence that antibiotic-loaded calcium sulfate pellets are a safe and effective alternative to PMMA beads, obviating the added morbidity of a subsequent procedure for removal of beads.

Calcium sulfate also has been used with other materials, such as calcium hydroxyapatite (HA), in composite carriers. The primary advantage of HA over other carriers is that it is slowly replaced by new-forming bone, which might reduce the requirement for additional reconstruction.[90] One study used equal quantities of calcium sulfate and HA in a composite delivery system and found, as compared with calcium sulfate alone, the addition of HA slowed down the resorption and maintained serum levels of antibiotic at 4 weeks better than calcium sulfate alone.[99] Korkusuz and colleagues[100] also found that an HA-ceramic composite had consistently higher serum levels of gentamicin than antibiotic-loaded PMMA and resulted in infection eradication at 7 weeks in a rat osteomyelitis model. It is hypothesized that the porous structure of HA allows the infiltration of calcium sulfate, allowing a more sustained release as compared with the carriers in isolation.[90]

The disadvantages of calcium sulfate include potential cytotoxicity, high rate of resorption, and rapid elution rates, all of which have been studied in vitro.[90] Furthermore, calcium sulfate has a low mechanical strength, rendering it unsuitable where load bearing is required.[101,102] Calcium sulfate is known to generate an inflammatory and osmotic response that may result in increased fluid in the wound bed, and may result in opaque drainage from the incision that can be mistaken for purulence or recurrence of infection.[103] This has been reported in the literature; however, this is most commonly inconsistent with infection, and more likely an osmotic effect, as bacterial cultures are typically negative and wound healing occurs with standard dressing changes. For these reasons, this material should be used carefully in the setting of inadequate soft tissue envelope.

Natural Polymers

As discussed, biodegradable carriers are theoretically advantageous for their reduced risk of secondary infection and lack of need for a secondary surgery for removal. Furthermore, in instances in which there is little potential space to manage following irrigation and debridement, space-occupying carriers such as beads are not desirable and can make closure more difficult. This clinical scenario is typical in osteomyelitis, where the maintenance of a soft tissue envelope

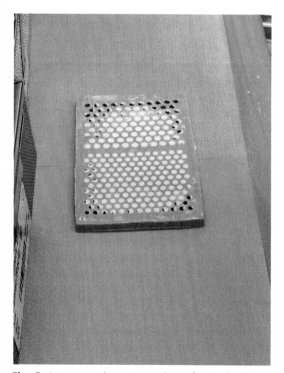

Fig. 5. Intraoperative preparation of mixed calcium sulfate beads setting in tray.

and long-term dead-space management is not required.[90] The most widely used and studied biodegradable natural polymer is the collagen sponge.[11,90] It is most commonly composed of a solid mesh of collagen-based material produced from sterile animal skin or the Achilles tendon.[90] In Europe, for example, it has been commercially available for more than a decade and is produced from sterilized bovine tendon in which gentamicin is suspended.[11] Collagen is a major component of the native connective tissue and is a structural component of virtually all organs, which makes the implant both biocompatible and nontoxic.[90] Furthermore, its variable drug-release profile and ability to attract and stimulate the proliferation of osteoblasts and promote mineralization make it an ideal delivery vehicle.[104,105] Collagen fleece kinetic studies have demonstrated a three-phase release of antibiotics.[106] This elution profile is largely due to the distinct structure of the collagen and the porosity of the fleece. Rapid release occurs soon after implantation due to the porous structure of the fleece with an intermediate release phase following due to the partially closed pores to which the antibiotic is enclosed, and finally a prolonged release phase due to the encasement of the drug within the fibrillar collagen structure.[107] Kinetic studies have quantified that 95% of gentamicin can be released in the first 1.5 hours compared with 8% from PMMA beads over the same time period.[106] Elution can be elongated by slowing the degradation rate of the fleece or sponge by macrophages. This can be accomplished by using hydrophilic gentamicin sulfate in combination with hydrophobic gentamicin crobefate resulting in prolonged release over 10 days.[108]

As compared with other biodegradables, antibiotic-loaded collagen delivery systems have been evaluated in several clinical studies.[109–113] Ascherl and colleagues[110] demonstrated a 94% infection-eradication rate in 67 patients with post-traumatic and postoperative osteomyelitis treated with a gentamicin-loaded collagen sponge. Other studies have reported infection-eradication rates of 93% to 100% with the addition of intravenous antibiotics.[109,111–113]

Gentamicin-loaded collagen sponge shows up to 600 times the minimum inhibitory concentration (MIC) as compared with PMMA beads at 300 MIC, and has been noted to be an effective delivery vehicle for up to 28 days in a rabbit model.[10,11] In a comparison study, Hettfleisch and Schottle[114] demonstrated a superior pharmacokinetic profile with complete elution of the antibiotic in collagen fleece as compared with PMMA. In the broader literature, a recent meta-analysis was conducted investigating nearly 7000 patients who had gentamicin-loaded collagen sponges placed for the prophylaxis of surgical site infections in several different surgical settings. The study concluded that the implants decreased the rate of surgical site infections.[115] Further investigation and characterization of the efficacy and safety of collagen sponges in orthopedic surgery are under way so they can be recommended and approved as a delivery vehicle in the United States.

Synthetic Polymers

More recent developmental work has focused on bioabsorbable gels as antibiotic delivery vehicles. Advantages of a gel include release of 100% of the carried antibiotics as it is degraded, and improved and more immediate distribution of antibiotic throughout the wound as opposed to discrete pockets around beads.

A recent in vitro study tested a sterile phospholipid gel containing 1.88% vancomycin and 1.68% gentamicin by weight. The study demonstrated local delivery of antibiotic by a bioabsorbable gel achieved complete wound coverage and was more effective in reducing bacteria than the commonly used antibiotic-PMMA bead depot in a contaminated defect study in a rat model.[87] The results of the study showed high initial concentrations that slowly declined over several days, and, in a supplemental unpublished study using a rabbit model, maintained persistent local tissue levels of antibiotics greater than the MIC for more than 14 days. The proposed strength of the gel is the ability of local antibiotic levels to rapidly exceed the MIC and minimum biofilm, eradicating concentrations of bacteria within the wound followed by a sustained release to combat and eradicate quiescent cells that are not as susceptible to the antibiotics at subtherapeutic levels.[43,87] The gel also provides immediate drug delivery to the entire wound contact area, with no need for the active drug to elute and diffuse through the wound bed.[87] Bioabsorbable gel shows promise as a capable delivery vehicle and translational research is currently under way to further evaluate its safety and efficacy.

Administrations in Aqueous Solution

Antibiotics can be effectively administered in aqueous solution as well. Although antibiotic (as well as antiseptic) solutions have been used for many years, there are clinical data that suggest this method of delivery is effective. A significant positive impact was shown in a series of patients with shoulder arthroplasty, where the rate of infection was decreased by 1 order of magnitude with intra-articular injection of aqueous gentamicin performed after wound closure.[116] This method of administration also has been effective in a rat model, where aqueous gentamicin was significantly better for infection prophylaxis after placement of a metal implant and contamination with *S aureus*, and this effect was further improved by concomitant administration of systemic antibiotics.[117,118] This method of delivery is distinct from antibiotic solution for irrigation, as the aqueous antibiotic is injected into the surgery site after the wound is closed. An 18-gauge needle is used adjacent to the incision to inject the solution throughout the wound. This technique allows the solution to ideally infiltrate the interstices or depths of the wound. In practice, the solution has been made in a concentration of 2 mg/mL (80 mg aminoglycoside in 40 mL injectable saline). Recent data, which suggested lower local cytotoxicity with tobramycin compared with gentamicin,[113] has prompted the switch to tobramycin in this application.

The advantages of delivering antibiotic in aqueous form are several, including cost, as there is no need for a specialized vehicle of delivery. The antibiotic drugs are approved and ready for use. Also, the wound encounters a higher maximum antibiotic concentration, potentially improving antibiotic efficacy.

Drawbacks to this method may include poor sustained antibiotic level; however, other vehicles for delivery, such as collagen sponge, have been shown to elute the drug very quickly, then potentially become a foreign body at the surgical site. Thus, this method of antibiotic delivery may be more effective in a situation in which sustained delivery is not required, such as prophylaxis of surgical site infections.

Local Antibiotic Pharmacokinetics and Safety

As stated previously, local antibiotics have the advantage of high local concentrations (thus efficacy at the surgical site), and low systemic concentrations (less risk of systemic side effects). Each of the carriers described previously elutes antibiotic at a different rate, resulting in variable potential risk for local cytotoxicity.[119] In an in vitro model, bone graft and demineralized bone matrix (DBM) were shown to elute 70% and 45% of their antibiotic load by 24 hours, and negligible amounts were detected at 1 week. In this study, PMMA cement was shown to elute 7% at 24 hours, with continued elution detected at 14 days. Calcium sulfate was shown to release 17% of its antibiotic by 24 hours, with trace amounts detected at 3 weeks. In other calcium sulfate elution studies, approximately 58% of the contained antibiotic is released during the first 24 hours in in vitro elution studies, and 20% released within the first 24 hours in an in vivo rabbit model.[60,120] Thus, bone graft and DBM may be best if only short duration of antibiotic coverage is needed, where calcium sulfate or bone cement may provide more prolonged coverage. Aqueous antibiotic solution would be expected to provide the shortest duration of coverage in the local tissue, as there is no vehicle of delivery.

Local levels as measured in wound exudate have been shown to be up to 300 µg/mL with gentamicin in PMMA.[121] Anagnostakos and colleagues[122] demonstrated that peak antibiotic levels for gentamicin and vancomycin from PMMA beads and spacers as measured in the drainage is highest on day 1, which then decreases significantly; however, antibiotic levels did persist through the 13 days tested. They concluded that beads eluted antibiotics more quickly and with higher peak concentration than spacers due to greater surface area, but that there was considerable variability between subjects for a given method of delivery, noting a lack of consistency in the elution profile.

Regarding local toxicity and safety, Rathbone and colleagues[123] demonstrated levels of toxicity for many commonly used antibiotics. These data are helpful for determining appropriate concentrations that are acceptable in the wound cavity, regardless of the delivery method. On evaluating osteogenic cell viability and activity as measured by alkaline phosphatase activity, wide variability was noted, even within families of antibiotics (**Fig. 6**). Rifampin, tetracyclines, and ciprofloxacin were noted to be particularly cytotoxic, with considerable decrease in cell number and activity at concentrations of even 100 µg/mL. Tobramycin, vancomycin, and amikacin were noted to be least cytotoxic. Of note, cell number and activity were measured at time points of 10 and 14 days for various concentrations of each antibiotic. Although the response of osteogenic cells to these concentrations of antibiotics is useful information, it should be noted that these are measured in response to sustained levels of antibiotics, and in the clinical setting, the antibiotic levels are highest at early time points and then often decrease rapidly.

Regarding the systemic levels achieved after local administration, Livio and colleagues[124] showed calcium sulfate with 4% tobramycin (262 or 524 mg tobramycin per 10 or 20 g calcium sulfate, respectively) resulted in systemic levels of tobramycin that fell well below the accepted safe serum level (2 mg/L) within 24 hours. However, based on their projected data, sustained

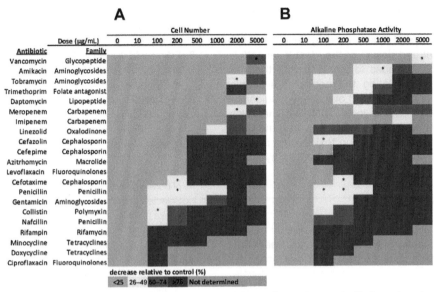

Fig. 6. Effects of different antibiotic treatments on osteoblast cell number and alkaline phosphatase activity (ALP). They are described in mean % decreases in osteoblast cell number (*A*) and ALP (*B*) activity as compared with a control after incubation with varying doses of antibiotic. Decreases in osteoblast cell number and ALP activity greater than 25% were significant, *P*<.05, whereas those marked with an *asterisk* were not significantly different from the control. (*From* Rathbone CR, Cross JD, Brown KV, et al. Effect of various concentrations of antibiotics on osteogenic cell viability and activity. J Orthop Res 2011;29(7):1072; with permission.)

potentially toxic concentrations were predicted by simulations with these doses at renal failure stages 4 and 5. Thus, even standard doses of tobramycin-loaded calcium sulfate should be used with caution in the setting of advanced renal failure.

Future Directions

Current treatment algorithms of prolonged systemic intravenous antibiotic treatment are becoming increasingly less effective with increasing bacterial resistance in addition to increasing patient costs and morbidity. A multidisciplinary approach with the application of various techniques will be required to treat orthopedic-related infections. At the forefront of this initiative are biofilm-disrupting treatments that break up biofilm layers into a single-celled planktonic form that are more susceptible to antibiotic treatment. Laser-generated shockwaves have been tested in vitro that use mechanical energy have been found to remove 97.9% of *P aeruginosa* biofilms on nitinol stents.[125,126] Furthermore, electrical stimulation on orthopedic implants is being studied to enhance detachment of the biofilm. Studies have shown that electrical current is able to enhance the detachment of biofilms growing on stainless steel implants infected with *S aureus* and *Staphylococcus epidermis*.[127–129] One study reported that the MIC of *S epidermidis* to gentamicin was decreased by 50% when infected

stainless steel pegs were pulsed with electromagnetic energy.[130] Thus, applying an electric current in combination with antibiotic therapy may help patients avoid the morbidity and cost of going through major revision surgeries and chronic suppressive antibiotic regimens.

The use of rifampin has been evaluated, including both local and systemic routes of administration. It has been demonstrated effective at penetrating bacterial biofilm in both in vitro and animal models.[131,132] One problem is that rifampin is relatively cytotoxic, resulting in a decreased osteoblast cell number and alkaline phosphatase activity at a concentration of less than 100 µg/mL.[123] Further research is required to determine local versus systemic efficacy, use with other antibiotics, and safe local concentrations.

Use of nonantibiotic agents, such as ᴅ-amino acids, may result in degradation of biofilms and make them more susceptible to antibiotic activity.[133,134] *Bacillus subtilis* has been found to produce this combination of ᴅ-amino acids as a signal to trigger break down of biofilms. However, this ᴅ-amino acid combination is not specific to *Bacillus*. In an in vitro setting, Losick[135] demonstrated increased biofilm breakdown, and Wenke and colleagues[136] showed that antibiotics were more effective against *S aureus* and *P aeruginosa* biofilm when administered with ᴅ-amino acids. Although only investigated in vitro at this point, the development of ᴅ-amino acids may be an effective adjunct in the treatment of biofilms and established infections.

The interest and research being devoted to the development and design of the ideal local antibiotic delivery continues to increase with the ultimate goal of obviating the need for systemic antibiotics for the treatment of many musculoskeletal infections. These local antibiotic therapies theoretically spare the morbidity and mortality associated with system drug toxicity and may be more effective at their targeted site than systemic therapies.

SUMMARY

Local antibiotics have a role in orthopedic trauma for both infection prophylaxis and treatment. They provide the advantage of high local antibiotic concentration without excessive systemic levels. The ideal delivery material and technique have not yet been completely established. The potential for the delivery vehicle to act as a foreign body must be considered. For established infections, such as osteomyelitis, a combination of surgical debridement with local and systemic antibiotics seems to represent the most effective treatment at this time. Further investigation of more effective local antibiotic utilization is currently under way.

REFERENCES

1. Pitt D, Aubin JM. Joseph Lister: father of modern surgery. Can J Surg 2012;55(5):E8–9.
2. Fleming A. The action of chemical and physiological antiseptics in a septic wound. Br J Surg 1920;7:99–129.
3. Jensen NK, Johnsrud LW, Nelson MC. The local implantation of sulfonamide in compound fractures. Surgery 1939;6:1–12.
4. Anderson DJ, Sexton DJ, Kanafani ZA, et al. Severe surgical site infection in community hospitals: epidemiology, key procedures, and the changing prevalence of methicillin-resistant *Staphylococcus aureus*. Infect Control Hosp Epidemiol 2007;28(9): 1047–53.
5. Schwarzkopf R, Takemoto RC, Immerman I, et al. Prevalence of *Staphylococcus aureus* colonization in orthopaedic surgeons and their patients: a prospective cohort controlled study. J Bone Joint Surg Am 2010;92(9):1815–9.
6. Obremskey WT, Bhandari M, Dirschl DR, et al. Internal fixation versus arthroplasty of comminuted fractures of the distal humerus. J Orthop Trauma 2003;17(6):463–5.
7. McGraw JM, Lim EV. Treatment of open tibial-shaft fractures. External fixation and secondary intramedullary nailing. J Bone Joint Surg Am 1988;70(6):900–11.
8. Raahave D. Postoperative wound infection after implant and removal of osteosynthetic material. Acta Orthop Scand 1976;47(1):28–35.
9. Eckman JB Jr, Henry SL, Mangino PD, et al. Wound and serum levels of tobramycin with the prophylactic use of tobramycin-impregnated polymethylmethacrylate beads in compound fractures. Clin Orthop Relat Res 1988;(237):213–5.
10. Humphre JS, Mehta S, Seaber AV, et al. Pharmacokinetics of a degradable drug delivery system in bone. Clin Orthop Relat Res 1998;(349):218–24.
11. Tsourvakas S. Local antibiotic therapy in the treatment of bone and soft tissue infections. In: Danilla S, editor. Selected Topics in Plastic Reconstructive Surgery. Rijeka (Croatia): InTech; 2012. p. 17–44.
12. Burdon DW. Principles of antimicrobial prophylaxis. World J Surg 1982;6:262–7.
13. Berend KR, Lombardi AV Jr, Morris MJ, et al. Two-stage treatment of hip periprosthetic joint infection is associated with a high rate of infection control but high mortality. Clin Orthop Relat Res 2013; 471(2):510–8.
14. Lazzarini L, Mader JT, Calhoun JH. Osteomyelitis in long bones. J Bone Joint Surg Am 2004;86-A(10): 2305–18.
15. Edin ML, Miclau T, Lester GE, et al. Effect of cefazolin and vancomycin on osteoblasts in vitro. Clin Orthop Relat Res 1996;(333):245–51.
16. Chang Y, Goldberg VM, Caplan AI. Toxic effects of gentamicin on marrow-derived human mesenchymal stem cells. Clin Orthop Relat Res 2006;(452):242–9.
17. Holtom PD, Pavkovic SA, Bravos PD, et al. Inhibitory effects of the quinolone antibiotics trovafloxacin, ciprofloxacin, and levofloxacin on osteoblastic cells in vitro. J Orthop Res 2000;18(5):721–7.
18. Hall-Stoodley L, Stoodley P, Kathju S, et al. Towards diagnostic guidelines for biofilm-associated infections. FEMS Immunol Med Microbiol 2012;65(2): 127–45.
19. Zoubos AB, Galanakos SP, Soucacos PN. Orthopedics and biofilm–what do we know? A review. Med Sci Monit 2012;18(6):RA89–96.
20. Arnold WV, Shirtliff ME, Stoodley P. Bacterial biofilms and periprosthetic infections. Instr Course Lect 2014;63:385–91.
21. Renner LD, Weibel DB. Physicochemical regulation of biofilm formation. MRS Bull 2011;36(5):347–55.
22. Berbari EF, Hanssen AD, Duffy MC, et al. Risk factors for prosthetic joint infection: case-control study. Clin Infect Dis 1998;27(5):1247–54.
23. Costerton JW, Post JC, Ehrlich GD, et al. New methods for the detection of orthopedic and other biofilm infections. FEMS Immunol Med Microbiol 2011;61(2):133–40.
24. Trampuz A, Piper KE, Jacobson MJ, et al. Sonication of removed hip and knee prostheses for

diagnosis of infection. N Engl J Med 2007;357(7):654–63.

25. Rodrigues L. Inhibition of bacterial adhesion on medical devices. In: Linke D, Golman A, editors. Bacterial Adhesion: Chemistry, Biology, and Physics. Dordrecht (The Netherlands): Springer; 2011. p. 351–67.

26. Shapiro IM, Hickok NJ, Parvizi J, et al. Molecular engineering of an orthopaedic implant: from bench to bedside. Eur Cell Mater 2012;23:362–70.

27. Stewart S, Barr S, Engiles J, et al. Vancomycin-modified implant surface inhibits biofilm formation and supports bone-healing in an infected osteotomy model in sheep: a proof-of-concept study. J Bone Joint Surg Am 2012;94(15):1406–15.

28. Nelson CL. The current status of material used for depot delivery of drugs. Clin Orthop Relat Res 2004;(427):72–8.

29. Decoster TA, Bozorgnia S. Antibiotic beads. J Am Acad Orthop Surg 2008;16(11):674–8.

30. Diefenbeck M, Muckley T, Hofmann GO. Prophylaxis and treatment of implant-related infections by local application of antibiotics. Injury 2006;37(Suppl 2):S95–104.

31. van de Belt H, Neut D, Schenk W, et al. *Staphylococcus aureus* biofilm formation on different gentamicin-loaded polymethylmethacrylate bone cements. Biomaterials 2001;22(12):1607–11.

32. Ensing GT, van Horn JR, van der Mei HC, et al. Copal bone cement is more effective in preventing biofilm formation than Palacos R-G. Clin Orthop Relat Res 2008;466(6):1492–8.

33. Snir N, Meron-Sudai S, Deshmukh AJ, et al. Antimicrobial properties and elution kinetics of linezolid from polymethylmethacrylate. Orthopedics 2013;36(11):e1412–7.

34. Duncan CP, Masri BA. The role of antibiotic-loaded cement in the treatment of an infection after a hip replacement. Instr Course Lect 1995;44:305–13.

35. Cui Q, Mihalko WM, Shields JS, et al. Antibiotic-impregnated cement spacers for the treatment of infection associated with total hip or knee arthroplasty. J Bone Joint Surg Am 2007;89(4):871–82.

36. Bistolfi A, Massazza G, Verne E, et al. Antibiotic-loaded cement in orthopedic surgery: a review. ISRN Orthop 2011;2011:290851.

37. Popham GJ, Mangino P, Seligson D, et al. Antibiotic-impregnated beads. Part II: factors in antibiotic selection. Orthop Rev 1991;20(4):331–7.

38. Sasaki T, Ishibashi Y, Katano H, et al. In vitro elution of vancomycin from calcium phosphate cement. J Arthroplasty 2005;20(8):1055–9.

39. Henry SL, Ostermann PA, Seligson D. The prophylactic use of antibiotic impregnated beads in open fractures. J Trauma 1990;30(10):1231–8.

40. Greene N, Holtom PD, Warren CA, et al. In vitro elution of tobramycin and vancomycin polymethylmethacrylate beads and spacers from Simplex and Palacos. Am J Orthop (Belle Mead NJ) 1998;27(3):201–5.

41. Anagnostakos K, Kelm J, Regitz T, et al. In vitro evaluation of antibiotic release from and bacteria growth inhibition by antibiotic-loaded acrylic bone cement spacers. J Biomed Mater Res B Appl Biomater 2005;72(2):373–8.

42. Nelson CL, Griffin FM, Harrison BH, et al. In vitro elution characteristics of commercially and non-commercially prepared antibiotic PMMA beads. Clin Orthop Relat Res 1992;(284):303–9.

43. Barton AJ, Sagers RD, Pitt WG. Measurement of bacterial growth rates on polymers. J Biomed Mater Res 1996;32(2):271–8.

44. Hendriks JG, van Horn JR, van der Mei HC, et al. Backgrounds of antibiotic-loaded bone cement and prosthesis-related infection. Biomaterials 2004;25(3):545–56.

45. Jiranek WA, Hanssen AD, Greenwald AS. Antibiotic-loaded bone cement for infection prophylaxis in total joint replacement. J Bone Joint Surg Am 2006;88(11):2487–500.

46. Elson RA, Jephcott AE, McGechie DB, et al. Antibiotic-loaded acrylic cement. J Bone Joint Surg Br 1977;59(2):200–5.

47. Hendriks JG, Neut D, van Horn JR, et al. Bacterial survival in the interfacial gap in gentamicin-loaded acrylic bone cements. J Bone Joint Surg Br 2005;87(2):272–6.

48. Torholm C, Lidgren L, Lindberg L, et al. Total hip joint arthroplasty with gentamicin-impregnated cement. A clinical study of gentamicin excretion kinetics. Clin Orthop Relat Res 1983;(181):99–106.

49. Wahlig H, Dingeldein E. Antibiotics and bone cements. Experimental and clinical long-term observations. Acta Orthop Scand 1980;51(1):49–56.

50. Prasarn ML, Zych G, Ostermann PAW. Wound management for severe open fractures: use of antibiotic bead pouches and vacuum-assisted closure. Am J Orthop (Belle Mead NJ) 2009;38(11):559–63.

51. Keating JF, Blachut PA, O'Brien PJ, et al. Reamed nailing of open tibia fractures: does the antibiotic bead pouch reduce the deep infection rate? J Orthop Trauma 1996;10(5):298–303.

52. Henry SL, Ostermann PA, Seligson D. The antibiotic bead pouch technique. The management of severe compound fractures. Clin Orthop Relat Res 1993;(295):54–62.

53. Stinner DJ, Hsu JR, Wenke JC. Negative pressure wound therapy reduces the effectiveness of traditional local antibiotic depot in a large complex musculoskeletal wound animal model. J Orthop Trauma 2012;26(9):512–8.

54. Warner M, Henderson C, Kadrmas W, et al. Comparison of vacuum-assisted closure to the antibiotic bead pouch for the treatment of blast injury of the extremity. Orthopedics 2010;33(2):77–82.

55. Chen NT, Hong HZ, Hooper DC, et al. The effect of systemic antibiotic and antibiotic-impregnated polymethylmethacrylate beads on the bacterial clearance in wounds containing contaminated dead bone. Plast Reconstr Surg 1993;92(7):1305–11 [discussion: 1312–3].

56. Fitzgerald RH. Experimental osteomyelitis: description of a canine model and the role of depot administration of antibiotics in the prevention and treatment of sepsis. J Bone Joint Surg Am 1983; 65A:371–80.

57. Ostermann PA, Henry SL, Seligson D. The role of local antibiotic therapy in the management of compound fractures. Clin Orthop Relat Res 1993;(295): 102–11.

58. Ostermann PA, Seligson D, Henry SL. Local antibiotic therapy for severe open fractures. A review of 1085 consecutive cases. J Bone Joint Surg Br 1995;77(1):93–7.

59. Evans RP, Nelson CL. Gentamicin-impregnated polymethylmethacrylate beads compared with systemic antibiotic therapy in the treatment of chronic osteomyelitis. Clin Orthop Relat Res 1993;(295):37–42.

60. Nelson CL, McLaren SG, Skinner RA, et al. The treatment of experimental osteomyelitis by surgical debridement and the implantation of calcium sulfate tobramycin pellets. J Orthop Res 2002;20(4):643–7.

61. Patzakis MJ, Mazur K, Wilkins J, et al. Septopal beads and autogenous bone grafting for bone defects in patients with chronic osteomyelitis. Clin Orthop Relat Res 1993;(295):112–8.

62. Calhoun JH, Henry SL, Anger DM, et al. The treatment of infected nonunions with gentamicin-polymethylmethacrylate antibiotic beads. Clin Orthop Relat Res 1993;(295):23–7.

63. Evans RP. Successful treatment of total hip and knee infection with articulating antibiotic components: a modified treatment method. Clin Orthop Relat Res 2004;(427):37–46.

64. Koo KH, Yang JW, Cho SH, et al. Impregnation of vancomycin, gentamicin, and cefotaxime in a cement spacer for two-stage cementless reconstruction in infected total hip arthroplasty. J Arthroplasty 2001;16(7):882–92.

65. Masri BA, Duncan CP, Beauchamp CP. Long-term elution of antibiotics from bone-cement: an in vivo study using the prosthesis of antibiotic-loaded acrylic cement (PROSTALAC) system. J Arthroplasty 1998; 13(3):331–8.

66. Riel RU, Gladden PB. A simple method for fashioning an antibiotic cement-coated interlocking intramedullary nail. Am J Orthop (Belle Mead NJ) 2010;39(1):18–21.

67. Thonse R, Conway J. Antibiotic cement-coated interlocking nail for the treatment of infected nonunions and segmental bone defects. J Orthop Trauma 2007;21(4):258–68.

68. Kim JW, Cuellar DO, Hao J, et al. Custom-made antibiotic cement nails: a comparative study of different fabrication techniques. Injury 2014;45(8): 1179–84.

69. Masquelet AC, Fitoussi F, Begue T, et al. Reconstruction of the long bones by the induced membrane and spongy autograft. Ann Chir Plast Esthet 2000;45(3):346–53.

70. Masquelet AC, Begue T. The concept of induced membrane for reconstruction of long bone defects. Orthop Clin North Am 2010;41(1):27–37 [table of contents].

71. Karger C, Kishi T, Schneider L, et al. Treatment of posttraumatic bone defects by the induced membrane technique. Orthop Traumatol Surg Res 2012;98(1):97–102.

72. Kendall RW, Duncan CP, Smith JA, et al. Persistence of bacteria on antibiotic loaded acrylic depots. A reason for caution. Clin Orthop Relat Res 1996;(329):273–80.

73. von Eiff C, Bettin D, Proctor RA, et al. Recovery of small colony variants of *Staphylococcus aureus* following gentamicin bead placement for osteomyelitis. Clin Infect Dis 1997;25(5):1250–1.

74. Wininger DA, Fass RJ. Antibiotic-impregnated cement and beads for orthopedic infections. Antimicrob Agents Chemother 1996;40(12):2675–9.

75. Granchi D, Ciapetti G, Savarino L, et al. Effects of bone cement extracts on the cell-mediated immune response. Biomaterials 2002;23(4):1033–41.

76. Salvati EA, Callaghan JJ, Brause BD, et al. Reimplantation in infection. Elution of gentamicin from cement and beads. Clin Orthop Relat Res 1986;(207):83–93.

77. Neut D, van de Belt H, van Horn JR, et al. Residual gentamicin-release from antibiotic-loaded polymethylmethacrylate beads after 5 years of implantation. Biomaterials 2003;24(10):1829–31.

78. McKee MD, Wild LM, Schemitsch EH, et al. The use of an antibiotic-impregnated, osteoconductive, bioabsorbable bone substitute in the treatment of infected long bone defects: early results of a prospective trial. J Orthop Trauma 2002;16(9):622–7.

79. McLaren AC. Alternative materials to acrylic bone cement for delivery of depot antibiotics in orthopaedic infections. Clin Orthop Relat Res 2004;(427): 101–6.

80. McLaren AC. Antibiotic impregnated bone graft. J Orthop Trauma 1989;3:171.

81. Chan YS, Ueng SW, Wang CJ, et al. Management of small infected tibial defects with antibiotic-impregnated autogenic cancellous bone grafting. J Trauma 1998;45(4):758–64.

82. Chan YS, Ueng SW, Wang CJ, et al. Antibiotic-impregnated autogenic cancellous bone grafting is an effective and safe method for the management of small infected tibial defects: a comparison study. J Trauma 2000;48(2):246–55.

83. Khoo PP, Michalak KA, Yates PJ, et al. Iontophoresis of antibiotics into segmental allografts. J Bone Joint Surg Br 2006;88(9):1149–57.

84. Mackey D, Varlet A, Debeaumont D. Antibiotic loaded plaster of Paris pellets: an in vitro study of a possible method of local antibiotic therapy in bone infection. Clin Orthop Relat Res 1982;(167): 263–8.

85. Beardmore AA, Brooks DE, Wenke JC, et al. Effectiveness of local antibiotic delivery with an osteoinductive and osteoconductive bone-graft substitute. J Bone Joint Surg Am 2005;87(1):107–12.

86. Borrelli J Jr, Prickett WD, Ricci WM. Treatment of nonunions and osseous defects with bone graft and calcium sulfate. Clin Orthop Relat Res 2003;(411):245–54.

87. Turner TM, Urban RM, Gitelis S, et al. Radiographic and histologic assessment of calcium sulfate in experimental animal models and clinical use as a resorbable bone-graft substitute, a bone-graft expander, and a method for local antibiotic delivery. One institution's experience. J Bone Joint Surg Am 2001;83-A(Suppl 2(Pt 1)):8–18.

88. Urban RM, Turner TM, Hall DJ, et al. Healing of large defects treated with calcium sulfate pellets containing demineralized bone matrix particles. Orthopedics 2003;26(5 Suppl):s581–5.

89. Blaha JD. Calcium sulfate bone-void filler. Orthopedics 1998;21(9):1017–9.

90. El-Husseiny M, Patel S, MacFarlane RJ, et al. Biodegradable antibiotic delivery systems. J Bone Joint Surg Br 2011;93-B:151–7.

91. Anagnostakos K, Schroder K. Antibiotic-impregnated bone grafts in orthopaedic and trauma surgery: a systematic review of the literature. Int J Biomater 2012;2012:538061.

92. Chen CE, Ko JY, Pan CC. Results of vancomycin-impregnated cancellous bone grafting for infected tibial nonunion. Arch Orthop Trauma Surg 2005; 125(6):369–75.

93. Wilson KJ, Cierny G, Adams KR, et al. Comparative evaluation of the diffusion of tobramycin and cefotaxime out of antibiotic-impregnated polymethylmethacrylate beads. J Orthop Res 1988;6(2): 279–86.

94. Scott CP, Higham PA, Dumbleton JH. Effectiveness of bone cement containing tobramycin. An in vitro susceptibility study of 99 organisms found in infected joint arthroplasty. J Bone Joint Surg Br 1999;81(3):440–3.

95. Gitelis S, Brebach GT. The treatment of chronic osteomyelitis with a biodegradable antibiotic-impregnated implant. J Orthop Surg (Hong Kong) 2002;10:53–60.

96. Sulo I. Gentamycin impregnated plaster beads in the treatment of bone infection. Rev Chir Orthop Reparatrice Appar Mot 1993;79(4):299–305.

97. McKee MD, Li-Bland EA, Wild LM, et al. A prospective, randomized clinical trial comparing an antibiotic-impregnated bioabsorbable bone substitute with standard antibiotic-impregnated cement beads in the treatment of chronic osteomyelitis and infected nonunion. J Orthop Trauma 2010;24:483–90.

98. McConoughey SJ, Howlin RP, Wiseman J, et al. Comparing PMMA and calcium sulfate as carriers for the local delivery of antibiotics to infected surgical sites. J Biomed Mater Res B Appl Biomater 2015;103(4):870–7.

99. Sato S, Koshino T, Saito T. Osteogenic response of rabbit tibia to hydroxyapatite particle-Plaster of Paris mixture. Biomaterials 1998;19(20):1895–900.

100. Korkusuz F, Uchida A, Shinto Y, et al. Experimental implant-related osteomyelitis treated by antibiotic-calcium hydroxyapatite ceramic composites. J Bone Joint Surg Br 1993;75(1):111–4.

101. Rauschmann MA, Wichelhaus TA, Stirnal V, et al. Nanocrystalline hydroxyapatite and calcium sulphate as biodegradable composite carrier material for local delivery of antibiotics in bone infections. Biomaterials 2005;26(15):2677–84.

102. Sanicola SM, Albert SF. The in vitro elution characteristics of vancomycin and tobramycin from calcium sulfate beads. J Foot Ankle Surg 2005;44(2):121–4.

103. Cai X, Han K, Cong X, et al. The use of calcium sulfate impregnated with vancomycin in the treatment of open fractures of long bones: a preliminary study. Orthopedics 2010;33(3). http://dx.doi.org/10.3928/01477447-20100129-17.

104. Rao KP. Recent developments of collagen-based materials for medical applications and drug delivery systems. J Biomater Sci Polym Ed 1995;7(7): 623–45.

105. Reddi AH. Implant-stimulated interface reactions during collagenous bone matrix-induced bone formation. J Biomed Mater Res 1985;19(3):233–9.

106. Sorensen TS, Sorensen AI, Merser S. Rapid release of gentamicin from collagen sponge. In vitro comparison with plastic beads. Acta Orthop Scand 1990;61(4):353–6.

107. Uludag H, Friess W, Williams D, et al. rhBMP-collagen sponges as osteoinductive devices: effects of in vitro sponge characteristics and protein pI on in vivo rhBMP pharmacokinetics. Ann N Y Acad Sci 1999;875:369–78.

108. Stemberger A, Grimm H, Bader F, et al. Local treatment of bone and soft tissue infections with the collagen-gentamicin sponge. Eur J Surg Suppl 1997;(578):17–26.

109. Chaudhary S, Sen RK, Saini UC, et al. Use of gentamicin-loaded collagen sponge in internal fixation of open fractures. Chin J Traumatol 2011; 14(4):209–14.

110. Ascherl R, Stemberger A, Lechner F, et al. Treatment of chronic osteomyelitis with a collagen-antibiotic compound–preliminary report. Unfallchirurgie 1986; 12(3):125–7.

111. von Hasselbach C. Clinical aspects and pharmacokinetics of collagen-gentamicin as adjuvant local therapy of osseous infections. Unfallchirurg 1989; 92(9):459–70.

112. Ipsen T, Jorgensen PS, Damholt V, et al. Gentamicin-collagen sponge for local applications. 10 cases of chronic osteomyelitis followed for 1 year. Acta Orthop Scand 1991;62(6):592–4.

113. Wernet E, Ekkernkamp A, Jellestad H, et al. Antibiotic-containing collagen sponge in therapy of osteitis. Unfallchirurg 1992;95(5):259–64.

114. Hettfleisch J, Schottle H. Local preventive antibiotic treatment in intramedullary nailing with gentamycin impregnated biomaterials. Aktuelle Traumatol 1993;23(2):68–71.

115. Chang WK, Srinivasa S, MacCormick AD, et al. Gentamicin-collagen implants to reduce surgical site infection: systematic review and meta-analysis of randomized trials. Ann Surg 2013; 258(1):59–65.

116. Lovallo J, Helming J, Jafari SM, et al. Intraoperative intra-articular injection of gentamicin: will it decrease the risk of infection in total shoulder arthroplasty? J Shoulder Elbow Surg 2014;23(9):1272–6.

117. Yarboro SR, Baum EJ, Dahners LE. Locally administered antibiotics for prophylaxis against surgical wound infection. An in vivo study. J Bone Joint Surg Am 2007;89(5):929–33.

118. Cavanaugh DL, Berry J, Yarboro SR, et al. Better prophylaxis against surgical site infection with local as well as systemic antibiotics. An in vivo study. J Bone Joint Surg Am 2009;91(8):1907–12.

119. Miclau T, Dahners LE, Lindsey RW. In vitro pharmacokinetics of antibiotic release from locally implantable materials. J Orthop Res 1993;11(5): 627–32.

120. McLaren AC, McLaren SG, Nelson CL, et al. The effect of sampling method on the elution of tobramycin from calcium sulfate. Clin Orthop Relat Res 2002;(403):54–7.

121. Wahlig H, Dingeldein E, Bergmann R, et al. The release of gentamicin from polymethylmethacrylate beads. An experimental and pharmacokinetic study. J Bone Joint Surg Br 1978;60-B(2): 270–5.

122. Anagnostakos K, Wilmes P, Schmitt E, et al. Elution of gentamicin and vancomycin from polymethylmethacrylate beads and hip spacers in vivo. Acta Orthop 2009;80(2):193–7.

123. Rathbone CR, Cross JD, Brown KV, et al. Effect of various concentrations of antibiotics on osteogenic cell viability and activity. J Orthop Res 2011;29(7): 1070–4.

124. Livio F, Wahl P, Csajka C, et al. Tobramycin exposure from active calcium sulfate bone graft substitute. BMC Pharmacol Toxicol 2014;15:12.

125. Hansen EN, Zmistowski B, Parvizi J. Periprosthetic joint infection: what is on the horizon? Int J Artif Organs 2012;35(10):935–50.

126. Kizhner V, Krespi YP, Hall-Stoodley L, et al. Laser-generated shockwave for clearing medical device biofilms. Photomed Laser Surg 2011;29(4):277–82.

127. Ercan B, Kummer KM, Tarquinio KM, et al. Decreased Staphylococcus aureus biofilm growth on anodized nanotubular titanium and the effect of electrical stimulation. Acta Biomater 2011;7(7): 3003–12.

128. Del Pozo JL, Rouse MS, Euba G, et al. The electricidal effect is active in an experimental model of Staphylococcus epidermidis chronic foreign body osteomyelitis. Antimicrob Agents Chemother 2009;53(10):4064–8.

129. van der Borden AJ, van der Mei HC, Busscher HJ. Electric block current induced detachment from surgical stainless steel and decreased viability of Staphylococcus epidermidis. Biomaterials 2005; 26(33):6731–5.

130. Pickering SA, Bayston R, Scammell BE. Electromagnetic augmentation of antibiotic efficacy in infection of orthopaedic implants. J Bone Joint Surg Br 2003;85(4):588–93.

131. Peck KR, Kim SW, Jung SI, et al. Antimicrobials as potential adjunctive agents in the treatment of biofilm infection with Staphylococcus epidermidis. Chemotherapy 2003;49(4):189–93.

132. Saginur R, Stdenis M, Ferris W, et al. Multiple combination bactericidal testing of staphylococcal biofilms from implant-associated infections. Antimicrob Agents Chemother 2006;50(1):55–61.

133. Kolodkin-Gal I, Romero D, Cao S, et al. D-amino acids trigger biofilm disassembly. Science 2010; 328(5978):627–9.

134. Sanchez CJ Jr, Akers KS, Romano DR, et al. D-amino acids enhance the activity of antimicrobials against biofilms of clinical wound isolates of Staphylococcus aureus and Pseudomonas aeruginosa. Antimicrob Agents Chemother 2014;58(8): 4353–61.

135. Losick R, Kolodkin-Gal I, Romero D, et al. D-amino acids trigger biofilm disassembly. Science 2010; 328(5978):627–9.

136. Wenke JC, Sanchez CJ Jr, Akers KS, et al. D-amino acids enhance the activity of antimicrobials against biofilms of clinical wound isolates of Staphylococcus aureus and Pseudomonas aeruginosa. Antimicrob Agents Chemother 2014;58(8):4353–561.

Percutaneous Sacroiliac Screw Fixation of the Posterior Pelvic Ring

Justin A. Iorio, MD[a],*, Andre M. Jakoi, MD[b], Saqib Rehman, MD[a]

KEYWORDS

- Percutaneous fixation • Pelvic ring • Sacroiliac screws • Imaging • Complications
- Preoperative planning • Technique

KEY POINTS

- Percutaneous sacroiliac (SI) screws are indicated for the treatment of unstable posterior pelvic ring injuries, sacral fractures, SI joint disruptions, or as adjunctive posterior pelvic fixation after anterior pelvic fixation.
- SI screws are associated with a shorter operating time, less blood loss, and less soft tissue injury compared with open surgical fixation of the posterior pelvis.
- The iliac cortical density (ICD) parallels the anterior border of the SI joint and represents the alar slope in a normal pelvis. In the case of an abnormal alar slope (dysmorphic pelvis), the ICD is located posteriorly and caudal; failure to recognize this may result in incorrect screw placement.
- The lumbosacral nerve roots, superior gluteal artery, and iliac vessels are at risk during screw insertion and should be managed with screw revision, embolization, ligation, or surgical consult.
- Malunion and malreduction are common complications. Posterior displacement of the pelvic ring greater than 1 cm is associated with a higher incidence of chronic pain and poorer functional outcomes.

INTRODUCTION

Pelvic injuries account for 3% of all skeletal fractures[1] and about 40% are unstable because of posterior ring disruption.[2] Injury to the sacroiliac (SI) joint is associated with significant morbidity, including chronic pain, sexual dysfunction, bowel and bladder impairment, and failure to return to work.[3–7] Surgical fixation of unstable pelvic injuries provides improved fracture reduction, early weight bearing and mobilization, lower mortalities, shorter hospital stays, and superior functional outcomes compared with nonoperative treatment.[6,8–10]

The classic method of surgical fixation of the SI joint consisted of open reduction and internal fixation (ORIF) by sacral bars or posterior plating. These implants carried a substantial risk of large dissection, prominent implants, iatrogenic nerve injury, infection, and blood loss to the already traumatized patient.[6,11–13] The development of percutaneous fixation via SI screws has decreased operating time, soft tissue injury, and blood loss compared with an open procedure.[14] SI screws are versatile; they can be used to treat a variety of sacral fracture patterns or SI joint dislocation; and can be placed in the supine, prone, or lateral

Conflicts of interest and sources of funding: None.
a Department of Orthopaedic Surgery, Temple University Hospital, 3401 North Broad Street, Zone B, 6th Floor, Philadelphia, PA 19140, USA; b Department of Orthopaedic Surgery, Drexel University, 240 North Broad Street, Mail Stop 420, Philadelphia, PA 19102, USA
* Corresponding author.
E-mail address: justiniorio@gmail.com

orthopedic.theclinics.com

position regardless of soft tissue injury. In addition, for placement in large fragments, cannulated screws are safe[15–17] even in patients with sacral dysmorphism.[18,19]

Various imaging modalities, including fluoroscopy and computed tomography (CT), are used for aiding screw insertion. Conventional fluoroscopy is the standard for intraoperative screw placement. However, acceptable reduction of the SI joint and proper implantation of screws without perforation of the neural foramina is challenging, especially when coupled with the difficulties of fluoroscopic imaging and variations in pelvic anatomy. Incorrect placement of SI screws may result in iatrogenic neurovascular complications.[20–22] The rate of screw malposition has been reported to approach 25%[23] and the incidence of neurologic injury is as high as 18%.[6,24,25] However, thorough preoperative planning and an understanding of SI screw placement technique minimize complications.

INDICATIONS/CONTRAINDICATIONS

SI screws can be used alone[26] or as supplemental fixation[27] for the treatment of pelvic fractures. SI screws were originally described for SI dislocations and fracture-dislocations.[28] Their applications were expanded to internal fixation of unstable posterior pelvic ring injuries, spinal-pelvic dissociation, incomplete sacral fractures (Denis zones 1–3) with or without pelvic instability, and sacral fractures with persistent gapping after anterior osteosynthesis (**Table 1**).[26,27] SI screws are advantageous in the setting of extensive soft tissue trauma, such as open fractures and degloving injuries, because of the limited dissection and minimal implant prominence compared with plates.[16,29] Unstable anterior-posterior compression (APC) injuries with bladder injury or contaminated, anterior soft tissue injuries can be treated by external fixation of the anterior pelvis and posterior SI screws. APC type IIb (posterior SI ligament attenuation with sagittal plane instability) injuries are indicated for SI screws in conjunction with anterior, symphyseal plating.[30]

Contraindications to closed reduction and percutaneous SI fixation include the inability to obtain closed reduction and active infection of the surgical site. Delay to fixation of greater than 5 days is a relative contraindication because organized hematoma may prohibit accurate reduction.[31] Open reduction must be performed if closed reduction is not possible. Horizontal sacral fractures are not well suited for SI screws because the implant is inserted parallel to the fracture line. Historically, transitional lumbosacral variants were considered relative contraindications,[16] but later studies have shown that most patients with sacral anomalies can safely undergo percutaneous SI fixation.[18,19] However, severe sacral dysmorphism may prevent safe placement of SI screws. U-shaped sacral fractures with sacral kyphosis or narrowing of neural foramina may require a posterior, open procedure for sacral reduction and nerve root decompression[17] in addition to SI screws. In these cases, in-situ, percutaneous SI fixation does not improve neurologic function. Morbidly obese patients may not be suitable for percutaneous techniques because of difficulties obtaining adequate fluoroscopic imaging and placement of screws.

SURGICAL TECHNIQUE/PROCEDURE
Preoperative Planning

A comprehensive physical examination and radiographic evaluation of the patient is necessary. Soft tissue injuries about the pelvis are important for surgical planning, especially if adjunctive ORIF of fractures is required. Other injuries, such as head, chest, abdomen, spine, or extremity trauma, may require procedures before pelvic fixation, affect patient positioning, or delay treatment. All patients with trauma should receive chest, anteroposterior (AP) pelvis, and C-spine radiographs. Advanced pelvic imaging, such as a CT scan with axial slices taken perpendicular to the sacral slope,[32] is recommended for operative planning and for identification of sacral fractures, which are missed on 30% of plain radiographs.[27] CT scans also provide information regarding body habitus, bone quality, soft tissue integrity, neural

Table 1 Indications and contraindications for percutaneous SI screw insertion	
Indications	Unstable posterior pelvic ring injuries
	SI joint dislocation
	Spinopelvic dissociation
	Incomplete sacral fractures ± pelvic ring instability
	Vertical posterior pelvic fractures
	Sacral fractures with gapping after symphyseal plating
Contraindications	Delayed fixation
	Active infection
	Severe sacral dysmorphism
	Morbid obesity
	Horizontal sacral fractures

foramina, and blood vessels.[32] Identifying the type of pelvic and/or sacral injury is important because unstable pelvic injuries may require binders, external fixation, or ORIF before SI screws. Characterizing the sacral disorder is important because guidewire orientation can be increased in the posterior-to-anterior plane for compression of SI dislocations or inserted in the transverse plane for sacral fractures.[30] Comminuted sacral fractures involving the neural foramina can be treated with static, fully threaded SI screws rather than a compression screw because of the risk of overcompression and nerve root entrapment.[17] Pelvic binders must remain in position to avoid clot disruption. In such cases, a large hole can be cut in the binder and the exposed skin sterilely prepped and draped.

Successful SI screw placement requires accurate SI joint reduction, identification of sacral dysmorphism, and adequate intraoperative imaging.[19] Sacral and pelvic injuries with an intact posterior tension band are typically good candidates for closed reduction.[33] Identifying the deformity in displaced fractures is imperative for obtaining closed reduction. Cephalad migration of the affected hemipelvis, with or without posterior displacement, may be improved by distal femoral traction. In contrast, caudal migration of the unaffected hemipelvis can be counterbalanced by placing the ipsilateral extremity in a traction boot. Alternative reduction techniques include internal rotation of the bilateral lower extremities, in which tape is wrapped around the thighs and feet, pelvic binders or sheets for reduction of external rotation deformities, pelvic C-clamps, and Schanz pins for percutaneously manipulating multiplanar deformities.[33] An open reduction can be performed in the supine or prone positions and must be done if closed reduction is unsuccessful.

Sacral dysmorphism affects 35% to 58% of adults and is a recognized predictor of aberrant SI screw insertion.[18,19,34] Dysmorphism refers to a variety of abnormal features affecting cranial fusion of the sacrum to L5 (sacralization); development of transverse processes and pedicles; and formation of disk spaces, SI joints, and neural foramina (**Fig. 1**).[18,19,35] Most variations are readily visible on pelvic and sacral radiographs. The pelvic outlet view may show proximal positioning of S1, such that it becomes collinear with the iliac crests; mammillary bodies, representing underdeveloped transverse processes; acute sacral ala sloping in the coronal plane; and large, irregular S1 foramina.[32] Lateral views of the pelvis and sacrum are also useful for identifying angulated sacral ala as well as residual sacral disks.[32] The iliac cortical density (ICD) parallels the anterior border of the SI

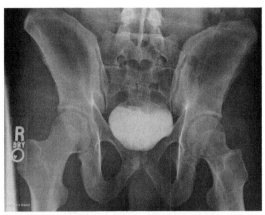

Fig. 1. AP pelvis radiograph showing features of sacral dysmorphism, including atrophic, residual transverse processes (mammillary bodies); abnormal sacral alar slope; and a sacral vertebra articulating with the ilium.

joint and represents the alar slope in a normal pelvis. However, the ICD is located posteriorly and caudal in the case of an abnormal alar slope and failure to recognize this may result in incorrect screw insertion.[18,32] The inlet view is useful for identifying irregularities in the ventral cortical sacrum, such as an indentation. More detailed identification of aberrant anatomy, including undulating SI joint spaces, is visible on CT. Both normal and dysmorphic sacrum can accommodate screws of at least 75 mm and the safe zones for screw insertion are the same.[18]

The details of intraoperative imaging are discussed earlier in this article.

Prep and Patient Positioning

A general anesthetic and a first-generation cephalosporin are administered in the operating room. Spinal precautions are used to protect the patient during transfer from the bed to a radiolucent operating table. A soft lumbosacral support made of towels or blankets is placed under the patient by elevating the patient's body and then placing the patient directly onto the bolster (if supine positioning is chosen for the procedure). Elevating the patient's pelvis from the operating room table is necessary to allow posterior pelvic percutaneous access. If needed, distal femoral traction is applied through the use of a pulley system that is attached to the operating room table. Neurodiagnostic monitoring may be helpful in patients with transforaminal sacral fractures undergoing closed reduction, or patients with neurologic deficits or cognitive impairment.[29]

Insertion of SI screws can be performed with the patient in the lateral, prone, or supine position. The lateral position complicates both anterior and posterior pelvic surgical exposures and is not recommended for patients with potential spinal injuries. Prone positioning allows posterior surgical exposures but prohibits direct visualization of SI joint reduction if an open reduction is required and may worsen fracture deformity.[30,33] Anterior pelvic external fixation frames further complicate prone and lateral patient positioning for surgery. Advantages of placing the patient supine include familiarity of positioning by anesthesia and nursing, ability of multiple teams to work simultaneously on polytrauma patients, and access to the anterior pelvis if additional reduction methods are required. Supine positioning may also be preferred in patients with pulmonary injuries and may improve closed-reduction techniques.

Surgical Approach

In the supine position, the anterior superior iliac spine (ASIS) is palpated and a line is drawn from the ASIS and directed perpendicularly to the floor. A second line, drawn in line with the femoral shaft, intersects the first line and thus forms 4 quadrants. The posterosuperior quadrant represents the starting zone for SI screw insertion (**Fig. 2**). A stab incision is made with a scalpel. Next, a Kirschner wire (K-wire) is inserted through the incision until the outer table of the ilium is contacted. Instrumentation should be directed toward the area of bone between the anterior sacral ala and the S1 neural foramina. In the prone position, the starting point is the intersection of a line drawn from the posterior superior iliac spine and a second line extending proximally, in line with the greater trochanter and femur.

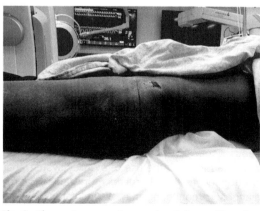

Fig. 2. The posterosuperior quadrant, formed by a line drawn from the ASIS and another in line with the femoral shaft, is the ideal starting point for SI screw placement. However, this location needs to be confirmed with lateral sacral imaging intraoperatively.

Imaging

- Position the fluoroscope on the side opposite from the injured posterior hemipelvis.
- Initial AP fluoroscopic imaging is used to assess proper patient positioning.
- Customize the inlet and outlet view for each patient.
  - The ideal inlet image of the pelvis superimposes the upper-sacral vertebral bodies as concentric circles (**Figs. 3** and **4**).
  - The ideal outlet image is obtained when the superior aspect of the symphysis pubis is superimposed on the S2 vertebral body (**Figs. 5** and **6**).
  - For dysmorphic upper-sacral segments, the fluoroscope is adjusted to focus on the segment that will receive the SI screw.
- If an upper-sacral-segment screw is chosen for a dysmorphic patient, the surgeon must understand that the anterior borders of the sacrum at S1 and S2 are different and therefore unique fluoroscopic markers highlight each specific site.
  - The outlet view highlights the nerve root tunnels for each segment.
  - On the true lateral view of the sacrum, the alar slope may be more acute and nonlinear with the ICD.
  - Screw orientation is directed from a posterior-caudal starting point with an anterior-cephalad directional aim.
  - These screws rarely extend beyond midline because of the abnormal anatomy.
- Last, obtain a lateral sacral view by adjusting the fluoroscope to superimpose the greater sciatic notches (**Figs. 7** and **8**).
  - On this image, the iliac cortical densities are identified and correlated with the preoperative CT scan, and should be collinear with the alar slope. Iliac cortical densities mark the alar locations according to the preoperative CT scan information.
  - A true lateral sacral image is possible only after accurate posterior pelvic fracture reduction or in those patients with minimal posterior pelvic deformities.

Fixation

- After closed reduction is confirmed, a smooth or drill bit–tipped 0.62-mm K-wire is inserted under triplanar, fluoroscopic control through the stab incision and onto the lateral ilium. Threaded wires are not preferred because tactile feedback for detecting a bony tunnel breach is limited.

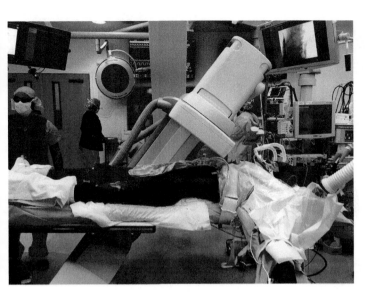

Fig. 3. For a pelvic inlet view, the fluoroscope is aimed approximately 45° caudad and is correctly positioned when S1 overlaps the S2 vertebral body.

- The starting point is best maintained by gently tapping the wire to engage the lateral, iliac cortical bone.
- After the appropriate starting point is confirmed, the skin incision is elongated around the wire and blunt deep dissection is accomplished with a narrow periosteal elevator or a drill guide.
- The guide pin is inserted with a power drill through the lateral iliac cortex using fluoroscopy to confirm placement into the safe zone.
- Frequent inlet and outlet images of the pelvis are used as the pin is inserted from the ilium across the SI articulation and into the lateral aspect of the sacral ala.
  - On the outlet view, the screw is angled approximately 20° cranially in normal sacra and 30° cranially in dysmorphic sacra.[18]

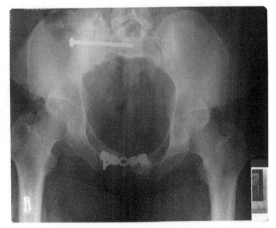

Fig. 4. The ideal inlet view permits visualization of the anterior sacral cortex and identification of screw breach through the ventral cortex.

- On the inlet view, the screw is angled approximately 5° anteriorly in normal sacra and 15° in dysmorphic sacra.[18]
- A drill bit–tipped guide pin rather than a threaded pin is preferred. The drill bit–tipped wire provides better tactile feedback to sense impending cortical perforation.
- For SI joint dislocation, the SI screw trajectory is posterior to anterior, whereas for sacral fractures the screw should be inserted transversely.[30]
- The guide pin is halted within the ala when the tip is located just cephalad to the upper-sacral corticated tunnel edge as seen on the outlet image.
- The outlet image identifies the corticated edge of the osseous tunnel of the upper-sacral nerve root that is immediately superior and medial relative to the ventral foramen.
- The surgeon must appreciate that the nerve root passes from posterior to anterior, midline to peripheral, and superior to inferior (**Figs. 9 and 10**). Tactile feedback and three-dimensional imaging may provide more information.
- Once the guide pin has reaches the sacral nerve root foramen, a true lateral sacral image should be obtained by fluoroscopically superimposing the greater sciatic notches of each reduced hemipelvis.
  - If the posterior pelvic reduction is accurate and the patient has a nondysmorphic pelvis, then the true lateral sacral image identifies the guide pin tip and its relation to the ICD.
  - The preoperative CT scan should reflect the relation between the ICD and the sacral ala,

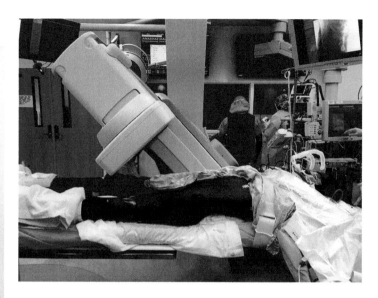

Fig. 5. For a pelvic outlet view, the fluoroscope is aimed approximately 45° cephalad and is correctly positioned when the pubic symphysis overlies the S2 body.

which, coupled with the intraoperative ICD, indicates whether the pin tip is safely placed.

- The tip of the guide pin should be caudal to the ICD and cephalad to the interosseous path of the upper-sacral nerve root; this can also be seen on the true lateral sacral image.
- The guide pin is then advanced to the midline of the upper-sacral vertebral body.
- The guide pin depth is measured with the reverse ruler and a cannulated drill is advanced over the guide pin.
  ○ A cannulated tap is used to prepare the pathway when necessary.
  ○ A 7.0-mm cancellous screw is used when compression is not desired, such as after accurate reductions of transforaminal sacral fractures.
  ○ Fully threaded screws are used to supplement compression screws.

- Obtain frequent fluoroscopic images during cannulated drilling, tapping, and screw insertion to confirm that the guide pin is not inadvertently advancing.
- A 20° to 30° obturator oblique image is used to visualize the tangential posterior ilium as the screw is tightened.
- Using a washer and rollover imaging, the surgeon prevents inadvertent screw penetration into the posterior ilium.
  ○ It is important to not over tighten the screw and penetrate the lateral iliac cortex, which is a concern in older patients with thin cortical bone.
- Next, remove the guide pin.
- The fixation construct is stressed under fluoroscopic imaging.
  ○ Additional screws or supplementary fixation are used if residual instability is noted on the fluoroscopic stress examination.
- Irrigate the percutaneous wound and close the skin.

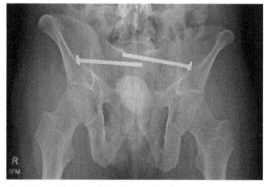

Fig. 6. In this outlet view, ideal screw placement (angled 20° cranially) and the corticated edges of the foramina are visualized.

SI screws are usually obliquely oriented in order to be perpendicular to the articulate joint surfaces, whereas sacral screws are more horizontally directed to be perpendicular to the fracture surfaces but also to increase the screw length for balance. Lag screws are used for SI joint compression, whereas fully threaded screws avoid overcompression of sacral fractures, particularly those involving the nerve root pathways, although nonunion can be a concern with this position-screw technique. SI screw length for most adults, if oriented perpendicular to the joint surfaces, ranges from 70 to 90 mm. Sacral fracture screws should be longer because the disorder is more

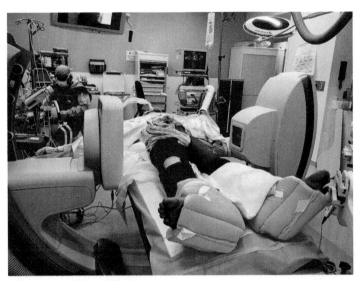

Fig. 7. Direct lateral positioning of the fluoroscope.

medial than for SI joint injury and to achieve a balanced implant. SI screws usually avoid the SI articular surface because of their oblique path, whereas sacral screws typically pass through the SI joint surfaces because of their orientation.

COMPLICATIONS AND MANAGEMENT

Percutaneous SI screw insertion is safe and effective[15–17,36] even for dysmorphic sacra[18,19] if the surgeon has an in-depth understanding of sacral osteology, fluoroscopic imaging, and preoperative planning. However, neurologic and vascular complications may occur with small deviations in screw trajectory; as little as 4° of screw misdirection may direct the screw into the S1 foramina or through the ventral sacrum.[37] In a cadaveric study by Mirkovic and colleagues,[38] the distance from the anterior cortex of the sacral ala to the internal iliac vein measured 2.4 mm and the L5 nerve root was as close as 1 mm. The incidence of screw malposition may be as high as 24%[23,37] and the

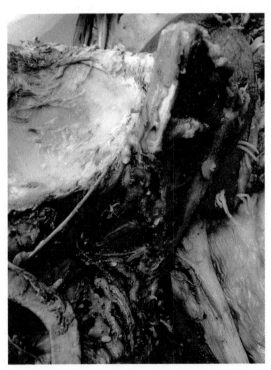

Fig. 9. An oblique view of bisected lumbosacral vertebral bodies. The L5 vertebral body is separated from S1 by the intervertebral disc. The L5 nerve root can be seen draping over the anterior ala and the sacral nerve roots are coursing over the ventral sacrum.

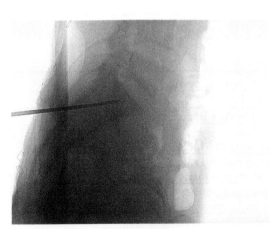

Fig. 8. The ICD, representing the alar slope, is the ventral border of the safe zone. On this view, the guide pin tip and its relation to the ICD can be seen.

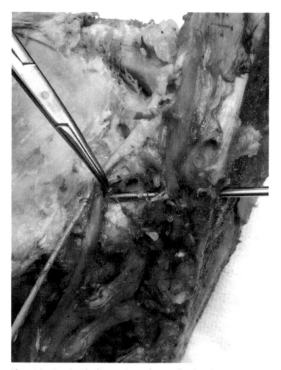

Fig. 10. Sagittal dissection through the lumbosacral vertebral bodies. An implant can be seen entering the S1 body and breaching ventrally to the sacral ala. The L5 nerve is retracted to show the relationship of the implant to the nerve. Even with perfect fluoroscopic imaging, an anterior cortical perforation may not be visualized.

rates of neurologic sequelae have approached 18% as a result of complex pelvic osteology and sacral dysmorphism.[6,23,39–41]

Complications include injury to the superior gluteal artery, iliac vessels, and lumbosacral nerves; malreduction; malunion; nonunion; implant failure; and infection (**Table 2**). Damage to the superior gluteal artery may occur during the initial trauma or the procedure. Specifically, the deep superior branch of the superior gluteal artery is most at risk despite placing screws in the desired starting location. Collinge and colleagues[42] performed a cadaveric study evaluating the proximity of percutaneously placed SI screws to the superior gluteal artery and nerve. Ten of 58 screws (18%) either impaled or entrapped the neurovascular bundle, and the mean distance from the screw to the superior gluteal bundle measured 9.1 ± 6.8 mm. Tamponade is unlikely to be effective, but angiographic embolization has been successful.[20,21] The common and internal iliac veins lie on the ventral surface of the sacral ala at the level of S1, either anterior to the SI joint or immediately medial.[38] Injury to these structures is serious and vascular or surgical consultation is warranted. Treatments include ligation or repair, retroperitoneal packing, and endovascular stent placement. Neurologic injury may occur to the lumbosacral nerves and should be treated by screw revision. In one study, 7 of 88 patients (7.9%) underwent screw revision for neurologic injury and all patients had complete resolution of their symptoms.[25] Malreduction and malunion are common complications.[6,14,43] In one study of vertically unstable pelvic fractures, malunion occurred in 36% of pelvic fractures treated by anterior plate fixation and SI screws versus 44% of pelvises treated by SI screws only. Although the numbers were not large enough to achieve statistical significance, the investigators postulated that anterior fixation in conjunction with SI screws reduces late displacement. Posterior displacement of the pelvic ring greater than 1 cm is associated with a higher

Table 2
Complications and management options of percutaneous SI screw insertion

Complication	Management
Iliac vessel injury	Emergent surgery consult
Neurologic injury to lumbosacral trunk	Screw revision
Superior gluteal artery injury	Ligation or angiographic embolization
Postoperative malreduction	Observation Revision with ORIF or SI joint fusion
Missed anterior pelvic or contralateral SI joint instability	Adjunctive symphyseal plating or joystick reduction of contralateral SI joint with fixation
Wound complications	Antibiotics (superficial) Incision and Drainage ± implant removal (deep)
Implant failure	Observation (asymptomatic union) Revision (symptomatic, loss of reduction)
Sacral nonunion	Debridement, bone grafting, and fixation

incidence of chronic pain and poorer functional outcomes than near-anatomic alignment[7]; revision fixation and SI joint fusion may provide partial pain relief in this setting.[6] Implant failure and nonunion are infrequent complications.[14] Treatment consists of debridement, bone grafting, and revision fixation. Infection rates after percutaneous SI screw insertion are very low, with some studies reporting 0%,[3,6,14,25] which is in contrast with open procedures.

POSTOPERATIVE CARE

- Intravenous antibiotics are administered for 24 hours after surgery.
- Chemical prophylaxis is initiated the day after surgery and continues for 30 days postoperatively.
- A licensed physical therapist supervises the rehabilitation.
  - Rehabilitation schedules depend on the overall condition of the patient and associated injuries.
- The stabilized hemipelvis is protected by partial weight bearing, which the patient accomplishes with the assistances of crutches or a walker for 6 weeks after surgery.
- Progressive weight bearing follows after the 6 weeks are completed, with the goal of crutch-free ambulation 12 weeks after surgery.
- Nonimpact aerobic and water activities are allowed 6 weeks after the operation.
- Inlet and outlet radiographs of the pelvis are obtained in the recovery room and generally at the 6-week and 12-week postoperative visits.
- Often, a postoperative CT scan is used to assess the reduction and implant location.
- Patients are seen in the clinic at 2, 6, and 12 weeks after the operation.
  - The follow-up pattern after this cycle usually depends on individual factors.
- Most adult patients can return to employment 4 to 6 months after surgery.
  - Patients with less physically demanding jobs may return sooner and others may require modifications.

Heavy lifting and working at heights are avoided until the patient's strength and conditioning goals are achieved.

OUTCOMES

Assessing outcomes after fixation of unstable pelvic injuries is difficult for several reasons. Studies are weakened by small cohorts; variable timing to surgery; poorly documented outcomes; lack of follow-up; heterogeneity of polytrauma injuries; variable fixation techniques, preoperative neurologic deficits, employment status, and activity level; and lack of systematic outcomes measures.[3,6,27,29] Neurologic injury in sacral fractures depends on zone of injury, with zone 3 fractures having the highest association with bowel, bladder, and sexual dysfunction (76%).[4] However, improvement of neurologic symptoms is variable.[17,29,44] Gibbons and colleagues[5] reported a 34% incidence of neurologic deficits in 44 patients with sacral fractures. Seven of 8 patients who were treated operatively with reduction and fixation, and 11 of 15 patients who were managed conservatively, had neurologic improvement. In another study of 15 transverse sacral fractures with bowel and bladder symptoms, all patients who were treated operatively and nonoperatively improved,[45] which is in contrast with a study by Denis and colleagues[4] in which none of the patients treated nonoperatively had improvement in bowel and bladder function. In a study by Nork and colleagues,[17] all 13 patients with U-shaped sacral fractures who underwent stabilization with SI screws showed clinical and radiographic union. Of the 9 patients with preoperative neurologic injury, 2 (22%) had persistent deficits at an average follow-up of 14 months: 1 patient had recovery of bowel and bladder control but has weakness consistent with his lumbar burst fractures, and the other patient has persistent bowel and bladder dysfunction. Chronic pain after fixation of pelvic fractures is common, with rates up to 85%.[6,27] Function and pain are more likely related to residual pelvic displacement than type of fixation. In a retrospective review of 43 patients, residual deformity of the pelvic ring, defined as more than 1 cm of posterior displacement, resulted in a significantly higher rate of chronic pain and poorer functional outcomes compared with patients without residual deformity.[7] Keating and colleagues[6] noted postoperative malunion in 50% of their 32 patients who had percutaneous SI fixation for unstable pelvic fractures. Of the 26 patients available at long-term follow-up, 22 reported pain related to their injury and 3 of these patients underwent SI fusion for pain relief, which provided only partial relief in 2 patients. Other sequelae of unstable pelvic ring injuries have also been reported. In a study of outcomes after fixation of pelvic ring injuries, urinary function was affected in 37%, sexual function in 29%, and work status in 35%.[3] However, the investigators opined that assessing patients' abilities to return to previous activities was challenging because of difficulties quantifying ability to work, performing household activities, and engaging in recreational activities.

SUMMARY

Percutaneous SI screws can be used to stabilize posterior pelvic ring instability, sacral fractures, and SI joint injuries, especially in the setting of extensive soft tissue trauma. SI screws can be safely inserted in both normal and dysmorphic sacra; however, identification of anomalies on preoperative imaging is crucial because radiographic landmarks and screw trajectories vary from those of normal sacra. Obtaining the appropriate intraoperative fluoroscopic views minimizes neurovascular injury and malreduction, which may negatively affect outcomes. Obtaining near-anatomic alignment of the posterior pelvic ring and treating concomitant pelvic injuries, such as anterior pelvis diastasis, improve long-term function.

REFERENCES

1. Failinger MS, McGanity PL. Unstable fractures of the pelvic ring. J Bone Joint Surg Am 1992;74:781–91.
2. Nelson DW, Duwelius PJ. CT-guided fixation of sacral fractures and sacroiliac joint disruptions. Radiology 1991;180:527–32.
3. Cole JD, Blum DA, Ansel LJ. Outcome after fixation of unstable posterior pelvic ring injuries. Clin Orthop Relat Res 1996;(329):160–79.
4. Denis F, Davis S, Comfort T. Sacral fractures: an important problem. Retrospective analysis of 236 cases. Clin Orthop Relat Res 1988;227:67–81.
5. Gibbons KJ, Soloniuk DS, Razack N. Neurological injury and patterns of sacral fractures. J Neurosurg 1990;72:889–93.
6. Keating JF, Werier J, Blachut P, et al. Early fixation of the vertically unstable pelvis: the role of iliosacral screw fixation of the posterior lesion. J Orthop Trauma 1999;13:107–13.
7. McLaren AC, Rorabeck CH, Halpenny J. Long-term pain and disability in relation to residual deformity after displaced pelvic ring fractures. Can J Surg 1990;33:492–4.
8. Burgess AR, Eastridge BJ, Young JW, et al. Pelvic ring disruptions: effective classification system and treatment protocols. J Trauma 1990;30:848–56.
9. Smith HE, Yuan PS, Sasso R, et al. An evaluation of image-guided technologies in the placement of percutaneous iliosacral screws. Spine 2006;31: 234–8.
10. Latenser BA, Gentilello LM, Tarver AA, et al. Improved outcome with early fixation of skeletally unstable pelvic fractures. J Trauma 1991;31:28–31.
11. Tile M. Pelvic ring fractures: should they be fixed? J Bone Joint Surg Br 1988;70:1–12.
12. Judet R, Judet J, Letournel E. Fractures of the acetabulum: classification and surgical approaches for open reduction. preliminary report. J Bone Joint Surg Am 1964;46:1615–46.
13. Kellam JF, McMurtry RY, Paley D, et al. The unstable pelvic fracture. Operative treatment. Orthop Clin North Am 1987;18:25–41.
14. Routt ML Jr, Kregor PJ, Simonian PT, et al. Early results of percutaneous iliosacral screws placed with the patient in the supine position. J Orthop Trauma 1995;9:207–14.
15. Routt ML Jr, Simonian PT, Swiontkowski MF. Stabilization of pelvic ring disruptions. Orthop Clin North Am 1997;28:369–88.
16. Routt ML Jr, Nork SE, Mills WJ. Percutaneous fixation of pelvic ring disruptions. Clin Orthop Relat Res 2000;(375):15–29.
17. Nork SE, Jones CB, Harding SP, et al. Percutaneous stabilization of U-shaped sacral fractures using iliosacral screws: technique and early results. J Orthop Trauma 2001;15:238–46.
18. Gardner MJ, Morshed S, Nork SE, et al. Quantification of the upper and second sacral segment safe zones in normal and dysmorphic sacra. J Orthop Trauma 2010;24:622–9.
19. Routt ML Jr, Simonian PT, Agnew SG, et al. Radiographic recognition of the sacral alar slope for optimal placement of iliosacral screws: a cadaveric and clinical study. J Orthop Trauma 1996;10:171–7.
20. Altman DT, Jones CB, Routt ML Jr. Superior gluteal artery injury during iliosacral screw placement. J Orthop Trauma 1999;13:220–7.
21. Stephen DJ. Pseudoaneurysm of the superior gluteal arterial system: an unusual cause of pain after a pelvic fracture. J Trauma 1997;43:146–9.
22. Stockle U, Konig B, Hofstetter R, et al. Navigation assisted by image conversion. An experimental study on pelvic screw fixation. Unfallchirurg 2001; 104:215–20 [in German].
23. Tonetti J, Carrat L, Blendea S, et al. Clinical results of percutaneous pelvic surgery. Computer assisted surgery using ultrasound compared to standard fluoroscopy. Comput Aided Surg 2001;6:204–11.
24. Routt ML Jr, Simonian PT, Mills WJ. Iliosacral screw fixation: early complications of the percutaneous technique. J Orthop Trauma 1997;11:584–9.
25. van den Bosch EW, van Zwienen CM, van Vugt AB. Fluoroscopic positioning of sacroiliac screws in 88 patients. J Trauma 2002;53:44–8.
26. Matta JM, Saucedo T. Internal fixation of pelvic ring fractures. Clin Orthop Relat Res 1989;(242):83–97.
27. Mehta S, Auerbach JD, Born CT, et al. Sacral fractures. J Am Acad Orthop Surg 2006;14:656–65.
28. Letournel E. Pelvic fractures. Injury 1978;10:145–8.
29. Vaccaro AR, Kim DH, Brodke DS, et al. Diagnosis and management of sacral spine fractures. Instr Course Lect 2004;53:375–85.
30. Langford JR, Burgess AR, Liporace FA, et al. Pelvic fractures: part 2. Contemporary indications and

techniques for definitive surgical management. J Am Acad Orthop Surg 2013;21:458–68.

31. Routt ML Jr, Simonian PT. Closed reduction and percutaneous skeletal fixation of sacral fractures. Clin Orthop Relat Res 1996;(329):121–8.

32. Miller AN, Routt ML Jr. Variations in sacral morphology and implications for iliosacral screw fixation. J Am Acad Orthop Surg 2012;20:8–16.

33. Ilyas A, Rehman S, Jupiter JB. Contemporary surgical management of fractures and complications. Philadelphia (PA): Jaypee Brothers, Medical Publishers; 2012.

34. Wu LP, Li YK, Li YM, et al. Variable morphology of the sacrum in a Chinese population. Clin Anat 2009;22:619–26.

35. Ziran BH, Smith WR, Towers J, et al. Iliosacral screw fixation of the posterior pelvic ring using local anaesthesia and computerised tomography. J Bone Joint Surg Br 2003;85:411–8.

36. Simonian PT, Routt ML Jr, Harrington RM, et al. Biomechanical simulation of the anteroposterior compression injury of the pelvis. An understanding of instability and fixation. Clin Orthop Relat Res 1994;(309):245–56.

37. Templeman D, Schmidt A, Freese J, et al. Proximity of iliosacral screws to neurovascular structures after internal fixation. Clin Orthop Relat Res 1996;(329): 194–8.

38. Mirkovic S, Abitbol JJ, Steinman J, et al. Anatomic consideration for sacral screw placement. Spine 1991;16:S289–94.

39. Barrick EF, O'Mara JW, Lane HE 3rd. Iliosacral screw insertion using computer-assisted CT image guidance: a laboratory study. Comput Aided Surg 1998;3:289–96.

40. Webb LX, de Araujo W, Donofrio P, et al. Electromyography monitoring for percutaneous placement of iliosacral screws. J Orthop Trauma 2000;14:245–54.

41. Ebraheim NA, Coombs R, Jackson WT, et al. Percutaneous computed tomography-guided stabilization of posterior pelvic fractures. Clin Orthop Relat Res 1994;(307):222–8.

42. Collinge C, Coons D, Aschenbrenner J. Risks to the superior gluteal neurovascular bundle during percutaneous iliosacral screw insertion: an anatomical cadaver study. J Orthop Trauma 2005;19:96–101.

43. Shuler TE, Boone DC, Gruen GS, et al. Percutaneous iliosacral screw fixation: early treatment for unstable posterior pelvic ring disruptions. J Trauma 1995;38:453–8.

44. Sabiston CP, Wing PC. Sacral fractures: classification and neurologic implications. J Trauma 1986; 26:1113–5.

45. Schmidek HH, Smith DA, Kristiansen TK. Sacral fractures. Neurosurgery 1984;15:735–46.

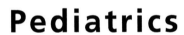

Pediatrics

Preface
Skeletal Dysplasia and Congenital Malformation

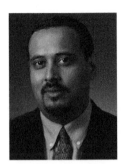

Shital N. Parikh, MD, FACS
Editor

In the article, "Evaluation of the Child with Short Stature," Mehlman and Ain provide an overview on the assessment of a child with skeletal dysplasia, including prenatal diagnosis. Short stature is a frequent cause of anxiety for patients and their families. Proportionate short stature, where limbs and trunk are proportionately affected, is either familial or due to a systemic cause like metabolic disorder, chronic illness, or endocrinopathy, and is usually treated by our medical colleagues. Disproportionate short stature, on the other hand, is usually due to skeletal dysplasia, is genetic in origin, and is frequently seen by the pediatric orthopedic surgeon. It could be either short-limb or short-trunk type. Fetal ultrasound and, recently, fetal MRI can identify lethal skeletal dysplasias, including achondrogenesis and osteogensis imperfecta type II as well as several nonlethal skeletal dysplasias. At birth and then after, the mainstays of diagnosis are clinical examination and radiographic evaluation. The authors summarize the important aspects of physical and radiographic examination, citing examples, to evaluate for skeletal dysplasias. The review is not meant to be all-inclusive but provides valuable points that can help establish a preliminary diagnosis for the common dysplasias. The knowledge about characteristic dysmorphic features, short limb versus short trunk dysplasia, and radiographic structural abnormalities of the bone can help with the initial evaluation of a child with short stature. Appropriate referrals and genetic evaluation can then help establish a definitive diagnosis and aid in further management and prognosis.

For the article, "Discoid Meniscus: Diagnosis and Management," Kushare and colleagues review the literature and discuss the methods of diagnosis and decision-making factors that are important in the management of discoid meniscus. Discoid meniscus should be ideally labeled as lateral meniscus variant because it encompasses variation in the size, shape, and attachments of the lateral meniscus. It is debatable as to what part of the anomaly is congenital and what is developmental. Traditionally, the discoid meniscus has been classified as complete, incomplete, and Wrisberg-type meniscus. The newer classification system that the authors discuss is based on peripheral rim stability of the meniscus, size of the meniscus, and presence or absence of a tear. Though many children with discoid meniscus are asymptomatic, symptoms attributable to discoid meniscus are due to either underlying tear or instability. The popping of the knee complaint, for which

Orthop Clin N Am 46 (2015) xix–xx
http://dx.doi.org/10.1016/j.ocl.2015.07.003
0030-5898/15/$ – see front matter © 2015 Published by Elsevier Inc.

orthopedic.theclinics.com

the parents frequently seek medical attention for their child, is usually due to the underlying insta-bility of the meniscus. If and when the child needs surgical treatment, the principle of treatment is to reshape the meniscus, stabilize the unstable part of the meniscus, and avoid total menisectomy.

I hope the readers will find both these articles useful and applicable in their clinical practice.

Shital N. Parikh, MD, FACS
Cincinnati Children's Hospital Medical Center
University of Cincinnati School of Medicine
3333 Burnet Avenue
Cincinnati, OH 45229, USA

E-mail address:
Shital.Parikh@cchmc.org

Evaluation of the Child with Short Stature

Charles T. Mehlman, DO, MPH[a],*, Michael C. Ain, MD[b]

KEYWORDS

• Prenatal evaluation • Children • Short stature • Differential diagnosis • Physical examination

KEY POINTS

• Orthopedic surgeons frequently encounter short statured patients. A systematic approach is needed for proper evaluation of these children.
• The differential diagnosis includes both proportionate and disproportionate short stature types.
• A proper history and physical examination and judicious use of plain film radiography will establish the diagnosis in most cases.
• In addition to the orthopedic surgeon, most of these patients will also be evaluated by other specialists, including endocrinologists and geneticists.

INTRODUCTION

Normal growth and development usually proceed quite smoothly from single-celled zygote all the way to an approximately one hundred trillion–celled adult human being.[1] Three discernable growth spurts occur, with the first being intrauterine (and arguably the most dramatic), the second involving the first 2 years of life (with about a 100% increase in size of the child), and the third is the adolescent (also known as pubescent) growth spurt. The amazing thing may not be that growth aberrations occur, but that they do not occur more frequently. When a child falls 2 standard deviations or more below the average height for age, sex, and ethnic group established norms, they are considered to have short stature.[2]

Short statured humans have been well-recognized by others within society all the way back to antiquity. For instance, the ancient Egyptian sarcophagus carving of Djeho offers a detailed picture of a prominent citizen with achondroplasia[3] (Fig. 1). Djeho lived around 360 BC and worked with the chief financial officer of Upper Egypt. There also were powerful short statured Egyptian gods with the god Bes (god of music and warfare) and the god Ptah (a god of creation and master architect of the universe) serving as excellent examples.[4]

In 1951 when Sir Harold Arthur Thomas Fairbank (at 75 years of age) published his classic *Atlas of General Affections of the Skeleton*, he helped bring order to the chaos of this complex mixture of musculoskeletal entities. This article focuses on important orthopedic aspects in the evaluation of short stature in children with a particular focus on skeletal dysplasia. It does not focus on each and every diagnostic entity, but rather the options that must be considered and the process one may undertake to arrive at the most precise diagnosis.

DIFFERENTIAL DIAGNOSIS

The differential diagnosis for short stature is exhaustive and includes what have been referred to as proportionate and disproportionate types.[5–8] Comprehensive evaluation often includes referrals to pediatric subspecialists like

a Division of Pediatric Orthopaedic Surgery, Cincinnati Children's Hospital Medical Center, MLC 2017, 3333 Burnet Avenue, Cincinnati, OH 45229, USA; b Department of Orthopaedic Surgery, The Johns Hopkins University, 1800 Orleans street, Baltimore, MD 21287, USA
* Corresponding author.
E-mail address: charles.mehlman@cchmc.org

Orthop Clin N Am 46 (2015) 523–531
http://dx.doi.org/10.1016/j.ocl.2015.06.006
0030-5898/15/$ – see front matter © 2015 Elsevier Inc. All rights reserved.

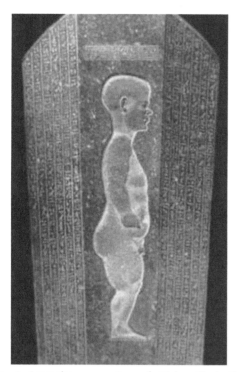

Fig. 1. Sarcophagus carving of Djeho illustrating typical features of achondroplasia.

endocrinology and genetics.[9] Proportionate short stature may be owing to familial short stature, intrauterine growth retardation (commonly owing to smoking), constitutional delay of growth, occult medical diseases (including endocrinopathy),

and idiopathic short stature.[10,11] Multiple evaluations over time may be quite valuable, because skeletal dysplasia may be later confirmed in up to 20% of patients previously labeled as idiopathic short stature or small for gestational age.[12] This paper does not focus on these proportionate short stature types because it is extremely rare for such patients to present undiagnosed to the orthopedic surgeon.

Disproportionate short stature relates to an improper balance between standing height and sitting height. In normal populations, the sitting height/standing height ratio has been shown to be approximately 0.7 at birth and closer to 0.5 at skeletal maturity.[13] Standing height has contributions from both limb length as well as trunk length, whereas sitting height is effectively all about trunk length. One broad (and imperfect) generalization is that disproportionate short stature can be divided into those characterized mainly by shortened limbs and those mainly characterized by a shortened trunk. In the past, these have been referred to as short limb dwarfism and short trunk dwarfism.[14] **Fig. 2** illustrates the striking contrast that can be seen when assessing standing height and sitting height. The sitting height/standing height ratio has been shown to be of significant clinical value.[15,16] In addition to many other more sophisticated methods, the relative femoral and tibial contributions to lower limb length discrepancy can be determined by instantaneous limb length assessment (**Fig. 3**).[17]

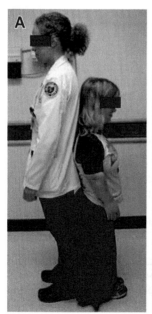
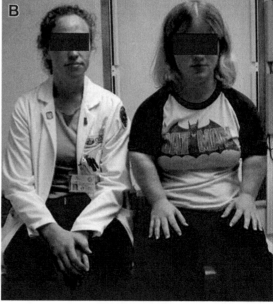

Fig. 2. Standing height versus sitting height. (A) A normal statured female standing back to back with a female with skeletal dysplasia. This illustrates a significant difference in standing height. (B) The same normal statured female and female with skeletal dysplasia sitting side by side, illustrating nearly identical sitting height.

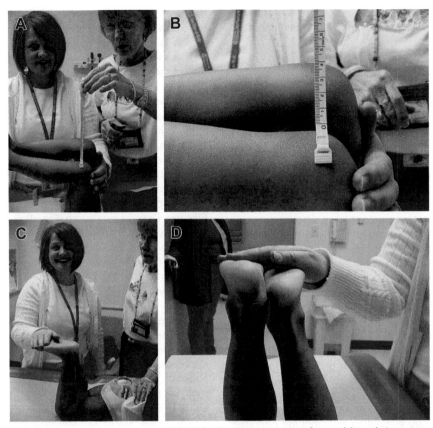

Fig. 3. Instantaneous leg length assessment. (*A*) With the patient supine femoral length is assessed with knees and hips flexed to 90°. (*B*) Measurement of knee height inequality with a ruler. (*C*) With the patient prone tibial (lower leg) length is assessed with knees flexed 90° and hips neutral. (*D*) Visualization of lower leg difference, which also clearly accounts for any difference in foot size.

PRENATAL EVALUATION

Various imaging techniques (most commonly ultrasonography) may be used to assess the unborn child suspected of having skeletal dysplasia.[18,19] It should be remembered that as many as 80% of prenatally detected skeletal dysplasias are lethal, and thus the prenatal cohort and the live birth cohort are epidemiologically distinct.[20] Understanding this allows one to properly interpret the differential prevalence between live births and still births (3.0 per 10,000 vs 20.0 per 10,000).[21] A powerful rule of thumb is that until proven otherwise, age-adjusted fetal femoral length of less than 40% indicates achondrogenesis, 40% to 60% is consistent with osteogenesis imperfecta type II or thanotophoric dysplasia, and greater than 80% of femoral length points to osteogenesis imperfecta type III or achondroplasia.[22,23] Additional prenatal cytogenetic and molecular genetic analysis may also be undertaken as indicated.[24] Situations where such studies are felt to be

appropriate include a parent with a known skeletal dysplasia, significant family history, and micomelic or hypoplastic thorax ultrasound findings.[25]

Although more firmly established for congenital central nervous system and cardiac anomalies, the role of fetal MRI continues to evolve in the setting of prenatal evaluation of skeletal dysplasias.[26,27] It should also be remembered that ultrasound remains the only recommended imaging in the first trimester.[28] Information from fetal MRI may be considered complementary to that obtained from ultrasound, adding additional findings in about 30% of cases and changing the diagnosis more than 50% of the time when considering all fetal diagnoses.[29] However, when focusing on musculoskeletal system fetal MRI, it is less likely to show diagnostic advantages over ultrasound.[29] Researchers from the Cincinnati Children's Hospital have recently shown that fetal MRI can play a significant role in predicting lethal skeletal dysplasias based on fetal lung volume.[30] Until these various applications mature and clinical utility becomes clear, the overall indications for fetal MRI for suspected skeletal dysplasia remain limited.

PHYSICAL EXAMINATION

Of the more than 450 known skeletal dysplasias, only about 100 are discernable at birth. The remainder may not manifest until after 2 to 3 years of age.[31] Height, weight, head circumference, and growth velocity are all important parameters that must be measured. There are significant rates of hearing impairment among skeletal dysplasia patients and it is reasonable for the orthopedist to ask about prior hearing assessment.[32] Airway and pulmonary compromise are also common in these patients and at times require sophisticated assessment.[33,34]

The impact on health-related quality of life caused by pain and decreased physical function can be substantial in skeletal dysplasia patients.[32,35,36] Many validated instruments are available to measure this in the clinical setting.[36] In the most common skeletal dysplasia, achondroplasia, low back pain and lower extremity pain have been shown to be brutally progressive over time.[37] An increased rate of sleep apnea and sudden infant death syndrome have also been identified in newborns with achondroplasia. Multidisciplinary evaluation may include pediatric otolaryngology as well as pediatric pulmonology and sleep studies of even very young children are often indicated.[38–40]

There are several important points regarding the history and physical examination of short statured patients during the newborn and early childhood periods. The craniofacial region should be inspected for a wide variety of abnormalities including clouding of the cornea (eg, mucopolysaccharidoses), calcification of or overall thickening of the ears (eg, diastrophic dwarfism), and midface hypoplasia (eg, achondroplasia). Nasal depression may be a prominent feature of achondroplasia, whereas broadening of the same nasal region is characteristic of mucopolysaccharidoses, like Hunter and Hurler syndromes. Abnormalities of the teeth and gums are common in Ellis van Crevald syndromes and cleft palate has been associated with diastrophic dysplasia and many other skeletal dysplasias.

In addition to anthropomorphic measurements of the trunk and extremities, particular attention should be paid to several other areas. A markedly abducted thumb (hitchhiker's thumb) is consistent with disastrohic dysplasia. Exceptionally well-formed polydactyly is strongly associated with Ellis van Crevald syndrome (**Fig. 4**). A trident hand (relatively abducted index and long finger one way and abducted ring and small finger the other way) is one of the hallmarks of achondroplasia.

Examination of the patient's trunk and axial skeleton may also yield important findings. A dysmorphic or otherwise distorted thoracic cage is associated with certain severe skeletal dysplasias like Jeune syndrome. Evidence of spinal deformity should be sought as a broad spectrum of scoliosis, kyphosis, excessive lumbar lordosis, and kyphoscoliosis may manifest. Kyphotic spinal deformity may be particularly striking when the patient is seated, while the appearance improves significantly while standing. Metatropic dysplasia is particularly famous for its associated coccygeal tail. It also behooves the pediatric orthopedist to remember that inguinal hernia is especially common in individuals with skeletal dysplasia.

RADIOGRAPHIC EVALUATION

The evaluation of disproportionate short stature always involves plain radiography.[31] Alanay and Lachman have described this as a 3-step radiographic process (**Box 1**). The skeletal survey is firmly rooted in the evaluation of both child

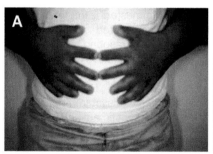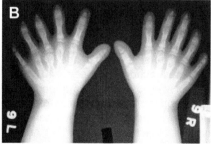

Fig. 4. Clinical and radiographic illustration of Ellis van Crevald associated polydactyly. (*A*) Clinical photo showing remarkably functional and well-formed polydactyly (6 digits on each hand). (*B*) Radiographic appearance of the same patient.

abuse and skeletal dysplasia, but skeletal dysplasia patients require fewer views.[11,41] Recommended skeletal survey views established by the American College of Radiology for skeletal dysplasias and syndromes are listed in **Box 2**. An interactive digital atlas of the most common skeletal dysplasias has also recently been created.[42] Now we will highlight some of the classic radiographic findings associated with skeletal dysplasias.

It has been said that the key radiographic feature of achondroplasia is the characteristic caudal narrowing of lumbar interpedicular

distance.[43,44] Thoracolumbar kyphosis with associated vertebral body wedging is also a common finding in patients with achondroplasia (**Fig. 5**).[45] In most instances, this kyphosis resolves spontaneously, although in a minority of cases it demonstrates relentless progression.[46] Varus lower extremity alignment is also common.[47–49] Midface hypoplasia is associated with radiographically underdeveloped facial structure. Stenosis of the foramen magnum is a particularly important radiographic problem to identify, because if left untreated, devastating neurologic consequences may occur. It has been recommended that all infants be screened for foramen magnum stenosis.[50]

A cluster of other radiographic findings including rhizomelic shortening, flaring of the metaphyses, and the so-called inverted V shape of the physis of the distal femur are all explained by the genetic root cause of achondroplasia. The FGF receptor 3 defect leads to a dysfunctional proliferative zone of the physis, thus disrupting proper endochondral ossification. Therefore, the fastest growing growth plates, which lie in the proximal limb segments (like the proximal humerus and that of the distal femur) take a disproportionate hit leading to the rhizomelic effect. It must also be remembered that intramembranous ossification proceeds relatively undisturbed, and this leads to the metaphyseal flaring and inverted V aspects of the observed radiography.

Spondyloepiphyseal dysplasia (SED) is notorious for its associated atlantoaxial instability (**Fig. 6**). An autosomal-dominant form of SED presenting with atlantoaxial instability and neurologic compromise has been reported by researcher from the Hospital for Sick Children in London, England.[51] The vertebral body involvement in SED has been variably described as the pear-shaped appearance in infancy (posterior vertebral body narrowing) to the extensive platyspondyly and flame-shaped vertebra of older individuals. The classic finding (which SED shares with multiple epiphyseal dysplasia) is the markedly delayed and irregular ossification of the capital femoral epiphyses.

The mucopolysaccharide disorders also may present with a vast array of radiographic findings.[52,53] Collectively, these have been referred to as dysostosis multiplex. White and Sousa[54] have provided a fine list of these abnormalities (**Box 3**), noting that they vary based on both the age of the patient and the specific mucopolysaccharide disorder. Modern medical therapies have significantly improved the lives and life spans of many mucopolysaccharide patients, but not to the point that these bony abnormalities are prevented.[55,56]

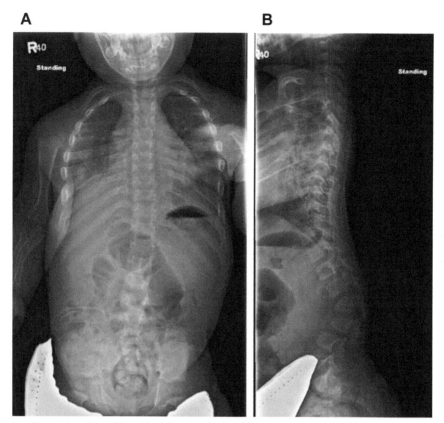

Fig. 5. Spinal radiographs of a child with achondroplasia. (*A*) Anteroposterior radiograph demonstrating progressive narrowing of L1 to L5 lumbar pedicle distance. (*B*) Standing lateral radiograph illustrating commonly seen wedging of L2 vertebra along with thoracolumbar kyphosis.

GENETIC/CHROMOSOMAL EVALUATION

Consultation with a clinical geneticist is a vital step in establishing an accurate diagnosis and prognosis.[57,58] In 2009, the American College of Medical Genetics published their practice guideline for the genetic evaluation of short stature.[11] These authors assert the importance of the history and physical examination in short stature patients,

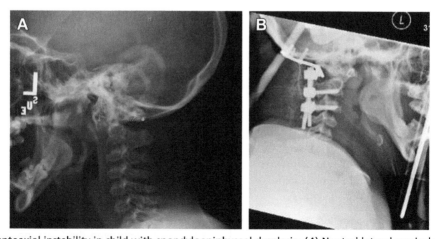

Fig. 6. Atlantoaxial instability in child with spondyloepiphyseal dysplasia. (*A*) Neutral lateral cervical spine radiograph showing increase in atlantodens interval and decrease in space available for cord. (*B*) Postoperative radiograph after C1 decompressive laminectomy and occipitocervical fusion (occiput to C3) with autogenous iliac crest bone graft. Halo vest immobilization was also utilized.

Box 3
Radiographic findings in mucopolysaccharide disorders

Hip dysplasia

Coarsened long bones

Shortened ulna

Madelung deformity of distal radius

Shortened metacarpals

Platyspondyly

Broad clavicles

Broad (oar-shaped) ribs

Enlarged skull/thickened calavaria

J-shaped sella tursica

Data from White KK, Sousa T. Mucopolysaccharide disorders in orthopedic surgery. J Am Acad Orthop Surg 2013;21:12–22.

---

and how a skeletal survey is indicated when faced with disproportionate short stature followed by selective use of genetic studies. They also state that in clinical situations where these initial measures do not indicate a clear diagnosis, chromosomal analysis may be of great value, particularly in identifying genetic mosaicism.[11]

SUMMARY

Short stature is not an uncommon concern. The aim of this article was to provide an overview of the evaluation of children presenting with this problem. Many other entities associated with short stature have not been discussed or illustrated in this article. The main points that the authors feel the reader should take away are the importance of the history and physical examination and plain film radiography as well as the importance of multidisciplinary care.

REFERENCES

1. Crawford AH. Orthopedics [Chapter 27]. In: Rudolph CD, Rudolph AM, Hostetter MK, et al, editors. Rudolph's pediatrics. 21st edition. New York: McGraw-Hill; 2003. p. 2419–20.
2. Wit JM, Clayton PE, Rogol AD, et al. Idiopathic short stature: definition epidemiology and diagnostic evaluation. Growth Horm IGF Res 2008;18:89–110.
3. Kozma C. Historical review: dwarfs in ancient Egypt. Am J Med Genet 2006;140-A:303–11.
4. Kozma C. Historical review: skeletal dysplasia in ancient Egypt. Am J Med Genet 2008;146-A: 3104–12.
5. Bailey JA. Orthopaedic aspects of achondroplasia. J Bone Joint Surg Am 1970;52-A:1285–301.
6. Kaufmann HJ. Classification of the skeletal dysplasias and the radiologic approach to their differentiation. Clin Orthop Relat Res 1976;114:12–7.
7. Silverman FN, Brunner S. Errors in the diagnosis of achondroplasia. Acta Radiol 1967;6:305–21.
8. Silverman FN. A differential diagnosis of achondroplasia. Radiol Clin North Am 1968;6:223–37.
9. Nampoothiri S, Yesodharan D, Sainulabdin G, et al. Eight years experience from a skeletal dysplasia referral center in a tertiary hospital in Southern India: a model for the diagnosis and treatment of rare diseases in a developing country. Am J Med Genet A 2014;164A(9):2317–23.
10. Lee MM. Idiopathic short stature. N Engl J Med 2006;354:2576–82.
11. Seaver LH, Irons M. ACMG practice guideline: genetic evaluation of short stature. Genet Med 2009; 11:465–70.
12. Flechtner I, Lambot-Juhan K, Teissier R, et al. Unexpected high frequency of skeletal dysplasia in idiopathic short stature and small for gestational age patients. Eur J Endocrinol 2014;170:677–84.
13. deArriba Munoz A, Dominguez Caja M, Rueda Caballero C, et al. Sitting height/standing height ratio in a Spanish population from birth to adulthood. Arch Argent Pediatr 2013;111:309–14.
14. Bailey JA. Disproportionate short stature: diagnosis and management. 1st edition. Philadelphia: WB Saunders; 1973. p. 5–25.
15. Fredriks AM, vanBuuren S, vanHeel WJM, et al. Nationwide age references for sitting height leg length and sitting height/height ratio and their diagnostic value for disproportionate growth disorders. Arch Dis Child 2005;90:807–12.
16. Malaquias AC, Scalco RC, Fontenele EG, et al. The sitting height/height ratio for age in healthy and short individuals and its potential role in selecting short children for SHOX analysis. Horm Res Paediatr 2013;80:449–56.
17. Smith CF. Instantaneous leg length discrepancy determination by the "thigh-leg" technique. Orthopedics 1996;19:955–6.
18. Krakow D, Lachman RS, Rimoin DL. Guidelines for the prenatal diagnosis of fetal skeletal dysplasias. Genet Med 2009;11:127–33.
19. Schramm T, Gloning KP, Minderer S, et al. Prenatal sonographic diagnosis of skeletal dysplasias. Ultrasound Obstet Gynecol 2009;34:160–70.
20. Yeh P, Saeed F, Paramasivam G, et al. Accuracy of prenatal diagnosis and prediction of lethality for fetal skeletal dysplasias. Prenat Diagn 2011; 31:515–8.
21. Stevenson DA, Carey JC, Byrne JLB, et al. Analysis of skeletal dysplasias in the Utah population. Am J Med Genet 2012;158:1046–54.

22. Dreyer SD, Ahou G, Lee B. The long and short of it: developmental genetics of the skeletal dysplasias. Clin Genet 1998;54:464–73.

23. Gonclaves L, Jeanty P. Fetal biometry of skeletal dysplasias: a multicentric study. J Ultrasound Med 1994;13:977–85.

24. Hatzaki A, Sifakis A, Apostolopoulou D, et al. FGFR3 related skeletal dysplasias diagnosed prenatally by ultrasonography and molecular analysis: presentation of 17 cases. Am J Med Genet A 2011;155-A: 2426–35.

25. Trujillo-Tiebas MJ, Fenollar-Cortea M, Lorda-Sanchez I, et al. Prenatal diagnosis of skeletal dysplasia due to FGFR3 gene mutations: a 9-year experience. J Assist Reprod Genet 2009;26:455–60.

26. Solopova A, Wisser J, Huisman TA. Osteogenesis imperfect type II: fetal magnetic resonance imaging findings. Fetal Diagn Ther 2008;24:361–7.

27. Yazici Z, Kline-Faith BM, Laor T, et al. Fetal MR imaging of Kniest dysplasia. Pediatr Radiol 2010;40: 348–52.

28. Pugash D, Brugger PC, Bettelheim D, et al. Prenatal ultrasound and fetal MRI: the comparative value of each modality in prenatal diagnosis. Eur J Radiol 2008;68:214–26.

29. Kul S, Korkmaz HAA, Cansu A, et al. Contribution of MRI to ultrasound in the diagnosis of fetal anomalies. J Magn Reson Imaging 2012;35:882–90.

30. Weaver KN, Johnson J, Kline-Faith B, et al. Predictive value of fetal lung volume in prenatally diagnosed skeletal dysplasia. Prenat Diagn 2014;32:1–6.

31. Alanay Y, Lachman RS. A review of the principles of radiological assessment of skeletal dysplasias. J Clin Res Pediatr Endocrinol 2011;3:163–78.

32. Tunkel D, Alade Y, Kerbavaz R, et al. Hearing loss in skeletal dysplasia patients. Am J Med Genet 2012; 158:1551–5.

33. Rodriguez ME, Mackenzie WG, Ditro C, et al. Skeletal dysplasias: evaluation with impulse oscillometery and thoracoabdominal motion analysis. Pediatr Pulmonol 2010;45:679–86.

34. Theroux MC, Nerker T, Ditro C, et al. Anesthetic care and perioperative complications of children with Morquio syndrome. Pediatr Anaesth 2012;22:901–7.

35. Alade Y, Tunkel D, Schulze K, et al. Cross-sectional assessment of pain and physical function in skeletal dysplasia patients. Clin Genet 2012;84: 237–43.

36. O'brien A, Bompadre V, Hale S, et al. Musculoskeletal function in patients with mucopolysaccharidosis using the pediatric outcomes data collection instrument. J Pediatr Orthop 2014;34:650–4.

37. Ain MC, Abdullah MA, Ting BL, et al. Progression of low back pain and lower extremity pain in a cohort of patients with achondroplasia. J Neurosurg Spine 2010;13:335–40.

38. Afsharpaiman S, Saburi A, Waters KA. Respiratory difficulties and breathing disorders in achondroplasia. Paediatr Respir Rev 2013;14:250–5.

39. Dessoffy KE, Modaff P, Pauli RM. Airway malacia in children with achondroplasia. Am J Med Genet A 2014;164-A:407–14.

40. Esteller E. Obstructive sleep apnea-hypopnea syndrome in children: beyond adenotonsillar hypertrophy. Acta Otorrinolaringol Esp 2015;66(2): 111–9.

41. Hansen KK, Keeshim BR, Flaherty E, et al. Sensitivity of the limited view follow-up skeletal survey. Pediatrics 2014;134(2):242–8.

42. Parnell SE, Wall C, Weinberger E. Interactive digital atlas of skeletal surveys for common skeletal dysplasias. Pediatr Radiol 2013;43:803–13.

43. Shirely ED, Ain MC. Achondroplasia: manifestations and treatment. J Am Acad Orthop Surg 2009;17: 231–41.

44. Srikumaran U, Woodard EJ, Leet AI, et al. Pedicle and spinal canal parameters of the lower thoracic and lumbar vertebrae in the achondroplast population. Spine 2007;32:2423–31.

45. Karikari IO, Mehta AI, Solakoglu C, et al. Sagittal spinopelvic parameters in children with achondroplasia: identification of 2 distinct groups. J Neurosurg Spine 2012;17:57–60.

46. Bethem D, Winter RB, Lutter L, et al. Spinal disorders of dwarfism: review of the literature and report of eighty cases. J Bone Joint Surg Am 1981;63: 1412–25.

47. Ain MC, Shirley ED, Pirouzmanesh A, et al. Genu varum in achondroplasia. J Pediatr Orthop 2006; 26:375–9.

48. Fraser SC, Neubauer PR, Ain MC. The role of arthrography in selecting an osteotomy for the correction of genu varum in pediatric patients with achondroplasia. J Pediatr Orthop B 2011;20:14–6.

49. Inan M, Thacker M, Church C, et al. Dynamic lower extremity alignment in children with achondroplasia. J Pediatr Orthop 2006;26:526–9.

50. Trotter TL, Hall JG. Health supervision for children with achondroplasia. Pediatrics 2005;116:771–83.

51. Reardon W, Hall CM, Shaw DG, et al. New autosomal dominant form of spondyloepiphyseal dysplasia presenting with atlanto-axial instability. Am J Med Genet 1994;52:432–7.

52. Dhawale AA, Church C, Henley J, et al. Gait pattern and lower extremity alignment in children with Morquio syndrome. J Pediatr Orthop B 2013;22:59–62.

53. Solanki GA, Martin KW, Theroux MC, et al. Spinal involvement in mucopolysaccharidosis IVA (Morquio-Brailsford or Morquio A syndrome): presentation diagnosis and management. J Inherit Metab Dis 2013;36:339–55.

54. White KK, Sousa T. Mucopolysaccharide disorders in orthopaedic surgery. J Am Acad Orthop Surg 2013;21:12–22.
55. Tomatsu S, MacKenzie WG, Theroux MC, et al. Current and emerging treatments and surgical interventions for Morquio A syndrome: a review. Res Rep Endocr Disord 2012;2:65–77.
56. White KK, Jester A, Bache CE, et al. Orthopedic management of the extremities in patients with Morquio A syndrome. J Child Orthop 2014;8: 295–304.
57. Rimon DL, Cohn D, Krakow D, et al. The skeletal dysplasias: clinical-molecular correlations. Ann N Y Acad Sci 2007;1117:302–9.
58. Unger S. A genetic approach to the diagnosis of skeletal dysplasia. Clin Orthop Relat Res 2002;(401): 32–8.

Discoid Meniscus
Diagnosis and Management

Indranil Kushare, MBBS, DNB, Kevin Klingele, MD, Walter Samora, MD*

KEYWORDS

- Discoid meniscus • Meniscus tears • Arthroscopy • Instability • Saucerization

KEY POINTS

- Discoid lateral meniscus is a common abnormal meniscal variant in children. A detailed history and physical examination, when combined with an MRI of the knee, can predictably diagnose a discoid meniscus. The discoid meniscus was typically classified as type I (complete), type II (incomplete), or type III (Wrisberg variant).
- It is now imperative to assess and determine the instability, and the newer classification based on stability of the peripheral rim is more relevant clinically and from the surgical perspective.
- The clinical presentation varies from being asymptomatic to snapping, locking, and causing severe pain and swelling of the knee. Because of the pathologic anatomy and instability, discoid menisci are more prone to tearing, which is often the cause of these presenting mechanical symptoms.
- Treatment options for symptomatic patients vary based on the type of anomaly, the age of the patient, stability, and the presence or absence of a tear. Most surgeons prefer arthroscopic partial central meniscectomy and stabilization to the capsule (if unstable) and repair of the tear if any rather than complete or subtotal meniscectomy.
- Improvements in arthroscopic equipment and technique have resulted in good to excellent short-term outcomes for saucerization and repair. Prospective studies with larger number of patients that assess the long-term outcome are required to define the perfect treatment strategy.

INTRODUCTION

The discoid lateral meniscus is the most common abnormal meniscal variant in children.[1] The morphology of a discoid meniscus varies but it typically covers a greater than normal area of the tibial plateau. The incidence of discoid lateral meniscus is estimated to be 0.4% to 17% in the lateral meniscus where it is most common.[2,3] Medial discoid menisci are extremely rare.[4] A discoid lateral meniscus can be unstable causing pain and mechanical symptoms in younger children and is more likely to present as a tear in older children.[5] Improvements in arthroscopic techniques have led to greater attempts to saucerize, repair, and stabilize the torn discoid lateral meniscus and recent literature suggests good

short-term results. This article reviews the anatomy, classification, clinical presentation, imaging studies, and management including surgical options for discoid lateral meniscus in the pediatric population.

ANATOMY AND CLASSIFICATION

The meniscus is completely vascular at birth with blood supply entering from the periphery of the meniscus. By the ninth month of life, the central third becomes avascular. Meniscal vascularity gradually diminishes to the peripheral 10% to 30% by age 10 years, at which time it resembles the adult meniscus.[6] Increased blood supply and recent evidence suggesting regeneration of a discoid meniscus after saucerization suggests

Disclosures: None of the authors received financial support for this study.
Department of Orthopedics, Nationwide Children's Hospital, 700 Childrens Drive, Columbus, OH 43205, USA
* Corresponding author.
E-mail address: Walter.Samora@nationwidechildrens.org

Orthop Clin N Am 46 (2015) 533–540
http://dx.doi.org/10.1016/j.ocl.2015.06.007
0030-5898/15/$ – see front matter

orthopedic.theclinics.com

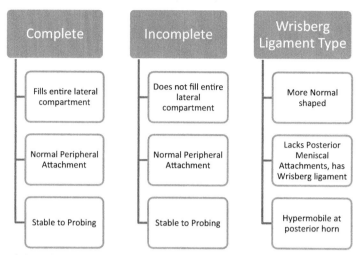

Fig. 1. Classification of discoid menisci.

increased potential for repair and regeneration of the meniscal tissue especially in the pediatric population and better reparative potential than the adult meniscus.[6,7]

Recent case reports discuss regeneration of discoid meniscus after partial meniscectomy in younger patients perhaps implying that a discoid meniscus arises through variant morphogenesis and also raises concerns of regrowth after partial meniscectomy.[7–9]

Normal menisci are fibrocartilaginous structures in the knee joint that are C-shaped in the axial plane and wedge-shaped in the coronal plane and help increase the contact surface area between the tibia and the femur. A discoid meniscus has a completely filled-in central area or a very small void in the central area in contrast to a normal semilunar-shaped meniscus. The outer rim of a discoid meniscus is also much thicker than a normal meniscal rim. These anatomic variations alter the normal mechanical relationship and predispose the meniscus to injury and tearing.[1] The exact cause of a discoid meniscus has not been determined, but is believed to be multifactorial. The normal meniscus is not formed from a discoid precursor. Because the menisci have a semilunar shape from the beginning of their formation, the discoid meniscus may likely represent a congenital anomaly.[6,10] There is also a genetic or familial factor that is believed to play a role in the development of discoid menisci.[1,11]

Watanabe classified the discoid menisci as complete, incomplete, or Wrisberg ligament type depending on the presence or absence of a normal posterior attachment and the degree of tibial plateau coverage (**Fig. 1**). The most common type of discoid meniscus is the complete type, which is characterized by a much thickened lateral meniscus

that fills the entire lateral compartment. The thickened cartilage, because of its anatomic properties, is more prone to tear with sports activities when compared with a normal meniscus (**Fig. 2**A). The second type is the incomplete type, because the meniscus is smaller than type I. Both type I and II have normal peripheral attachments and are stable to arthroscopic probing (see **Fig. 2**B).

The Wrisberg type (least common, type III) is a more normally shaped meniscus that lacks usual posterior meniscal attachments, including the meniscotibial (ie, coronary) ligament. It does have a ligament of Wrisberg that connects the posterior horn of the lateral meniscus to the lateral surface of the medial femoral condyle (see **Fig. 2**C). Hypermobility of the lateral meniscus at the posterior horn allows the meniscus to displace with knee extension and is postulated to cause the classic snapping knee syndrome.[10]

Although this is a frequently used classification, its utility for surgical decision making is questionable. Because of its variability, Klingele and colleagues[12] described the peripheral rim instability patterns in discoid menisci. In their series of 128 discoid lateral menisci, 62.1% were complete discoid and 37.9% were incomplete. Peripheral rim instability was noted in 28.1% of cases. Instability most commonly occurred in the anterior horn of the meniscus (47.2%), followed by the posterior third (38.9%), and the middle third (11.1%). These findings suggest a newer classification system based on the size, stability, and presence or absence of a meniscal tear (**Fig. 3**).

CLINICAL FEATURES

- Asymptomatic: Children often have no symptoms from a discoid lateral meniscus.

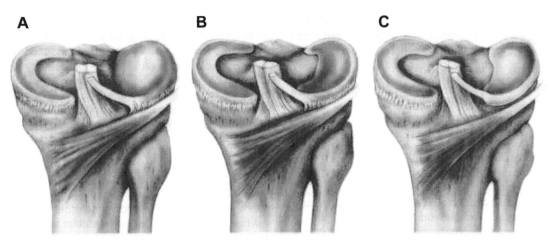

Fig. 2. (*A–C*) Watanabe classification of discoid lateral meniscus. (*From* Kramer DE, Micheli LJ. Meniscal tears and discoid meniscus in children: diagnosis and treatment. J Am Acad Orthop Surg 2009;17(11):703; with permission.)

- Symptoms referable to a discoid meniscus typically stem from either a tear of the meniscus or from an unstable discoid variant.
- The typical presentation in a young child with a symptomatic discoid meniscus is that of a popping or snapping of the knee that is heard and felt by the child or parent. The onset of the snapping or popping is usually insidious without any specific traumatic cause, classically between the ages of 5 and 10 years.
- The snapping knee may have associated pain, giving way, effusion, quadriceps atrophy, limitation of motion or asymmetric extension, clicking, or locking.
- The older child may also present with more acute symptoms, such as significant pain, knee locking, and inability to put weight on the affected extremity. These mechanical symptoms are more likely caused by tearing of the discoid meniscus. Physical examination findings include lateral joint line tenderness and snapping as the knee is flexed or extended. Frequently, McMurray test and Apley grinding test produce pain and an audible and palpable loud click or snap. This occurs because of the translation of the femoral condyle over a thickened posterior rim of the lateral meniscus.
- Patients with unstable discoid meniscus may present with complaints of knee instability because of a defect in the posterior meniscofemoral ligament.

INVESTIGATIONS

Plain radiographs of the knee should be obtained in all children with an acute injury. These views include the anteroposterior, lateral, tunnel, and sunrise or Merchant views.

- Tunnel views: to rule out osteochondritis dissecans (OCD) lesions as the source of knee pain. The typical anatomic location of an OCD lesion is the lateral aspect of the medial femoral condyle. However, lateral OCD lesions should raise the concern for a discoid meniscus as the underlying cause. Patellar dislocation may result in a chondral loose body displaced from the lateral trochlea, which can result in mechanical symptoms mimicking a meniscal tear.
- Sunrise or Merchant radiograph: to rule out patellar subluxation, trochlear dysplasia, and osteochondral loose bodies.
- Radiographs are often normal in patients with a discoid meniscus, but may show subtle widening of the lateral joint space especially when compared with the contralateral knee. A squared-off appearance of the lateral

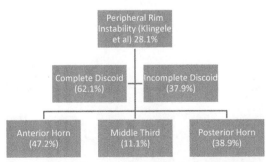

Fig. 3. Peripheral rim instability in discoid menisci. (*Data from* Klingele KE, Kocher MS, Hresko MT, et al. Discoid lateral meniscus: prevalence of peripheral rim instability. J Pediatr Orthop 2004;24(1):79–82.)

femoral condyle, cupping of the lateral tibial plateau, and tibial eminence flattening can also occasionally be seen indicating severe discoid menisci.[1,10]

MRI is the modality of choice for confirming the diagnosis of a discoid meniscus (**Fig. 4**).

MRI FEATURES OF A LATERAL DISCOID

- Ratio of the minimal meniscal width to maximal tibial width (on the coronal MRI slice) of more than 20%.[11]
- Three or more 5-mm thick consecutive sagittal sections demonstrate continuity of the meniscus between the anterior and posterior horns.[13]
- An abnormal, thickened, bow-tie appearance of the meniscus may also be suggestive of a discoid meniscus (**Fig. 5**).
- MRI can also show tears that are frequently associated with a discoid lateral meniscus. However, its ability to determine the type of tear is questionable.[14]
- It can be difficult to appreciate the stability a discoid meniscus on an MRI scan and some incomplete discoid menisci often look normal on MRI.[1,10]

Kocher and colleagues[15] found significant differences for sensitivity of lateral discoid meniscus (clinical examination, 88.9% vs magnetic resonance imaging, 38.9%) showing that MRI does not provide enhanced diagnostic utility over clinical examination, particularly in children. In some circumstances, a diagnostic arthroscopy might be needed to confirm the diagnosis of discoid meniscus especially in a symptomatic patient with an unstable or Wrisberg variant that has normal shape and normal MRI appearance.[16]

MANAGEMENT

Many children with discoid meniscus remain asymptomatic and require no treatment according to most authors.[16–18] Arthroscopic surgery is generally recommended if the discoid meniscus is associated with mechanical symptoms, such as pain, locking, swelling, giving way, or causing inability to participate in sports. Treatment recommendations for an asymptomatic, stable complete, or incomplete discoid lateral meniscus found during investigation or treatment of some other knee condition are still being debated.

Because of concerns about the development of degenerative arthritis following complete meniscectomy, arthroscopic partial central meniscectomy (ie, saucerization) is the usually recommended treatment with an attempt to convert meniscus back to a more normal shape and size.[1,3,5,10,16–23] The saucerization procedure is the resection of the central portion of the discoid meniscus until the remaining rim is established to the width of a normal meniscus, typically 6 to 8 mm.[17]

Recently, attention has been focused on peripheral instability seen in discoid menisci.[20] Peripheral rim instability was noted by Klingele and

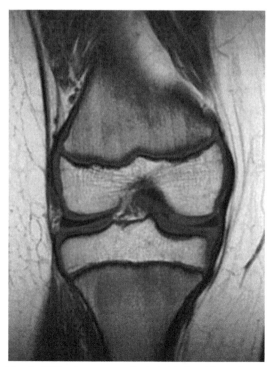

Fig. 4. MRI appearance of a lateral discoid meniscus.

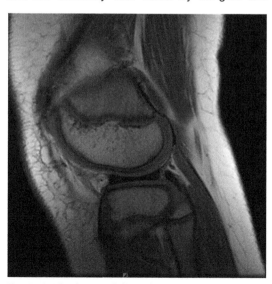

Fig. 5. Sagittal MRI of discoid meniscus.

colleagues[12] in 28.1% of cases, most commonly occurring in the anterior horn.

Discoid menisci are predisposed to meniscal tears. A common tear pattern in the discoid meniscus is the horizontal cleavage tear pattern. This pattern is thought to occur because of the shearing of the femoral condyle on the abnormally shaped meniscus. There may be some instances in which a torn discoid meniscus is unsalvageable and near complete excision might be the only possible surgical option. However, with 'the current advancement of arthroscopic meniscal repair techniques a reparable peripheral tear in the vascular zone can be repaired in conjunction with partial central meniscectomy.[17] Improvements in arthroscopic instrumentation, newer suture techniques, modification of arthroscopic portals, and increased surgeon experience have reduced the complexity of the surgical techniques.

SURGICAL TECHNIQUE

1. In the supine position, lateral and then medial infrapatellar portals are established using a 4-mm 30° oblique arthroscope.
2. Routine diagnostic arthroscopic inspection of the knee joint is performed.
3. Surgical assistant applies constant varus stress to the knee with the leg in a leg holder or in the figure-of-four position for better maneuverability and visualization of the lateral compartment (**Fig. 6**).
4. After visualization, probing of the discoid meniscus is an important step to check the stability and presence of tears if any.

5. Saucerization can be performed in a piecemeal fashion using arthroscopic instruments, such as a basket punch (**Fig. 7**). It is often better to begin the saucerization with the knee at 90° of flexion to allow one to enter the lateral compartment easier. Another technique of single piece excision using straight scissor punch with three unique portals (lateral patellofemoral axillary, far anteromedial, and low anterolateral) has also been described.[24]
6. Continuous reassessment of the peripheral rim is essential to avoid accidentally resecting too much meniscus.
7. An attempt should be made to leave normal width (6–8 mm) of the peripheral rim trying to create a normal contour of the free edge of the meniscus (**Fig. 8**).
8. In the horizontal cleavage tear pattern (**Fig. 9**) extending to the periphery, the inferior or superior leaf of the meniscus might need to be resected, leaving the rim, which maintains peripheral attachment.
9. For meniscus tears, depending on the type of tear and location, all inside, inside-out, or outside-in repairs can be done to stabilize the torn meniscus with the capsule after rasping the edges (**Fig. 10**).

POSTOPERATIVE PROTOCOL

For saucerization only, usually no brace is required. Range of motion can be started as soon as comfortable with pain and weight bearing is as tolerated.

For meniscal repair and peripheral rim stabilization, the same rehabilitation protocol applies as any other meniscal repair, which is typically

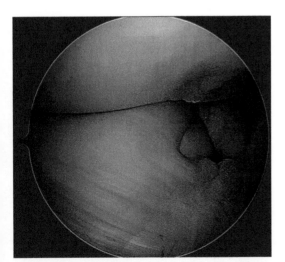

Fig. 6. Arthroscopic appearance of a complete lateral discoid meniscus.

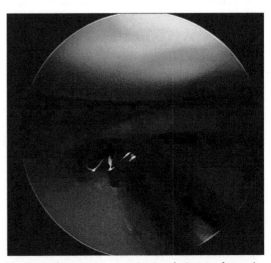

Fig. 7. Arthroscopic saucerization being performed.

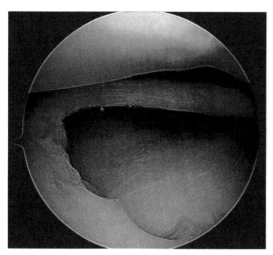

Fig. 8. Postsaucerization arthroscopic appearance of discoid meniscus.

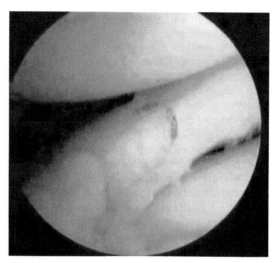

Fig. 10. Meniscus tear and instability stabilized with sutures.

restricting the range of motion from 0° to 90° and toe touch weight bearing for about 4 to 6 weeks.

SURGICAL OUTCOMES

There are few long-term outcome studies of discoid menisci treated with arthroscopy and saucerization. However, the few short-term studies that are available in the past decade that assess partial central meniscectomy, repair, and recontouring of the discoid meniscus are quite promising. In a study with a follow-up averaging 4.5 years, Ogut and colleagues[25] reviewed 10 knees with complete discoid lateral menisci that had undergone arthroscopic partial meniscectomy with excellent result in nine of the knees and no evidence of degenerative changes on radiographic examination. They also recommended leaving 5

to 6 mm of residual meniscal rim to normalize stability and function. Longer follow-up is needed, however, to assess for later development of osteoarthritis. Ahn and colleagues[20] had similar good results in their 23 patients treated similarly with 2 years follow-up. A total of 85% showed good or excellent results in a 5-year follow-up by Atay and colleagues,[18] but the lateral condyle showed radiographic flattening in a significant percentage of patients. Meniscal stabilization for peripheral instability did not lead to any increase in complications[26] and has good short-term efficacy.[21] Subtotal or total meniscectomy was more frequently performed in longitudinal or complex tears, whereas partial meniscectomy was carried out in radial and degenerative tears.[27]

COMPLICATIONS OF SURGERY

- Complications that are associated with knee arthroscopy for any meniscal surgery include premature osteoarthritis, incomplete resection of the torn unstable rim, injury to nerves/vessels, arthrofibrosis, persistent effusion, infection, and instrument breakage.
- It is important to remember that following partial meniscectomy and/or repair of a discoid meniscus, the cartilage remains thickened because it is not a normal meniscus to begin with. Thus, a discoid meniscus is still more likely to develop a tear when compared with a normal meniscus.[1]
- A complication unique to discoid meniscus surgery is OCD of the lateral femoral condyle following total or partial resection of a discoid lateral meniscus.[28] Studies have shown an

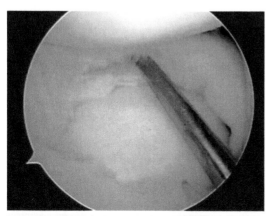

Fig. 9. Horizontal degenerative cleavage tear in a discoid meniscus.

association of OCD with discoid menisci variants.[29] Repeated impaction in sports activities on the immature osteochondral structures under altered mechanical force transmission after resection of the discoid meniscus might be predispose to the development of OCD in the lateral femoral condyle.[28] Valgus deviation of the knee after removal of the thick discoid meniscus and increased sporting activity in the young patient can lead to concentrated excessive stress on the lateral condyles because of change in the alignment in the standing position.[30] OCD of the lateral femoral condyle associated with discoid lateral meniscus has also been shown to heal after meniscoplasty.[11,31]

- Regrowth of the meniscus after excision has been described in two case reports in the pediatric population.[7,9] This might be of concern if excessive meniscal tissue is left behind during saucerization because of the fear of causing early osteoarthritis if too much tissue is resected.

SUMMARY

A discoid lateral meniscus is a common abnormal meniscal variant in children. A detailed history and physical examination, when combined with an MRI of the knee, can predictably diagnose a discoid meniscus. The discoid meniscus was typically classified as type I (complete), type II (incomplete), or type III (Wrisberg variant). It is now imperative to assess and determine the instability and the newer classification based on stability if the peripheral rim is more relevant clinically and from the surgical perspective. The clinical presentation varies from being asymptomatic to snapping, locking, and causing severe pain and swelling of the knee. Because of the pathologic anatomy and instability, discoid menisci are more prone to tearing, which is often the cause of these presenting mechanical symptoms. Treatment options for symptomatic patients vary based on the type of anomaly, the age of the patient, stability, and the presence or absence of a tear. Most surgeons prefer arthroscopic partial central meniscectomy and stabilization to the capsule (if unstable) and repair of the tear if any rather than complete or subtotal meniscectomy. Improvements in arthroscopic equipment and technique have resulted in good to excellent short-term outcomes for saucerization and repair. Prospective studies with larger number of patients that assess the long-term outcome are required to define the perfect treatment strategy.

REFERENCES

1. Hart ES, Kalra KP, Grottkau BE, et al. Discoid lateral meniscus in children. Orthop Nurs 2008;27(3):174–9 [quiz: 180–1].
2. Greis PE, Bardana DD, Holmstrom MC, et al. Meniscal injury: I. Basic science and evaluation. J Am Acad Orthop Surg 2002;10(3):168–76.
3. Ikeuchi H. Arthroscopic treatment of the discoid lateral meniscus. Technique and long-term results. Clin Orthop Relat Res 1982;(167):19–28.
4. Kini SG, Walker P, Bruce W. Bilateral symptomatic discoid medial meniscus of the knee: a case report and review of literature. Arch Trauma Res 2015;4(1): e27115.
5. Kocher MS, Klingele K, Rassman SO. Meniscal disorders: normal, discoid, and cysts. Orthop Clin North Am 2003;34(3):329–40.
6. Clark CR, Ogden JA. Development of the menisci of the human knee joint. Morphological changes and their potential role in childhood meniscal injury. J Bone Joint Surg Am 1983;65(4):538–47.
7. Stein MI, Gaskins RB 3rd, Nalley CC, et al. Regeneration of a discoid meniscus after arthroscopic saucerization. Am J Orthop (Belle Mead NJ) 2013; 42(1):E5–8.
8. Soejima T, Kanazawa T, Tabuchi K, et al. Regeneration of ring-shaped lateral meniscus after partial resection of discoid meniscus with anterior cruciate ligament reconstruction. Int J Surg Case Rep 2013; 4(12):1093–6.
9. Bisicchia S, Tudisco C. Re-growth of an incomplete discoid lateral meniscus after arthroscopic partial resection in an 11 year-old boy: a case report. BMC Musculoskelet Disord 2013;14:285.
10. Kramer DE, Micheli LJ. Meniscal tears and discoid meniscus in children: diagnosis and treatment. J Am Acad Orthop Surg 2009;17(11):698–707.
11. Yaniv M, Blumberg N. The discoid meniscus. J Child Orthop 2007;1(2):89–96.
12. Klingele KE, Kocher MS, Hresko MT, et al. Discoid lateral meniscus: prevalence of peripheral rim instability. J Pediatr Orthop 2004;24(1):79–82.
13. Silverman JM, Mink JH, Deutsch AL. Discoid menisci of the knee: MR imaging appearance. Radiology 1989;173(2):351–4.
14. Yilgor C, Atay OA, Ergen B, et al. Comparison of magnetic resonance imaging findings with arthroscopic findings in discoid meniscus. Knee Surg Sports Traumatol Arthrosc 2014;22(2):268–73.
15. Kocher MS, DiCanzio J, Zurakowski D, et al. Diagnostic performance of clinical examination and selective magnetic resonance imaging in the evaluation of intraarticular knee disorders in children and adolescents. Am J Sports Med 2001;29(3):292–6.
16. Kelly BT, Green DW. Discoid lateral meniscus in children. Curr Opin Pediatr 2002;14(1):54–61.

17. Adachi N, Ochi M, Uchio Y, et al. Torn discoid lateral meniscus treated using partial central meniscectomy and suture of the peripheral tear. Arthroscopy 2004;20(5):536–42.

18. Atay OA, Doral MN, Leblebicioğlu G, et al. Management of discoid lateral meniscus tears: observations in 34 knees. Arthroscopy 2003;19(4):346–52.

19. Bellisari G, Samora W, Klingele K. Meniscus tears in children. Sports Med Arthrosc 2011;19(1):50–5.

20. Ahn JH, Lee SH, Yoo JC, et al. Arthroscopic partial meniscectomy with repair of the peripheral tear for symptomatic discoid lateral meniscus in children: results of minimum 2 years of follow-up. Arthroscopy 2008;24(8):888–98.

21. Good CR, Green DW, Griffith MH, et al. Arthroscopic treatment of symptomatic discoid meniscus in children: classification, technique, and results. Arthroscopy 2007;23(2):157–63.

22. Youm T, Chen AL. Discoid lateral meniscus: evaluation and treatment. Am J Orthop (Belle Mead NJ) 2004;33(5):234–8.

23. Tachibana Y, Yamazaki Y, Ninomiya S. Discoid medial meniscus. Arthroscopy 2003;19(7):E12–8.

24. Kim SJ, Yoo JH, Kim HK. Arthroscopic one-piece excision technique for the treatment of symptomatic lateral discoid meniscus. Arthroscopy 1996;12(6): 752–5.

25. Ogut T, Kesmezacar H, Akgün I, et al. Arthroscopic meniscectomy for discoid lateral meniscus in children and adolescents: 4.5 year follow-up. J Pediatr Orthop B 2003;12(6):390–7.

26. Carter CW, Hoellwarth J, Weiss JM. Clinical outcomes as a function of meniscal stability in the discoid meniscus: a preliminary report. J Pediatr Orthop 2012;32(1):9–14.

27. Bin SI, Kim JC, Kim JM, et al. Correlation between type of discoid lateral menisci and tear pattern. Knee Surg Sports Traumatol Arthrosc 2002;10(4): 218–22.

28. Mizuta H, Nakamura E, Otsuka Y, et al. Osteochondritis dissecans of the lateral femoral condyle following total resection of the discoid lateral meniscus. Arthroscopy 2001;17(6):608–12.

29. Deie M, Ochi M, Sumen Y, et al. Relationship between osteochondritis dissecans of the lateral femoral condyle and lateral menisci types. J Pediatr Orthop 2006;26(1):79–82.

30. Hashimoto Y, Yoshida G, Tomihara T, et al. Bilateral osteochondritis dissecans of the lateral femoral condyle following bilateral total removal of lateral discoid meniscus: a case report. Arch Orthop Trauma Surg 2008;128(11):1265–8.

31. Yoshida S, Ikata T, Takai H, et al. Osteochondritis dissecans of the femoral condyle in the growth stage. Clin Orthop Relat Res 1998;(346):162–70.

Upper Extremity

Preface

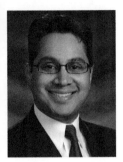

Asif M. Ilyas, MD
Editor

In this issue of the *Orthopedic Clinics of North America*, we present several interesting articles in the Upper Extremity section reviewing a broad range of topics.

As the population continues to grow and age, distal radius fractures are increasing in both prevalence and their association with osteoporosis. Subsequently, understanding fixation strategies of these fractures complicated by osteoporosis are paramount to successful treatment. Tulipan and colleagues provide a detailed review of osteoporosis and its effect on distal radius fracture treatment.

Scapholunate ligament injuries continue to be among the most challenging injuries managed by upper extremity surgeons. Many treatment options abound predicated on the extent and acuity of the symptoms. Ward and Fowler present a comprehensive review of these difficult wrist injuries.

Trigger fingers are among the most common conditions treated by upper extremity surgeons. However, treatment algorithms vary based on the patient's age and duration of symptoms. Giugale and Fowler review the current treatment options and controversies associated with trigger finger management.

Distal radius fractures remain an area of intense biomechanical research interest due to their high incidence and associated morbidity. Recently, the use of high-speed radiographs has been utilized to better understand pathomechanics of fractures. Gutowski and colleagues present their experience with the use of this research modality to better understand distal radius pathomechanics.

Asif M. Ilyas, MD
Hand & Upper Extremity Surgery
Rothman Institute
Thomas Jefferson University
925 Chestnut Street
Philadelphia, PA 19107, USA

E-mail address:
asif.ilyas@rothmaninstitute.com

Orthop Clin N Am 46 (2015) xxi
http://dx.doi.org/10.1016/j.ocl.2015.07.005
0030-5898/15/$ – see front matter © 2015 Published by Elsevier Inc.

The Effect of Osteoporosis on Healing of Distal Radius Fragility Fractures

Jacob Tulipan, MD[a],*, Christopher M. Jones, MD[b], Asif M. Ilyas, MD[b]

KEYWORDS

- Distal radius fracture • Osteoporosis • Volar locking plate • Biomechanics • Fracture healing

KEY POINTS

- Distal radius fractures are among the most common fractures seen and are increasing in incidence because of increased prevalence of osteoporosis and increasing age of our population.
- The osteoporotic distal radius is deficient in both cortical and trabecular bone, but early changes in cortical bone most predispose to fragility fractures.
- The fracture callus formed around an osteoporotic fracture is less stiff than a normal fracture callus, but it is unclear how this affects long-term function or biomechanics.
- Nonoperative management of osteoporotic distal radius fractures in low-demand patients remains well indicated and can lead to long-term clinical outcomes similar to operative management.
- There are multiple acceptable methods for operative management of osteoporotic distal radius fractures; but volar locking plates are most commonly used, safely and readily applied, allowing for early motion, and have an acceptable complication profile.

INTRODUCTION

Fractures of the distal radius are among the most common fragility fractures seen in clinical practice, with estimates of annual incidence ranging as high as 86,000 in the United States alone.[1] Given the aging population, this number is only expected to increase.

Although the surgical treatment of distal radius fractures has advanced significantly since the advent of the volar locking plate, recent studies, including Arora and colleagues,[2] Koval and colleagues,[3] and Young and Rayan,[4] have challenged the trend toward operative management and have prompted increased interest in nonoperative treatment of these fractures. Although the decision for operative versus nonoperative treatment still remains subjective and is performed on a case-by-case basis, evaluation and treatment of patients with a distal radius fragility fracture requires understanding of the behavior of this injury as a distinct subset of distal radius fractures. Age, infirmity, and osteoporosis affect every aspect of the fracture, from epidemiology and injury biomechanics to fixation mechanics and the biology of healing. Understanding what makes these fractures unique assists the surgeon in more effective and efficient treatment.

[a] Department of Orthopaedic Surgery, Thomas Jefferson University, 1015 Walnut Street, Curtis Building, Suite 810, Philadelphia, PA 19107, USA; [b] Department of Orthopaedic Surgery, Rothman Institute, Thomas Jefferson University, 925 Chestnut Street, Philadelphia, PA 19107, USA
* Corresponding author.
E-mail address: jacob.tulipan@gmail.com

Orthop Clin N Am 46 (2015) 541–549
http://dx.doi.org/10.1016/j.ocl.2015.06.012
0030-5898/15/$ – see front matter © 2015 Elsevier Inc. All rights reserved.

EPIDEMIOLOGY

Most distal radius fractures in the elderly are attributable to osteoporosis, with a correspondingly higher incidence in the female versus male population. A 2004 study of the French National Hospital Database found an incidence of 7.5 per 1000 in women and 2.3 per 1000 in men older than 45 years.[5] A later single-center British study estimated that these fractures compose 17.5% of adult fractures.[6] Other studies have confirmed the strong correlation between fracture incidence and displacement and patient age, especially for female patients, in whom incidence increases from 8.9 per 10,000 in patients aged 19 to 49 years to 119 per 10,000 in patients older than 80 years.[7]

Several risk factors for occurrence and severity of distal radius fragility fracture have been elucidated, with most relating directly or indirectly to bone quality. Known osteoporosis or decreased bone mineral density (BMD) as measured by a dual-energy x-ray absorptiometry (DEXA) scan is well established to increase the risk for distal radius fragility fracture[8,9]; but other studies have examined nutritional, lifestyle, and genetic predisposing factors. A case-control study demonstrated lower serum 25-hydroxyvitamin levels in fracture patients versus matched controls, independently of measured BMD, indicating a qualitative as well as quantitative bone deficit.[10] Although this has been posited as a potential explanation for prior studies finding increased incidence of distal radius fractures in the elderly during winter months, the studies have been unable to differentiate between vitamin D levels and variations in patient activity as causative factors.

BIOMECHANICS

Osteoporotic and normal distal radii differ in structural and mechanical properties. A cadaver study by Spadaro and colleagues[11] attempted to determine whether cortical or trabecular properties are the main contributors to biomechanical load to failure. The ultimate compressive strength of 21 osteopenic cadaver radii was found to correlate strongly with cortical cross-sectional area, indicating a major contribution by the cortical shell to the ultimate strength of distal radii. A correlation was also noted, however, between trabecular *density* (as opposed to area) and strength, leading to the conclusion that axial distal radius strength is affected by both quantity of cortex and quality of trabecular bone.

More recent studies have used high-resolution quantitative computed tomography (HR-QCT) to reveal in vivo changes associated with postmenopausal distal radius. A recent study of 51 women over 1 year by Kawalilak and colleagues[12] used this method and found that postmenopausal women experience a decrease in total density, accompanied by a reduction in number and an increase in thickness of trabeculae. Another recent study of 117 postmenopausal women by Stein and colleagues[13] demonstrated significantly altered trabecular morphology in women with fractures, including rodlike rather than platelike trabecular microarchitecture, and loss of axial trabecular orientation. Although BMD was lost in both cortex and trabeculae in this group, there were no measureable differences in cortical structure.

The difficulty in parsing these data is in determining the relative contribution of cortical and trabecular bone to total strength in the distal radius; although both are correlated to increase fracture risk, causality and contribution to weakness are difficult to determine. Among the studies that attempted to isolate cortical contribution is a case-control study of 138 postmenopausal women by Bala and colleagues[14], which found that dense cortical porosity of the distal radius as measured by HR-QCT is predictive of fracture independent of BMD. Although this study was unable to make a strong statement of cortical porosity's effect in osteoporotic individuals because of the high prevalence of this finding (approximately 90%) in this population, it did demonstrate that cortical architecture has an independent effect (odd ratio 4.00, confidence interval 1.15–13.90) on fracture risk in osteopenic women.

A more focused study by Bjørnerem and colleagues[15] in 2013 examined 345 women aged 40 to 61 years. Each 1-SD increase in cortical porosity of the distal radius, as measured by HR-QCT, was found to correlate with an increased risk of fracture, although the association was weak in the distal radius as compared with the tibia and fibula.

Taken as a whole, these studies make a convincing argument that, at least in the early stages of osteopenia, cortical rather than trabecular bone provides the most significant contribution to distal radius fracture resistance. Although further studies are certainly required to test this conclusion, it can inform our methods of treatment of these fractures.

EFFECTS OF OSTEOPOROSIS ON BONE HEALING

The effects of osteoporosis on the healing of fractures can be conceptualized as 2 separate processes: First is the effect of osteoporosis on the natural history of fracture healing. Second is the extent to which osteoporosis forces us to modify our treatment strategy.

Osteoporosis' effect on the natural history of fractures is a much-debated subject. Much of the major work in the field has been performed on hypogonadal animal models using biomechanical data as an outcome measure. A study by Thormann and colleagues[16] analyzed metaphyseal osteotomies in ovarectomized versus control rat femurs. After 6 weeks of healing with a noncompressive plate-screw construct, the femurs were biomechanically and histologically analyzed. Osteoporotic and control group callus was found to possess equivalent vascularity and ossified tissue percentage. Biomechanical testing revealed decreased shear rigidity in the osteoporotic group but found no difference in bending rigidity. Qualitatively, the callus in the osteoporotic group had a larger volume of unmineralized tissue and failed to demonstrate bony remodeling, a process well noted in the control. Taken together, this indicates a delay in fracture healing in the osteoporotic group but does not differentiate between delay caused by intrinsic bone properties versus inadequate bony fixation leading to increased micromotion at the fracture site.

These results seemed to validate the conclusions of an earlier trial, performed by Namkung-Matthai and colleagues[17] in 2001, which demonstrated decreased BMD and decreased load to failure at 21 days after injury in a rat femur model. Numerous other studies in rats and sheep demonstrated decreased BMD[18–21] and decreased stiffness[20,22,23] in osteoporotic versus control animals. These biomechanical studies in animals, which are well summarized in a review by Giannoudis and colleagues,[24] provide convincing evidence that osteoporotic fractures suffer from decreased mineralization and poor mechanical properties during the early healing period. They suffer, however, from a focus on the subacute period of fracture healing and a failure to examine the remodeling phase. Of the aforementioned studies, only one[23] studied the subjects beyond 18 weeks; this study found that both ovariectomized and control rats failed to regain normal mechanical properties in older subjects. This finding provided some indication that differences between osteoporotic and nonosteoporotic fractures may fade over the course of fracture remodeling. Further research is required to determine whether late fracture remodeling is significantly affected by osteoporosis.

Human data regarding the biomechanical changes wrought by osteoporosis on fracture healing are necessarily limited by the absence of noninvasive testing methods. A recent paper by Meyer and colleagues[25] examined postmenopausal distal radius fractures and found that early postfracture trabecular density and calculated torsional stiffness was related to outcomes at 12 weeks. This study, however, did not involve a control group; thus, it can only be inferred that the osteoporotic biomechanical and structural deficits in this group relate to outcome measures.

OSTEOPOROSIS AND DISTAL RADIUS FRACTURE MANAGEMENT

The treatment of osteoporotic distal radius fractures is governed by 3 major considerations. First, patients must be considered in toto, not only with regard to medical conditions and other injuries but also with regard to their functional goals and occupational/recreational demands. This determination helps guide the decision for operative versus nonoperative management. In low-demand elderly patients, a bias toward nonoperative treatment is appropriate. In contrast, in high-demand patients or patients living alone and independently, operative repair may better support their needs. The second consideration, in the event that operative management is chosen, is one of optimal fixation strategy. This strategy must take into account not only the fracture pattern but also bone quality, severity, optimal mobilization time, and surgeon experience. The third consideration is one of osteoporosis management as a whole, including secondary prevention of future fragility fractures using both pharmacologic and lifestyle measures.

Regardless of changes in fracture healing mechanics in osteoporotic individuals, the principles of fracture care remain the same in osteoporotic and nonosteoporotic individuals. The fracture must be immobilized internally or externally to provide pain relief and optimize fracture alignment. Motion must be instituted in the early postoperative period to prevent stiffness and loss of function, not only of the wrist but also of the fingers.

Patients with fragility fractures tend to be older, with lower functional demands than those with normal bone. As a result, acceptable levels of satisfaction may be achieved with imperfectly aligned fractures. However, in unstable fractures, open reduction internal fixation continues to be the mainstay of treatment, with goals of improved, immediate fracture stability, and earlier return to function. In recent years, volar locking plates have grown in popularity and have demonstrated good results in the treatment of unstable distal radius fragility fractures[26,27] (**Fig. 1**). This increased utilization of the volar locking plate can be attributed to several reasons, including a consistent and safe surgical approach,

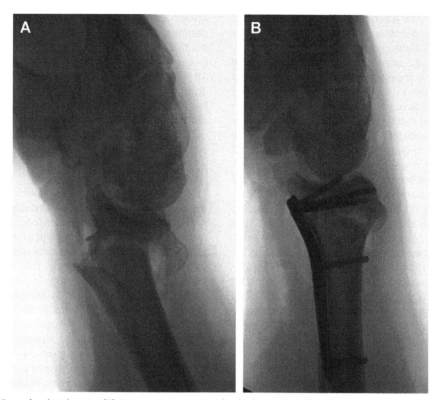

Fig. 1. (A) Prereduction image. (B) Image status post volar locking plate fixation of a displaced and angulated distal radius fracture in the dominant wrist of a woman with a DEXA-proven history of osteoporosis. These plates can improve fracture alignment, provide immediate fracture stability, and allow for earlier return to function and weight bearing.

applicability to a broad range of fracture patterns, ease of application, ability to institute early mobilization, and an acceptable complication profile.

Head-to-head comparisons of volar locking plates versus alternatives (dorsal plate fixation, external fixator, and pinning) have been performed,[28–31] demonstrating equivalent or superior results with volar locking plates versus the alternatives. Furthermore, biomechanical studies have specifically examined the utility of volar plates for the management of dorsally comminuted fractures, the pattern most commonly seen in distal radius fragility fractures. Kandemir and colleagues[32,33] using matched-pair radii demonstrated equivalent axial and torsional stiffness and load to failure in dorsal versus volar locking plates when used to fix a dorsally comminuted fracture. Similarly, Gondusky and colleagues[34] cyclically loaded plated distal radius constructs before testing load to failure and found no difference between volar and dorsal plating stability.

Clinical outcomes of volar versus dorsal plating have been directly compared in several retrospective studies. Rein and colleagues[28] examined 34 patients with intraarticular fractures treated by volar or dorsal plating and found that 4 of the 20

dorsal plating patients required tenosynovectomies or tenolyses and one suffered an extensor tendon rupture. In contrast, the complication rate was significantly lower in the volar plating group, and Gartland and Werley scores were also significantly better in that group. Similarly, Wichlas and colleagues[31] examined 285 distal radius fractures, 225 treated with volar locking plates and 60 with a dorsal locked plating. The complication rate was significantly higher in the dorsal plating group (17% vs 4%) with an increased incidence of pain and tenosynovitis. Although dorsal plates remain well indicated and also remain in regular use, particularly with newer lower-profile designs, ongoing concerns over long-term soft tissue complications have, among other things, led to the increased popularity of volar locking plates as the most common form of surgical fixation construct of distal radius fractures.

Although other surgical fixation techniques for distal radius fractures have been described, studies have generally found volar locking plates to have equivalent or better results as compared with alternatives.[28,30,31,35,36] One such prospective study examined intrafocal pinning versus volar locking plates in a prospectively gathered group of 62 patients older than 60 years. The study demonstrated improved range of motion, grip strength, and radiographic reduction in the volar locking plate group during the 12 weeks postoperatively and at the final follow-up.[30] A retrospective study of patients aged 50 to 70 years also compared percutaneous wire versus volar locking plate fixation and similarly demonstrated improved range of motion at the final follow-up in the volar plate group.[35] Of note, this study initiated range of motion at 2 weeks for the volar locking plate group versus 8 to 10 weeks in the pinning group, whereas the prior study initiated wrist motion at 4 to 5 days for volar locking plate (VLP) versus 3 weeks for pinning, highlighting another advantage of volar locking plate fixation, which is the ability to initiate early motion and return to function. Similarly, Karantana and colleagues[36] prospectively randomized 130 patients to volar locking plates versus Kirschner wire fixation with or without external fixator. The volar locking plate patients were mobilized at 2 weeks after surgery, whereas the percutaneous fixation group was mobilized at 6 weeks. Again, the volar plate group demonstrated early improved range of motion and grip strength. However, the differences equalized between the groups by 12 weeks; at 1 year, the patient-centered outcome scores were equivalent.

Intramedullary radial nailing has also emerged as an alternative to volar locking plating (**Fig. 2**). Purported benefits include minimally invasive insertion techniques and a zero-profile implant that can minimize long-term soft tissue complications.[37] Safi and colleagues[38] randomly assigned patients (average age of 55 years) to an intramedullary nail or a volar locking plate, mobilizing both groups immediately postoperatively. At 6 weeks, the disability score and range of motion were better in the intramedullary nailing group; but by 3 months the differences were minimal, and by 12 months the groups were equivalent.

Fracture-spanning fixation, including external fixation or bridge plating, is also a commonly used method for the fixation of osteopenic distal radius fractures (**Fig. 3**). These methods are especially appealing in badly comminuted fractures whereby they can serve to maintain overall reduction without extensive surgical dissection while also providing pain relief. This construct can also allow immediate weight bearing for assistive devices. A recent meta-analysis of volar locking plates versus external fixation reviewed 6 studies comparing the two methods. The meta-analysis found a significantly lower reoperation rate in the ex-fix group but a statistically significant (albeit clinically minor) better outcome at 3, 6, and 12 months in the volar plate group.[39] Although no

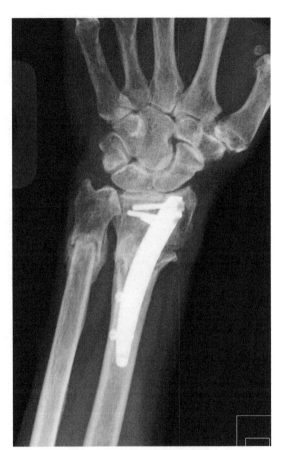

Fig. 2. Intramedullary nailing of a displaced osteoporotic distal radius fracture. This construct provides immediate stability using a load-sharing construct while leaving no prominent hardware and potentially avoiding late soft tissue complications.

direct head-to-head comparisons of bridge plating and volar locking plates exist, the technique has been well described for use in comminuted distal radius fractures. Richard and colleagues[40] retrospectively reviewed 33 patients older than 60 years with comminuted fractures treated with bridge plating. All fractures healed, and the DASH (disabilities of the arm, shoulder, and hand) score averaged 32 at 47 weeks (mean follow-up). Another study, performed on 62 patients, examined the use of this method in polytrauma and also found a 100% healing rate. Although the clinical follow-up is not as detailed in this study, it is noteworthy that these patients were allowed to bear weight through a bridged fracture at 1 month postoperatively with crutches or walkers.[41] Although this technique has a place in the treatment of comminuted fractures not amenable to volar locking plates, the requirement for a second surgery and the inability to perform early wrist range of motion renders it a second-line treatment.

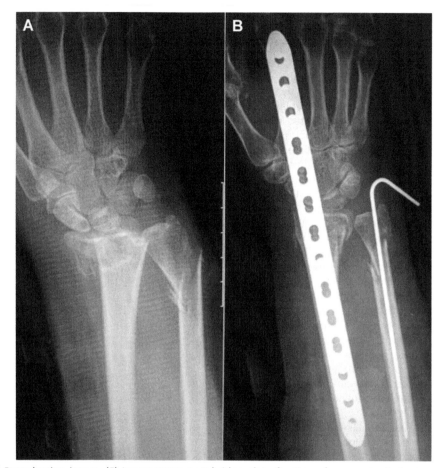

Fig. 3. (*A*) Prereduction image. (*B*) Image status post bridge plate fixation of a comminuted osteoporotic distal radius fracture. This construct provides immediate stability and weight bearing while minimizing surgical exposure and dissection. Removal of hardware is required once the fracture has healed.

Other recent trials, however, have cast into doubt the indications for surgical fixation of distal radius fractures in low-demand elderly patients. Egol and colleagues[42] randomized patients older than 65 years to operative treatment versus closed reduction and splinting and found equivalent disability scores in both groups, although grip strength and radiographic outcomes were better in the operative cohort. Although this study was lacking in randomization (patients were allowed to choose operative versus nonoperative treatment in cases of failure of closed reduction), its conclusions were borne out later by Arora and colleagues.[43] This latter study prospectively randomized patients 65 years of age or older with unstable, displaced distal radius fractures to operative versus nonoperative treatment and found that disability scores, although worse during early follow-up in the nonoperative group, also evened out by 6 months despite inferior radiographic outcomes in the nonoperative group. Of course, the findings of these studies must take into account the unknown long-term risk and significance of developing posttraumatic arthritis of the wrist with nonoperative treatment.[44,45] Moreover, despite expecting acceptable functional outcomes, patients must be informed early that with nonoperative treatment the appearance of their wrist will be altered permanently (**Fig. 4**).

DISCUSSION

Distal radius fragility fractures in osteoporosis present a unique and discrete subset of distal radius fractures, unique in both biology and in the population they affect. Given the large number of these injuries that occur each year, their management is of significant concern to all practicing orthopedic surgeons.

Given the wide variety of distal radius fractures sustained by the elderly, and the tremendous variation in functional requirements within this

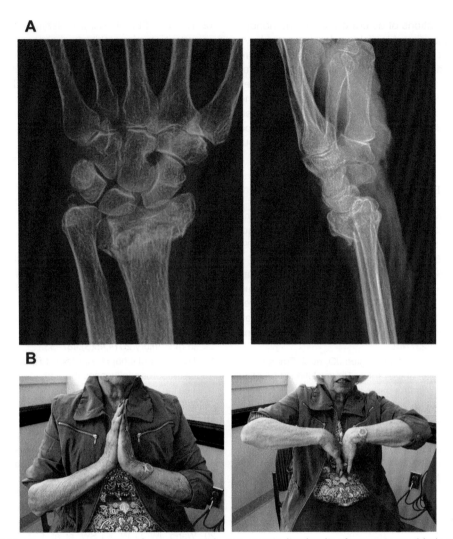

Fig. 4. (*A*) (1) AP and (2) lateral xrays of a comminuted osteoporotic distal radius fracture in an elderly woman. (*B*) Nonsurgical treatment was selected, despite poor radiographic alignment, the patient has regained good functional range of motion as demonstrated here in (1) extension and (2) flexion.

population, it is difficult to generalize regarding treatment of these fractures. Furthermore, osteoporosis tends to strike a population at risk for other illnesses as well as general deconditioning, complicating any study of outcomes within this group. An understanding of the basic biology and circumstances surrounding the fractures, in combination with an understanding of individual patient circumstance, can, however, inform the choice of treatment.

Osteopenic or osteoporotic bone, present by definition in these fragility-type fractures, suffers from qualitative and quantitative changes to both cortical and trabecular bone, resulting in a weaker shell of cortex surrounding a less-dense trabecular matrix. The advent of locking plates has allowed

for more secure fixation in these bones without requiring bicortical screws[46] and provided a means to avoid some of the soft tissue complications traditionally associated with dorsal plating while also facilitating early motion.

The biology of fragility fracture healing is incompletely understood, but current studies have demonstrated deficits in mechanical properties during the acute healing phase. The callus formed by osteoporotic bone has decreased stiffness and is less mineralized than that formed by normal bone. Although this mechanical insufficiency theoretically puts fragility fractures at risk for displacement with nonoperative treatment, the standard practice of immobilization with cast or splint allows the callus time to consolidate.

The implications of osteoporosis on the nonoperative management in distal radius fractures have been thrust into the spotlight given the literature demonstrating the equivalence of long-term results. As a result, the art of treating these fractures is the decision for or against surgery, of balancing a diminished healing capacity with decreased functional demands. In the end, such a question can never be fully answered by evidence but must take individual patients into account.

REFERENCES

1. Chung KC, Shauver MJ, Birkmeyer JD. Trends in the United States in the treatment of distal radial fractures in the elderly. J Bone Joint Surg Am 2009; 91(8):1868–73.
2. Arora R, Gabl M, Gschwentner M, et al. A comparative study of clinical and radiologic outcomes of unstable Colles type distal radius fractures in patients older than 70 years: nonoperative treatment versus volar locking plating. J Orthop Trauma 2009;23(4):237–42.
3. Koval KJ, Harrast JJ, Anglen JO, et al. Fractures of the distal part of the radius. The evolution of practice over time. Where's the evidence? J Bone Joint Surg Am 2008;90(9):1855–61.
4. Young BT, Rayan GM. Outcome following nonoperative treatment of displaced distal radius fractures in low-demand patients older than 60 years. J Hand Surg Am 2000;25(1):19–28.
5. Maravic M, Le Bihan C, Landais P, et al. Incidence and cost of osteoporotic fractures in France during 2001. A methodological approach by the national hospital database. Osteoporos Int 2005;16(12): 1475–80.
6. Court-Brown CM, Caesar B. Epidemiology of adult fractures: a review. Injury 2006;37(8):691–7.
7. Brogren E, Petranek M, Atroshi I. Incidence and characteristics of distal radius fractures in a southern Swedish region. BMC Musculoskelet Disord 2007;8:48.
8. Hung LK, Wu HT, Leung PC, et al. Low BMD is a risk factor for low-energy Colles' fractures in women before and after menopause. Clin Orthop Relat Res 2005;435:219–25.
9. Lofman O, Hallberg I, Berglund K, et al. Women with low-energy fracture should be investigated for osteoporosis. Acta Orthop 2007;78(6):813–21.
10. Øyen J, Apalset EM, Gjesdal CG, et al. Vitamin D inadequacy is associated with low-energy distal radius fractures: a case–control study. Bone 2011; 48(5):1140–5.
11. Spadaro JA, Werner FW, Brenner RA, et al. Cortical and trabecular bone contribute strength to the osteopenic distal radius. J Orthop Res 1994;12(2):211–8.
12. Kawalilak CE, Johnston JD, Olszynski WP, et al. Characterizing microarchitectural changes at the distal radius and tibia in postmenopausal women using HR-pQCT. Osteoporos Int 2014;25(8):2057–66.
13. Stein EM, Kepley A, Walker M, et al. Skeletal structure in postmenopausal women with osteopenia and fractures is characterized by abnormal trabecular plates and cortical thinning. J Bone Miner Res 2014;29(5):1101–9.
14. Bala Y, Zebaze R, Ghasem-Zadeh A, et al. Cortical Porosity Identifies Women with Osteopenia at Increased Risk for Forearm Fractures. Journal of bone and mineral research: the official journal of the American Society for Bone and Mineral Research 2014;29(6):1356–62.
15. Bjørnerem Å, Bui QM, Ghasem-Zadeh A, et al. Fracture risk and height: an association partly accounted for by cortical porosity of relatively thinner cortices. J Bone Miner Res 2013;28(9):2017–26.
16. Thormann U, El Khawassna T, Ray S, et al. Differences of bone healing in metaphyseal defect fractures between osteoporotic and physiological bone in rats. Injury 2014;45(3):487–93.
17. Namkung-Matthai H, Appleyard R, Jansen J, et al. Osteoporosis influences the early period of fracture healing in a rat osteoporotic model. Bone 2001; 28(1):80–6.
18. Kubo T, Shiga T, Hashimoto J, et al. Osteoporosis influences the late period of fracture healing in a rat model prepared by ovariectomy and low calcium diet. J Steroid Biochem Mol Biol 1999;68(5–6):197–202.
19. Xu SW, Wang JW, Li W, et al. Osteoporosis impairs fracture healing of tibia in a rat osteoporotic model. Zhonghua yi xue za zhi 2004;84(14):1205–9 [in Chinese].
20. Wang JW, Li W, Xu SW, et al. Osteoporosis influences the middle and late periods of fracture healing in a rat osteoporotic model. Chin J Traumatol 2005;8(2):111–6.
21. Qiao L, Xu KH, Liu HW, et al. Effects of ovariectomy on fracture healing in female rats. Sichuan da xue xue bao Yi xue ban 2005;36(1):108–11 [in Chinese].
22. Walsh WR, Sherman P, Howlett CR, et al. Fracture healing in a rat osteopenia model. Clin Orthop Relat Res 1997;(342):218–27.
23. Meyer RA Jr, Tsahakis PJ, Martin DF, et al. Age and ovariectomy impair both the normalization of mechanical properties and the accretion of mineral by the fracture callus in rats. J Orthop Res 2001; 19(3):428–35.
24. Giannoudis P, Tzioupis C, Almalki T, et al. Fracture healing in osteoporotic fractures: Is it really different?: a basic science perspective. Injury 2007;38(Suppl 1): S90–9.
25. Meyer U, de Jong JJ, Bours SGP, et al. Early changes in bone density, microarchitecture, bone resorption, and inflammation predict the clinical

outcome 12 weeks after conservatively treated distal radius fractures: an exploratory study. J Bone Miner Res 2014;29(9):2065–73.

26. Orbay JL, Fernandez DL. Volar fixed-angle plate fixation for unstable distal radius fractures in the elderly patient. J Hand Surg Am 2004;29(1):96–102.

27. Chung KC, Watt AJ, Kotsis SV, et al. Treatment of unstable distal radial fractures with the volar locking plating system. J Bone Joint Surg Am 2006;88(12):2687–94.

28. Rein S, Schikore H, Schneiders W, et al. Results of dorsal or volar plate fixation of AO type C3 distal radius fractures: a retrospective study. J Hand Surg Am 2007;32(7):954–61.

29. Wright TW, Horodyski M, Smith DW. Functional outcome of unstable distal radius fractures: ORIF with a volar fixed-angle tine plate versus external fixation. J Hand Surg Am 2005;30(2):289–99.

30. Oshige T, Sakai A, Zenke Y, et al. A comparative study of clinical and radiological outcomes of dorsally angulated, unstable distal radius fractures in elderly patients: intrafocal pinning versus volar locking plating. J Hand Surg 2007;32(9):1385–92.

31. Wichlas F, Haas NP, Disch A, et al. Complication rates and reduction potential of palmar versus dorsal locking plate osteosynthesis for the treatment of distal radius fractures. J Orthop Trauma 2014;15(4):259–64.

32. Kandemir U, Matityahu A, Desai R, et al. Does a volar locking plate provide equivalent stability as a dorsal nonlocking plate in a dorsally comminuted distal radius fracture?: a biomechanical study. J Orthop Trauma 2008;22(9):605–10.

33. Trease C, McIff T, Toby EB. Locking versus nonlocking T-plates for dorsal and volar fixation of dorsally comminuted distal radius fractures: a biomechanical study. J Hand Surg Am 2005;30(4):756–63.

34. Gondusky JS, Carney J, Erpenbach J, et al. Biomechanical comparison of locking versus nonlocking volar and dorsal t-plates for fixation of dorsally comminuted distal radius fractures. J Orthop Trauma 2011;25(1):44–50.

35. Lee YS, Wei TY, Cheng YC, et al. A comparative study of Colles' fractures in patients between fifty and seventy years of age: percutaneous K-wiring versus volar locking plating. Int Orthop 2012;36(4):789–94.

36. Karantana A, Downing ND, Forward DP, et al. Surgical treatment of distal radial fractures with a volar locking plate versus conventional percutaneous methods: a randomized controlled trial. J Bone Joint Surg Am 2013;95(19):1737–44.

37. Ilyas AM, Thoder JJ. Intramedullary fixation of displaced distal radius fractures: a preliminary report. J Hand Surg Am 2008;33(10):1706–15.

38. Safi A, Hart R, Těkněďžjan B, et al. Treatment of extra-articular and simple articular distal radial fractures with intramedullary nail versus volar locking plate. J Hand Surg Eur Vol 2013;38(7):774–9.

39. Li-Hai Z, Ya-Nan W, Zhi M, et al. Volar locking plate versus external fixation for the treatment of unstable distal radial fractures: a meta-analysis of randomized controlled trials. J Surg Res 2014;193(1):324–33.

40. Richard MJ, Katolik LI, Hanel DP, et al. Distraction plating for the treatment of highly comminuted distal radius fractures in elderly patients. J Hand Surg 2012;37(5):948–56.

41. Hanel DP, Lu TS, Weil WM. Bridge plating of distal radius fractures: the Harborview method. Clin Orthop Relat Res 2006;445:91–9.

42. Egol KA, Walsh M, Romo-Cardoso S, et al. Distal radial fractures in the elderly: operative compared with nonoperative treatment. J Bone Joint Surg Am 2010;92(9):1851–7.

43. Arora R, Lutz M, Deml C, et al. A prospective randomized trial comparing nonoperative treatment with volar locking plate fixation for displaced and unstable distal radial fractures in patients sixty-five years of age and older. J Bone Joint Surg Am 2011;93(23):2146–53.

44. Cannada LK. Commentary on an article by K.A. Egol, MD, et al.: distal radial fractures in the elderly: operative compared with nonoperative treatment. J Bone Joint Surg Am 2010;92(9):e11.

45. Lichtman DM, Bindra RR, Boyer MI, et al. Treatment of distal radius fractures. J Am Acad Orthop Surg 2010;18(3):180–9.

46. Wall LB, Brodt MD, Silva MJ, et al. The effects of screw length on stability of simulated osteoporotic distal radius fractures fixed with volar locking plates. J Hand Surg 2012;37(3):446–53.

Scapholunate Ligament Tears
Acute Reconstructive Options

Patrick J. Ward, MD, John R. Fowler, MD*

KEYWORDS

- Scapholunate advanced collapse • Capsulodesis • Scapholunate axis method
- Reduction and association of scaphoid and lunate • Scapholunate ligament

KEY POINTS

- Left untreated, scapholunate (SL) ligament tears can result in a predictable pattern of radiocarpal arthritis, termed *SL advanced collapse (SLAC)*.
- SL reconstruction is indicated in symptomatic patients without evidence of radiocarpal arthritis. Patients with established radiocarpal arthritis may be better served with a salvage procedure.
- Most current treatments have not been shown to reliably maintain reduction of the SL interval and SL angle at long-term follow-up.
- Currently there is no consensus on the optimal treatment method for patients with SL ligament tears.
- Several new treatment methods for SL ligament tears have been developed but need further clinical evaluation.

INTRODUCTION

The SL interosseous ligament (SLIL) is an important structure for maintaining normal carpal alignment and kinematics.[1] SL instability can be defined as a wrist that exhibits abnormal kinematics with motion and is symptomatic during weight-bearing activities and normal arc of motion.[1] Untreated, SL instability leads to a predictable pattern of radiocarpal arthritis referred to as SLAC. The decision to repair or reconstruct the SLIL is predicated on the absence of radiocarpal arthritis. Patients with evidence of established radiocarpal arthritis are better treated with salvage procedures. Ideally, an orthopedic surgeon can intervene and prevent the development of an SLAC wrist. The purpose of this article is to review the reconstructive treatment options for SL instability.

Epidemiology

The SLIL is the most commonly injured intercarpal ligament and it results in the most frequent pattern of carpal instability.[2] The prevalence of this injury is likely underestimated because it is commonly missed on initial presentation. Cadaveric studies have found tears in approximately one-third of wrists in elderly patients, many with no history of wrist injury.[3,4] These tears may represent a combination of acute and degenerative tears. In a clinical study, Jones[5] reviewed 100 cases of wrist injuries in which a sprained wrist was the initial diagnosis. Subsequently, a clenched fist radiograph was preformed and 19 of 100 patients had an increase in the SL interval. Significant SL instability was ultimately diagnosed in 5 patients. Intercarpal ligamentous injuries are also common in association with distal radius fractures and scaphoid fractures.

Department of Orthopaedic Surgery, University of Pittsburgh, Suite 1010, Kaufmann Building, 3471 Fifth Avenue, Pittsburgh, PA 15213, USA
* Corresponding author.
E-mail address: Johnfowler10@gmail.com

Orthop Clin N Am 46 (2015) 551–559
http://dx.doi.org/10.1016/j.ocl.2015.06.013
0030-5898/15/$ – see front matter © 2015 Elsevier Inc. All rights reserved.

SL ligament tears have been reported to occur in as high as 54% of displaced distal radius fractures[6] and instability can be seen in as many as 21.5% of cases.[7] Jorgsholm and colleagues[8] found SL ligament injuries in approximately 50% of scaphoid waist fractures and complete disruption in 24%. These findings point to the importance of maintaining a high index of suspicion when treating patients with wrist injuries.

Anatomy

The wrist joint is kinematically one of the most complex joints in the body. In actuality, it is the summation of several smaller joints, including the articulations between the carpals bones, radius, ulna, and metacarpals. It can be conceptually simplified into the distal row (trapezium, trapezoid, capitate, and hamate), proximal row (scaphoid, lunate, and triquetrum), and the surrounding articulations. The distal row is tightly bound by strong intercarpal ligaments with little motion between its constituents. The bones of the proximal row functionally are intercalary pieces because there are no tendinous insertions on them and their motion depends on their articulations, with the surrounding intrinsic and extrinsic ligaments restricting their motion.[9] The SLIL is one of these intrinsic ligaments. It is C-shaped, running between the dorsal, volar, and proximal thirds of the bones. It is generally subdivided based on anatomic location. The dorsal portion is the most robust and strongest, comprised primarily of collagen. It is the primary restraint to distraction, torsion, and translation.[10] The volar portion is also collagenous but thin and provides primarily rotational control. The proximal portion is comprised of fibrocartilage and is grossly membranous with little restraint to motion. Several extrinsic ligaments function as secondary stabilizers and their disruption in isolation do not cause frank SL instability.[11] Important volar ligaments are the radioscaphocapitate ligament, radiolunate ligaments, and the radioscapholunate ligament. Dorsally the dorsal intercarpal ligament and dorsal radiotriquetral ligament assist in SL stabilization.

Mechanism of Injury

Injury to the SLIL usually occurs with stress loading of extended carpus. It can occur with a fall onto an outstretched hand or with higher-energy trauma. The theorized mechanism for injury during a fall on an outstretched hand is wrist extension, intercarpal supination, and ulnar deviation, which cause failure of the SLIL.[12] In severe hyperextension, the injury continues causing, in succession, tears of the radiocapitate,

radiotriquetral, and dorsal radiocarpal ligaments. The lunate then falls into extension by virtue of is attachment to triquetrum, and dorsal intercalated segment instability (DISI) deformity occurs.

When the SLIL is injured, there is variable presentation based on the severity of the injury to the secondary stabilizing ligaments and surrounding soft tissues. Left unchecked this instability can progress in a stepwise succession to frank arthritis. Determination of the stage of SL instability is important because it can guide treatment. Geissler and colleagues[13] proposed a method to quantify SL injury by arthroscopic assessment with a probe. In grade I injury there is attenuation but no step-off. Grade II injuries have attenuation with incongruency between the scaphoid and lunate. Grades III and IV injuries have complete SLIL disruption but in grade III a 1-mm probe passes through the SL interval and in grade IV a 2.7-mm probe passes through.

The least severe presentation of SL instability is termed *occult instability*. In this pattern there is either a tear or attenuation of the SL ligament but generally no radiographic findings, even with stress radiographs. The only hint is pain with mechanical loading or painful clunks. The next step in progression occurs when patients have normal static radiographs but abnormal stress radiographs. These patients have dynamic instability and have subtotal or complete SL disruptions with partial disruption of the secondary stabilizers.[12] An anteroposterior (AP) grip film with 2 to 3 mm of increased gapping compared with the contralateral wrist, is suggestive of SL insufficiency.[14] Lateral full flexion radiographs show an SL angle greater than 60% and subluxation of the proximal pole of the scaphoid to contact the volar articular surface of the radius. Radial and ulnar deviation films may also show SL widening.

After dynamic instability is static instability in which there are abnormal static radiographs. These patients have complete disruption of the SLIL and 1 or more of the secondary stabilizing ligaments. Cadaveric studies have recognized the dorsal intercarpal (DIC) ligament as one of the most important stabilizing ligaments, allowing palmar subluxation of the lunate.[15,16] As the motions of the scaphoid and lunate are uncoupled, they rotate in opposite directions. The scaphoid rotates into increased flexion as the SL gap increases.[17] The lunate extends with mechanical loading due to the dorsally directed force of the capitate. With time, abnormal motion becomes a deformity and static radiographs are abnormal, termed *DISI with fixed flexion of the scaphoid and extension of the lunate and triquetrum*. The distal carpal row translates proximally and dorsally.[9] When a patient has demonstrated DISI deformity, soft tissue procedure alone is ineffective due to attenuation and degeneration of secondary stabilizers as well as surrounding soft tissue envelope. The abnormal kinematics of the wrist lead to degenerative changes found in SLAC wrists. Watson and colleagues[18,19] described the sequential arthritic evolution of an SLAC wrist in 1984. Initially the degenerative changes are limited to the articulation between the tip of the radial styloid and radial aspect of the distal pole of the scaphoid. Next they involve the entire radioscaphoid articulation. Later the changes progress to the capitolunate joint due to abnormal articular wear as the capitate migrates proximally between the capitate and lunate.[18,19]

In general, reconstructive options are indicated in cases of SL dissociation without evidence of degenerative changes.

TREATMENT
Capsulodesis

Acute surgical intervention is believed to improve outcomes with the goal of intervening before arthritic changes have set in. Capsulodesis is designed is to reinforce the extrinsic ligaments. Unfortunately, the procedure often sacrifices postoperative flexion. It is indicated in both chronic and subacute settings. It was classically described without SL ligament repair; however, when possible, a ligamentous repair should be done. Since the original description by Blatt in 1987,[20] multiple modifications have been described. Blatt capsulodesis was designed to limit palmar flexion of the scaphoid. It involves a straight dorsal capsulotomy, raising a radially-based capsular flap that is left attached to the radius. The scaphoid and lunate are reduced using Kirschner (K) wires as joysticks and the flap is then attached to the distal pole of the scaphoid via a bony trough and tied over a button. The scaphoid is pinned to the capitate for 3 months.[20] Short-term outcomes showed good symptomatic relief and patient satisfaction rates of 58%. There was, however, poor restoration of normal carpal relationships, in particular SL widening, and some patients developed SLAC wrists requiring further surgery.[21]

Several investigators have described combining the capsulodesis with suture and anchors repairing the SLIL. Lavernia and colleagues[22] evaluated 21 patients at an average follow-up of 33 months and found 11° loss of palmar flexion and similar grip strength to the contralateral side. Approximately 50% patients reported that wrist function still interfered with activities. The SL angle improved from 62° to 57° degrees and SL gap reduced from 3.2 mm to 1.9 mm. Uhl and colleagues[23] examined 35 patients at an average of 36 months finding an average loss of 15° flexion and 85% recovery of grip strength. A majority of patients (25/35) returned to their preinjury job. The SL gap recurred in all patients but the investigators noted that radiographic recurrence of the SL gap did not correlate with symptoms. Pomerance[24] evaluated 17 patients at an average follow-up of 66 months. Grip strength was 82% percent of the uninjured wrist and all patients reporting continued pain with activity (1 severe, 7 moderate, and 7 mild). SL angle on average progressed from 49° preoperatively to 54° at follow-up and 3 developed an SLAC wrist. The investigators noted that at long-term follow-up, initial clinical and radiographic gains deteriorated, especially in patients with a strenuous occupation.

Berger and colleagues[25] described a capsular-sparing approach in which the dorsal radiocarpal and DIC ligaments are split, creating a flap with the apex at the triquetrum (**Fig. 1**). To perform the capsulodesis (Mayo capsulodesis [MC]), the proximal strip of the flap is attached to dorsal lunate after the lunate is derotated from extension to a neutral position and held in place with K-wires. Moran conducted a retrospective review of 31 patients, at a mean follow-up of 54 months, who were treated with either a Blatt capsulodesis or MC. The investigators noted an average loss of wrist flexion of 20° and no improvement in grip strength after surgery. Pain was minimal or none in approximately 60% of patients, but more than 20% of patients continued to complain of severe pain with activities of daily living. Although the preoperative SL gap was corrected from 2.7 mm to 1.7 mm, the mean SL gap at final follow-up was 3.9 mm. The study did not analyze differences between the Blatt capsulodesis and MC techniques.[26] Wyrick and colleagues[27] reviewed 17 patients at mean follow-up of 30 months and found that no patients were pain-free and radiographic improvements obtained at the time of surgery were not maintained. The mean SL angle preoperatively was 78° and the final mean SL angle was 72°. Mean total wrist arc of motion was only 60% of the contralateral side and mean grip strength was 70% of the contralateral side.

Szabo described a technique of SL ligament repair with DIC reinforcement. A standard dorsal approach to the wrist is used and the DIC is dissected and isolated using umbilical tape (**Fig. 2**A). The SL interval is reduced and held in place with a scaphocapitate K-wire and an SL K-wire. The SLIL is then repaired with anchors. The DIC is sharply detached from the trapezium and trapezoid and transferred to a trough in the distal

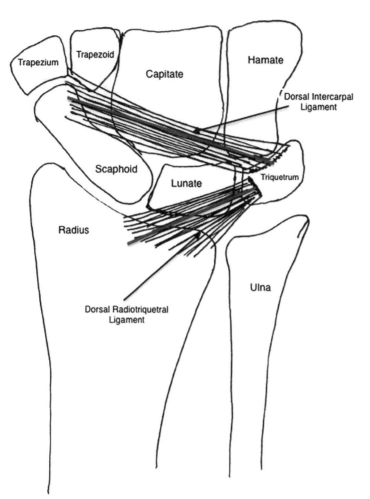

Fig. 1. Drawing depicting the Berger capsular-sparing approach to the wrist. (*Courtesy of* John R. Fowler, MD, Pittsburgh, PA.)

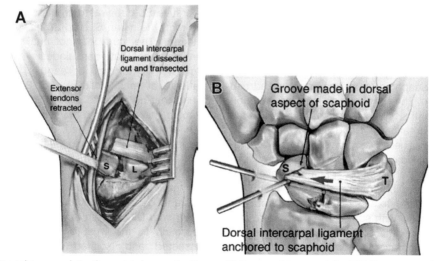

Fig. 2. (*A*) Dorsal approach to the wrist demonstrating an SL ligament tear and the DIC ligament and removal of the DIC from its radial insertion. (*B*) Repair of the SL ligament with a suture anchor, pinning of the scaphoid to the lunate and scaphoid to the capitate, and reattachment of the DIC to the distal pole of the scaphoid (*red arrow*) to prevent scaphoid flexion. L, lunate; S, scaphoid. (*From* Szabo RM. Scapholunate ligament repair with capsulodesis reinforcement. J Hand Surg Am 2008;33(9):1648–49; with permission.)

pole of the scaphoid (see **Fig. 2**B). The purpose of the transfer is to prevent flexion of the scaphoid. The pins are cut below the skin and removed at 8 weeks. Gajendran and colleagues[28] reviewed 15 patients, at an average of 86 months, who underwent this modification of the MC technique. The investigators noted that the procedure does not maintain SL angle or SL gap and that 50% of patients demonstrated radiographic arthritis. Given the poor results with capsulodesis, researchers have attempted to supplement SL repair with other methods.

Reduction and Association of the Scaphoid and Lunate

Reduction and association of the scaphoid and lunate (RASL) is a procedure that reduces an SL gap and places a temporary screw across the SL interval. The goal is to stabilize the 2 bones for a sufficient period of time to allow formation of a neoligament that would allow a small degree of motion between the 2 bones, reproducing natural biomechanics.[29] The theory is similar to syndesmotic screw fixation of the ankle. The technique involves a universal dorsal approach to the wrist. K-wires are inserted into the scaphoid and lunate and are used as joysticks. The joysticks are used to gap open the SL interval and the remnants of the SL ligament are excised. A burr is used to remove the cartilage between the scaphoid and lunate. A second incision is made on the radial side of the wrist and the 1st dorsal compartment is opened. A radial styloidectomy is performed to facilitate screw placement. The joysticks are used to reduce the SL interval and a cannulated screw is then placed. Rosenwasser and colleagues[29] described the use of a cannulated headless compression screw; however, standard partially threaded cancellous screws also may be used. Cognet and colleagues[30] reported partial destruction of the scaphoid and/or lunate in all 7 patients in their series. The investigators stated that they no longer use the procedure. Larson and Stern[31] reviewed 8 wrists at mean follow-up of 38 months. The investigators noted a loss of reduction in all patients with development of an SLAC wrist in 1 patient. Mean grip strength was 77% of the contralateral side and total arc of motion decreased 9° compared with preoperative values. Caloia and colleagues[32] studied 9 wrists undergoing arthroscopic RASL at mean follow-up of 35 months. Mean grip strength was 78% of the contralateral side and postoperative total arc of motion was 107°. The SL angle decreased from 70.5° to 59.3°. In 3 cases, screws were removed owing to loosening or symptoms.

Ligament Reconstruction

Several investigators have described various techniques for ligament reconstruction. In 1995, Brunelli and Brunelli[33] described a technique in which a slip of the flexor carpi radialis (FCR) tendon is used to stabilize the SL joint. In the original technique, both dorsal and palmar approaches to the wrist were used and a 7-cm slip of FCR tendon harvested while retaining its attachment to the volar 2nd metacarpal. A hole was then drilled in the distal pole of the scaphoid, parallel to its distal articular margin, and the tendon passed through the tunnel. When tightened, this corrects the palmar flexion of the scaphoid. Then tendon was then sutured into the dorsoulnar edge of the distal radius, the scaphoid pinned in place with K-wires, and dorsal capsule repaired. A majority of patients returned to their occupations and had good strength and pain resolution, but the average loss of flexion was 45°.[33] In response to poor postoperative wrist flexion, Van Den Abbeele and colleagues[34] modified the procedure so that the distal slip of FCR was no longer anchored in the radius. Instead, the tendon was looped under or though the dorsal radiolunotriquetral ligament (RLT) and secured to the lunate (**Fig. 3**). This procedure was termed *modified Brunelli tenodesis (MBT)*. Pain improved from an average of 7 preoperatively to an average of 3 at final follow-up of only 9 months. Grip strength and wrist function scores were unchanged from preoperative levels. Range of motion decreased after surgery, especially in flexion and extension. Talwalkar and

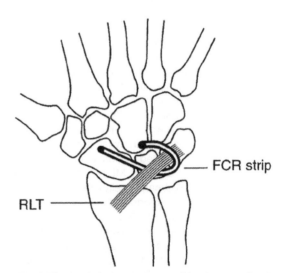

Fig. 3. The MBT. (*From* Van Den Abbeele KL, Loh YC, Stanley JK, et al. Early results of a modified Brunelli procedure for scapholunate instability. J Hand Surg Br 1998;23:260; with permission.)

colleagues[35] reviewed 162 patients who underwent MBT (55 patients for clinical evaluation and 117 with a questionnaire) at a mean follow-up of 4.1 years. The investigators found a 31% reduced flexion, 20% less grip strength then contralateral, 62% with little to no pain, and 79% satisfaction.

Nienstedt[36] reported on the long-term follow-up of patients who underwent MBT for treatment of SL instability. At an average follow-up of 14 years, the SL angle increased from 46° immediately postoperatively to 63° at final follow-up. The SL interval widened from an average of 2.4 mm immediately postoperatively to an average of 2.8 mm at final follow-up. Despite loss of radiographic parameters, patients reported an average Disabilities of the Arm, Shoulder and Hand (DASH) score of 9 and average Mayo wrist score of 83, indicating good outcomes. Chabas and colleagues[37] reviewed 19 patients treated with chronic SL instability who were treated with MBT. At an average of just over 36 months, 15 had minimal pain and 4 had constant pain. Mean wrist flexion was 41° and mean wrist extension was 50°. Only 1 patient went onto develop SLAC arthritis. Garcia-Elias and colleagues[38] reviewed 38 subjects at a mean follow-up of 46 months and found 74% had pain relief at rest and 76% could return to their previous occupations. Two patients had recurrence of DISI, 7 had arthritis at the radial styloid and 2 developed SLAC wrist. Sousa and colleagues[39] reported on 22 patients treated with the MBT technique at mean follow-up of 61 months. On average, patients lost approximately 20° of flexion and extension and grip strength return to only 67% of the contralateral side. Degenerative changes were noted in 3 of 22 patients at final follow-up.

Moran and colleagues[40] compared MBT (15 patients) with MC (14 patients). At a mean of approximately 36 months, these patients with chronic SL instability were compared. Grip strength (91% MC vs 87% MBT), average range of motion (64% MC vs 63% MBT) and Mayo wrist scores (77 MC vs 74 MBT) were not significantly different between the 2 groups. There was 1 frank failure in the tenodesis group resulting in wrist fusion. Pollock and colleagues[41] used cadaveric wrists to compare the MC and the MBT and found that MBT better restored carpal relationships on both static and dynamic radiographs.

Fook and Fernandex[42] described the use of an MBT with temporary screw fixation across the SL interval. The investigators reviewed 36 patients at a mean follow-up of 7.9 years and noted that 95% had mild or no pain. Mean wrist flexion was 51° and mean wrist extension 55°. Mean SL angle was 56°. Almquist and colleagues[43] described a "four-bone ligamentous weaver reconstruction"

for chronic SL dissociation. Drill holes are placed in the proximal neck of the capitate, nonarticular surface of the lunate, distal radius, and proximal pole of the scaphoid. Half of the extensor carpi radialis brevis is harvested and passed from dorsal to volar through the capitate, then from volar to dorsal through the lunate, from dorsal to volar through the proximal pole of the scaphoid, and finally from volar to dorsal through the radius (**Fig. 4**). The tendon graft is then sutured to the dorsal periosteum and/or wrist capsule. The investigators reviewed 36 patients at mean follow-up of 4.8 years. Average extension was 52° and flexion was 27°. Grip strength returned to 73% of the noninvolved side. The investigators noted no evidence of degenerative changes on radiographs.

Links[44] retrospectively compared 2 groups of patients with chronic SL dissociation. One group received an MBT with RASL (**Fig. 5**) and the other group received a 4-tendon weave as described by Almquist and colleagues.[43] The investigators reported better maintenance of the SL angle, less pain with grip strength, larger improvement in DASH scores, and improved grip strength when using the MBT with RASL technique.

Scapholunate Axis Method

The SL axis method (SLAM) has recently been developed by Lee and colleagues[45] for a more anatomic SLIL reconstruction (**Fig. 6**). A dorsal capsulotomy is made using either a ligament-sparing approach or inverted T. A second incision is made radially to visualize the scaphoid. A C-shaped reduction guide is placed on the proximal ulnar aspect of the lunate at its midpoint and a cannulated sleeve of the reduction guide is then applied to the lateral border of the scaphoid. A ratcheting mechanism is used to compress the SL while axial load of the carpus is performed. The SL interval is then pinned through the reduction guide to hold the alignment. A second K-wire is placed to control rotation. The reduction guide also functions as a drill guide and a cannulated drill bit is used to cross the SL interval into the lunate. A tendon autograft is harvested and threaded through the lunate bullet anchor. The anchor is then passed through the scaphoid and into the lunate. A mallet is used to secure the anchor in the lunate. The free ends of the tendon autograft are then pulled out the radial side of the scaphoid and an interference screw placed into the hole. The free tendon ends are passed over the dorsum of the scaphoid, and secured to the lunate using a suture anchor. An industry-sponsored cadaveric study has been conducted comparing

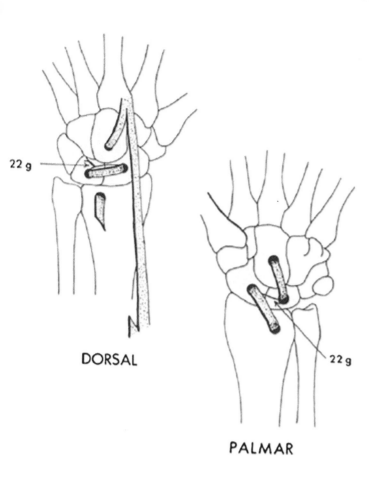

22 g

DORSAL

PALMAR

22 g

Fig. 4. The 4-bone ligament reconstruction. (*From* Almquist EE, Bach AW, Sack JT, et al. Four bone ligament reconstruction for treatment of chronic complete scapholunate separation. J Hand Surg 1991;16A:325; with permission.)

SLAM, Blatt capsulodesis, and the MBT. Twelve cadaveric limbs were randomized to 1 of the 3 procedures. Radiographs of the SLAM and MBT had improved SL interval and SLAM had the best restoration of the native SL angle. There were no complications; however, the article indicated that scaphoid fracture is a possible complication of SLAM.[45] At this point, no patient outcomes have been reported in the literature and further clinical validation is needed.

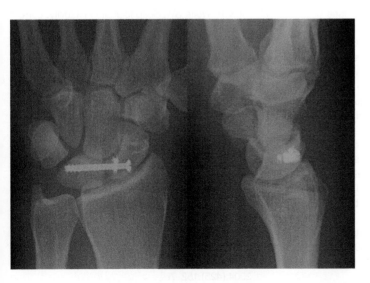

Fig. 5. Anteroposterior and lateral radiographs of the left wrist demonstrating MBT with supplemental cancellous screw. (*From* Links AC. Scapholunate interosseous ligament reconstruction: results with a modified Brunelli technique vs four-bone weave. J Hand Surg Am 2008;33: 853; with permission.)

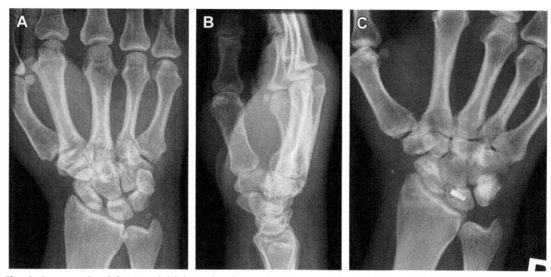

Fig. 6. Preoperative (*A*) AP and (*B*) lateral radiographs demonstrating SL interval widening and increased SL angle. (*C*) AP radiograph demonstrating correction of the SL gap after SLAM reconstruction. (*Courtesy of* John R. Fowler, MD, Pittsburgh, PA.)

SUMMARY

SL reconstruction is indicated in patients with symptomatic SL instability and absences of radiographic degenerative changes in the radiocarpal joint. Most current treatments fail to reliably maintain reduction of the SL interval and SL angle at long-term follow-up and result in decreased wrist range of motion and possibly pain. Further research is needed to determine the optimal treatment of this condition.

REFERENCES

1. Kitay, Wolfe JHS 2012 Definition of carpal instability. The Anatomy and Biomechanics Committee of the International Federation of Societies for Surgery of the Hand. J Hand Surg Am 1999;24:866–7.
2. Gelberman RH, Cooney WP III, Szabo RM. Carpal instability. J Bone Joint Surg 2000;82A:578–94.
3. Lee DH, Dickson KF, Bradley EL. The incidence of wrist interosseous ligament and triangular fibrocartilage articular disc disruptions: a cadaveric study. J Hand Surg Am 2004;29(4):676–84.
4. Wright TW, Del Charco M, Wheeler D. Incidence of ligament lesions and associated degenerative changes in the elderly wrist. J Hand Surg Am 1994;19:313–8.
5. Jones WA. Beware the sprained wrist. The incidence and diagnosis of scapholunate instability. J Bone Joint Surg Br 1988;70(2):293–7.
6. Lindau T, Arner M, Hagberg L. Intraarticular lesions in distal fractures of the radius in young adults. A descriptive arthroscopic study in 50 patients. J Hand Surg Br 1997;22:638–43.
7. Richards RS, Bennett JD, Roth JH, et al. Arthroscopic diagnosis of intra-articular soft tissue injuries associated with distal radial fractures. J Hand Surg Am 1997;22:772–6.
8. Jorgsholm P, Thomsen NO, Bjarkman A, et al. The incidence of intrinsic and extrinsic ligament injuries in scaphoid waist fractures. J Hand Surg Am 2010; 35(3):368–74.
9. Linscheid RL, Dobyns JH, Beabout JW, et al. Traumatic instability of the wrist. J Bone Joint Surg 1972;54A:1262–7.
10. Berger RA, Imeada T, Berglund L, et al. Constraint and material properties of the subregions of the scapholunate interosseous ligament. J Hand Surg Am 1999;24:953–62.
11. Kitay A, Wolfe SW. Scapholunate instability: current concepts in diagnosis and management. J Hand Surg Am 2012;37(10):2175–96.
12. Mayfield JK, Johnson RP, Kilcoyne RK. Carpal dislocations: pathomechanics and progressive perilunar instability. J Hand Surg Am 1980;5(3):226–41.
13. Geissler WB, Freeland AE, Savoie FH, et al. Intracarpal soft-tissue lesions associated with an intraarticular fracture of the distal end of the radius. J Bone Joint Surg Am 1996;78:357–65.
14. Schimmerl-Metz SM, Metz VM, Totterman SM, et al. Radiologic measurement of the scapholunate joint: implications of biologic variation in scapholunate joint morphology. J Hand Surg Am 1999;24: 1237–44.
15. Elsaidi GA, Ruch DS, Kuzma GR, et al. Dorsal wrist ligament insertions stabilize the scapholunate interval: cadaver study. Clin Orthop Relat Res 2004;(425):152–7.

16. Mitsuyasu H, Patterson RM, Shah MA, et al. The role of the dorsal intercarpal ligament in dynamic and static scapholunate instability. J Hand Surg Am 2004;29(2):279–88.

17. Drewniany JJ, Palmer AK, Flatt AE. The scaphotrapezial ligament complex: an anatomic and biomechanical study. J Hand Surg Am 1985;10:492–8.

18. Watson H, Ballet FL. The SLAC wrist: scapholunate advanced collapse pattern of degenerative arthritis. J Hand Surg Am 1984;9:358–65.

19. Watson HK, Weinzweig J, Guidera PM, et al. One thousand intercarpal arthrodeses. J Hand Surg Am 1999;24:307–15.

20. Blatt G. Capsulodesis in reconstructive hand surgery. Dorsal capsulodesis for the unstable scaphoid and volar capsulodesis following excision of the distal ulna. Hand Clin 1987;3:81–102.

21. Wintman BI, Gelberman RH, Katz JN. Dynamic scapholunate instability: results of operative treatment with dorsal capsulodesis. J Hand Surg Am 1995; 20:971–9.

22. Lavernia CJ, Cohen MS, Taleisnik J. Treatment of scapholunate dissociation by ligamentous repair and capsulodesis. J Hand Surg Am 1992;17(2): 354–9.

23. Uhl RL, Williamson SC, Bowman MW, et al. Dorsal capsulodesis using suture anchors. Am J Orthop 1997;26:547–8.

24. Pomerance J. Outcome after repair of the scapholunate interosseous ligament and dorsal capsulodesis for dynamic scapholunate instability due to trauma. J Hand Surg Am 2006;31(8):1380–6.

25. Berger RA, Bishop AT, Bettinger PC. New dorsal capsulotomy for the surgical exposure of the wrist. Ann Plast Surg 1995;35:54–9.

26. Moran SL, Cooney WP, Berger RA, et al. Capsulodesis for the treatment of chronic scapholunate instability. J Hand Surg Am 2005;30(1):16–23.

27. Wyrick JD, Youse BD, Kiefhaber TR. Scapholunate ligament repair and capsulodesis for the treatment of static scapholunate dissociation. J Hand Surg Br 1998;23:776–80.

28. Gajendran VK, Peterson B, Slater RR, et al. Long-Term Outcomes of Dorsal Intercarpal Ligament Capsulodesis for Chronic Scapholunate Dissociation. J Hand Surg Am 2007;32(9):1323–33.

29. Rosenwasser MP, Miyasaki KC, Strauch RJ. The RASL procedure: reduction and association of the scaphoid and lunate using the Herbert screw. Tech Hand Up Extrem Surg 1997;1(4):263–72.

30. Cognet JM, Levadoux M, Martinache X. The use of screws in the treatment of scapholunate instability. J Hand Surg Eur Vol 2011;36:690–3.

31. Larson TB, Stern PJ. Reduction and association of the scaphoid and lunate procedure: short-term clinical and radiographic outcomes. J Hand Surg Am 2014;39(11):2168–74.

32. Caloia M, Caloia H, Pereira E. Arthroscopic scapholunate joint reduction. Is an effective treatment for irreparable scapholunate ligament tears? Clin Orthop Relat Res 2012;470(4):972–8.

33. Brunelli GA, Brunelli GR. A new technique to correct carpal instability with scaphoid rotary subluxation: a preliminary report. J Hand Surg Am 1995;20:S82–5.

34. Van Den Abbeele KL, Loh YC, Stanley JK, et al. Early results of a modified Brunelli procedure for scapholunate instability. J Hand Surg Br 1998;23: 258–61.

35. Talwalkar SC, Edwards AT, Hayton MJ, et al. Results of tri-ligament tenodesis: a modified Brunelli procedure in the management of scapholunate instability. J Hand Surg Br 2006;31(1):110–7.

36. Nienstedt F. Treatment of static scapholunate instability with modified Brunelli tenodesis: results over 10 years. J Hand Surg Am 2013;38(5):887–92.

37. Chabas JF, Gay A, Valenti D, et al. Results of the modified Brunelli tenodesis for treatment of scapholunate instability: a retrospective study of 19 patients. J Hand Surg Am 2008;33(9):1469–77.

38. Garcia-Elias M, Lluch AL, Stanley JK. Three-ligament tenodesis for the treatment of scapholunate dissociation: indications and surgicaltechnique. J Hand Surg Am 2006;31(1):125–34.

39. Sousa M, Aido R, Freitas D, et al. Scapholunate ligament reconstruction using a flexor carpi radialis tendon graft. J Hand Surg Am 2014;39:1512–6.

40. Moran SL, Ford KS, Wulf CA, et al. Outcomes of dorsal capsulodesis and tenodesis for treatment of scapholunate instability. J Hand Surg Am 2006;31: 1438–46.

41. Pollock PJ, Sieg RN, Baechler MF, et al. Radiographic evaluation of the modified Brunelli technique versus the Blatt capsulodesis for scapholunate dissociation in a cadaver model. J Hand Surg Am 2010;35(10): 1589–98.

42. Fook MW, Fernandex FL. Chronic scapholunate instability treated with temporary screw fixation. J Hand Surg Am 2015;40(4):752–8.

43. Almquist EE, Bach AW, Sack JT, et al. Four bone ligament reconstruction for treatment of chronic complete scapholunate separation. J Hand Surg 1991; 16A:322–7.

44. Links AC. Scapholunate interosseous ligament reconstruction: results with a modified Brunelli technique versus four-bone weave. J Hand Surg Am 2008;33:850–6.

45. Lee SK, Zlotolow DA, Sapienza A, et al. Biomechanical comparison of 3 methods of scapholunate ligament reconstruction. J Hand Surg Am 2014;39(4): 643–50.

Trigger Finger
Adult and Pediatric Treatment Strategies

Juan M. Giugale, MD, John.R. Fowler, MD*

KEYWORDS

- Trigger finger • A1 pulley release • Trigger thumb • Corticosteroid injection • Percutaneous release

KEY POINTS

- Stenosing flexor tenosynovitis is a debilitating, common condition affecting both the adult and pediatric populations, causing catching, clicking, and locking of the digits.
- Several nonsurgical options are used, including anti-inflammatory medications, splinting, and/or local corticosteroid injections.
- Open A1 pulley release remains the gold standard of treatment, but percutaneous, in-office techniques have been established with similar success rates.
- Pediatric trigger finger and thumb have a distinct pathology, natural history, and treatment algorithm.

ADULT TRIGGER DIGIT

Stenosing flexor tenosynovitis of the hand, commonly known as trigger finger, is a potentially debilitating condition characterized by catching, clicking, or locking of the fingers. The etiology is any pathology between the flexor sheath and the underlying tendons that impedes smooth gliding during flexion. Early epidemiologic studies found a 2.6% lifetime risk of developing trigger finger, with an increased incidence in certain systemic conditions, such as diabetes mellitus and inflammatory arthritidies.[1] Women are more affected than men and the thumb is the most commonly involved digit.[2]

The flexor sheath, enveloping the flexor digitorum superficialis (FDS) and flexor digitorum profundus (FDP), is composed of 5 annular pulleys and 3 cruciate pulleys (**Fig. 1**). In-between the sheath and the underlying tendon is a thin synovial membrane that decreases the friction during gliding. The etiology of trigger finger is chronic repetitive friction between the tendon and the A1 pulley, which imparts a high angular load on the underlying tendon during flexion. In the thumb, the flexor pollicis longus (FPL) enters the tendon sheath at a more acute angle, in contrast to the FDP and FDS tendons, providing a mechanical strength advantage; however, this is likely the reason it has the highest incidence of stenosing flexor tenosynovitis.[3]

Histologic analysis of tissue biopsied from patients with trigger finger shows fibrocartilaginous metaplasia with positive staining for S-100 proteins, usually found in chondrocytes.[4] Similarly, biopsies of tendons diagnosed with trigger finger demonstrate disrupted fibers and hypercellularity, with an increased number of chondrocytes and glycoaminoglycans.[5] No significant amount of inflammatory cell or synoviocyte proliferation was discovered in these studies. These findings are consistent with tendinopathy and suggest that

Department of Orthopaedic Surgery, University of Pittsburgh, Suite 1010, Kaufmann Building, 3471 Fifth Avenue, Pittsburgh, PA 15213, USA
* Corresponding author.
E-mail address: Johnfowler10@gmail.com

Orthop Clin N Am 46 (2015) 561–569
http://dx.doi.org/10.1016/j.ocl.2015.06.014

orthopedic.theclinics.com

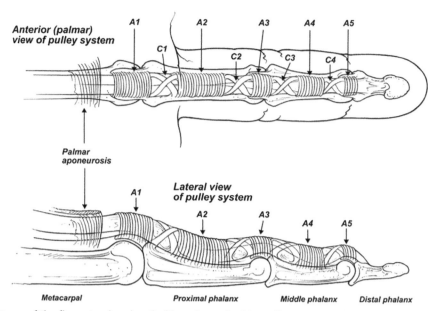

Fig. 1. Anatomy of the flexor tendon sheath. (*From* Ryzewicz M, Wolf JM. Trigger digits: principles, management, and complications. J Hand Surg Am 2006;31:136, with permission.)

the term, *flexor tenosynovitis*, is actually a misnomer because there is no evidence of synovial inflammation. The term, *flexor tendovaginosis*, has been proposed to more accurately reflect the disease process.

Ultrasound examination in patients with symptomatic trigger finger has found that the A1 pulley is significantly thicker and stiffer than normal controls.[6,7] Three weeks after corticosteroid injection, the thickness and stiffness return to values comparable with healthy A1 pulleys, whereas the cross-sectional area of the FDS and FDP tendons is unchanged.[7] Whether the instigating factor behind the development of digit triggering is a pathologic pulley system or a pathologic tendon remains unclear. By the time clinical symptoms become noticeable, both the tendon and the pulley are likely involved.

The diagnosis of trigger finger is made based on clinical findings. The natural progression of symptoms is painless clicking, followed by painful triggering, and ultimately a flexed, locked digit. With more-advanced disease, patients may report pain radiating retrograde to the forearm. Although a patient may present with advanced symptoms in a single digit, the clinician must astutely examine all other digits because severe symptoms in 1 finger may mask early signs of triggering in other digits. It is prudent to treat all affected digits simultaneously regardless of severity. Further imaging or diagnostic studies are not necessary, unless unusual examination findings warrant ruling out concomitant conditions.

The Quinnell grading system, based on mechanical symptoms, is commonly used to classify trigger finger severity (**Table 1**).[8] Freiberg and colleagues[9] proposed a 2-tier classification system based on the pattern of inflammation along the involved tendon – nodular or diffuse. The nodular group had a local, contained, palpable nodule within the tendon sheath and was found to have a much higher success rate with nonoperative management, 93%, compared with a diffuse inflammation group, 47%. The results between these 2 types of flexor tendon sheath inflammation, however, have not been reproduced in further investigations. As such, the Quinnell system is more frequently used in the clinical and research setting.

Table 1 Quinnell grading system	
Grade 0	Pain with flexion, no mechanical symptoms
Grade 1	Uneven motion during flexion/clicking
Grade 2	Locked digit that is actively corrected
Grade 3	Locked digit that is passively corrected
Grade 4	Locked digit, uncorrectable/fixed flexion contracture

Data from Quinnell R. Conservative management of trigger finger. Practitioner 1980;224:187–90.

NONSURGICAL TREATMENT

Noninvasive treatment modalities are used for mild or early cases of triggering and in patients who are opposed to injections. Activity modification, especially symptom-provoking activities, should be avoided. Although there is no scientific evidence to support the use of nonsteroidal anti-inflammatory drugs (NSAIDs), this drug class is commonly recommended to alleviate the local inflammatory response secondary to triggering. Prolonged use, however, may contribute to peptic ulcer disease and kidney failure.

Splinting is a commonly used conservative treatment option with the theoretic concept that limiting tendon gliding allows time for inflammation to resolve (**Fig. 2**). In a series of 28 patients placed in a metacarpophalangeal (MCP) blocking splint at 10° to 15° of flexion for a 6- to 10-week period, Colbourn and colleagues[10] found that 93% of patients reported improvement in symptoms. Rogers and colleagues[11] achieved 83% success with a distal interphalangeal joint blocking splint, limiting FDP excursion, in a small series of laborers. Tarbhai and colleagues[12] compared these 2 splinting techniques in a randomized trial and found a higher percentage of patients had complete or partial relief of symptoms with the MCP blocking splint (77% vs 43%), although it was subjectively reported as more cumbersome. Immobilization is most effective in mild cases of triggering, with short duration of symptoms, and requires high level of splint compliance.[9,13]

Local corticosteroids are routinely used as a first-line treatment of trigger finger of all severities. Although local steroid injections are more effective compared with a placebo injection, there is a significant number of patients who fail this modality or develop recurrence.[14] Castellanos and colleagues[15] performed a review of trigger fingers treated with corticosteroid injections with a mean follow-up of 8 years and found a success rate, defined as resolution of symptoms for at least 36 months, of 69%. A more recent review of the literature found that only 57% of patients had relief with corticosteroid injections.[16] Rozental and colleagues[17] found a recurrence of 56% up to 1 year after injections and found that younger age, type 1 diabetes mellitus, involvement of multiple digits, and history of other tendonopathies were associated with a higher rate of treatment failure. Patients with more than 6 months of symptoms are also less likely to have triggering resolution.[18] The type of steroid has not been shown to affect long-term outcomes. Triamcinolone, however, a non—water-soluble medication, has shown more effective in the short term (6 weeks after administration) when prospectively compared with dexamethasone, a water-soluble steroid.[19] Appropriate counseling should be provided to patients because patience may be required to see a beneficial effect from the steroid.

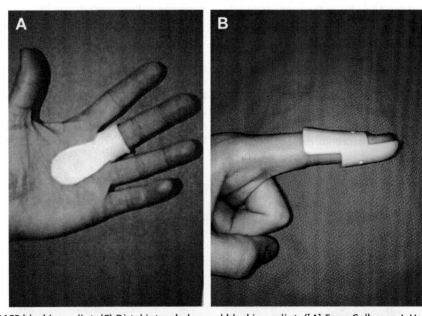

Fig. 2. (*A*) MCP blocking splint. (*B*) Distal interphalangeal blocking splint. ([*A*] *From* Colbourn J, Heath N, Manary S, et al. Effectiveness of splinting for the treatment of trigger finger. J Hand Ther 2008;21:338; with permission; and [*B*] *Courtesy of* Christopher Myer, MD, Pittsburgh, PA.)

Delivery of the steroid into the tendon sheath is classically thought critical for effectiveness of the treatment. The 2 most commonly used injection techniques are the palmar and midaxial needle trajectories (**Fig. 3**). The 2 techniques have been found equivalent in delivering medication into the sheath but have not been compared clinically.[20] Kamhim and colleagues[21] demonstrated that injections reach the intrasheath compartment in only 50% of attempts, giving rise to the notion that medication does not need to be in the sheath to be effective. Taras and colleagues[22] compared groups of intrasheath and extrasheath injections and, in contrast to popular belief, found that the extrasheath cohort had better outcomes. Whether to apply the steroid into the tendon sheath or subcutaneously continues to be a topic of debate and a focus for further investigation.

Minor complications associated with local corticosteroids include skin depigmentation and fat necrosis. Major complications, such as tendon attrition and rupture, are rare but have been reported.[23] Local steroid use may lead to transient fluctuation in blood glucose level that can last 5 days and should be used with caution in fragile diabetic patients.[24] For this reason, local NSAID injections have also been advocated, and, in the short term, 1 series demonstrated comparable benefit to local steroid 3 months after the injection with no difference in recurrence rates.[25]

SURGICAL TREATMENT

Open release of the A1 pulley is the gold standard for surgical treatment of trigger finger. Longitudinal, oblique, or transverse incisions are made over the A1 pulley of the involved digit. Blunt dissection is carried down to the tendon sheath and care is taken to protect the neurovascular bundles that travel on the ulnar and radial side of the tendon. When incising the A1 pulley, care must be exercised to avoid extension into the A2 pulley, because there is a theoretic risk of tendon

bowstringing if the A2 pulley is released. The procedure can be performed under local anesthesia with the benefit of an awake patient who can actively flex the involved digit, allowing a surgeon to observe triggering prior to wound closure. Turowski and colleagues[26] reviewed 97 patients and reported a 97% success of open A1 pulley release. In a much larger series, Bruijnzeel and colleagues[27] retrospectively reviewed 1598 cases using the standard open technique and found a 99.1% success rate with 0.9% recurrence or persistent triggering. In a review of 254 cases with an average of 14 year follow-up, Lange-Riess and colleagues[28] reported complete symptom resolution in all patients with open A1 pulley release.

The complication rate of open A1 pulley release ranges from 7% to 43%.[26,27,29] This wide spectrum is likely secondary to variety in opinion as to what classifies as a reportable adverse event. A vast majority of complications are considered minor, including superficial infection, wound dehiscence, persistent incision discomfort, and stiffness. Concomitant carpal tunnel surgery and diabetes have been found associated with higher incidence of these complications. Iatrogenic injury to the digital nerves is one of the most feared complications, but fortunately only a few cases have been reported.[30] Trigger finger release of the thumb is at particular risk of nerve injury because the digital nerve courses over the A1 pulley.[31] Flexor tendon bowstringing can occur with accidental release of the A2 pulley, leading to a painful protrusion of the flexor tendons into the palm and a decrease in flexion efficiency.[32]

Although open release is largely successful in alleviating symptoms, persistent triggering or unresolved flexion contracture can occur. In these rare situations, further surgical intervention is warranted. In patients with persistent flexion contracture after A1 pulley release or who present with advanced flexion contracture, FDS ulnar slip resection results in near-complete resolution of the deformity.[33,34] The ulnar slip can be transected

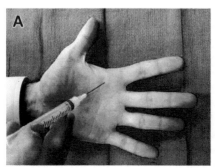 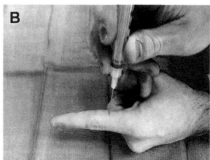

Fig. 3. (*A*) Palmar injection technique; (*B*) midaxial technique. (*Courtesy of* John R. Fowler, MD, Pittsburgh, PA.)

at the edge of the A3 border and excised in the A2-A3 interval. In rheumatoid arthritis patients, FDS slip resection decreases the recurrence of flexor tenosynovitis and should be considered as an adjunct to A1 pulley release in this subpopulation.[35]

Percutaneous release of the A1 pulley was first described in 1958 and has increased in popularity over the past 2 decades.[36] The procedure involves releasing the A1 pulley under local anesthesia with the use of a large bore needle or tenotome while the patient intentionally triggers the affected finger. Immediate symptom resolution should be directly observed with a successful procedure. Understanding anatomic landmarks is pivotal in avoiding injury to the neurovascular bundles (**Fig. 4**). Several guides based on cutaneous landmarks have been supported to determine the safest trajectory for insertion of a cutting guide.[37–39] Although the percutaneous technique has been shown effective and safe for the thumb, many advocates avoid performing the procedure on the thumb because the digital nerve courses over the A1 pulley.[40]

Ragoowansi and colleagues[41] performed percutaneous A1 release on 180 patients and 95% had symptom resolution. Ha and colleagues[42] had similar success in 185 patients, 94% success, after percutaneous release with a specially designed hooked knife. A recent meta-analysis of more than 2100 percutaneous A1 pulley releases found a success rate of 94% with only 4 major complications: 2 infections, 1 fixed flexion deformity, and 1 permanent digital nerve injury.[43] In this review, there was no difference in results found when comparing a large bore needle to a cutting instrument or if cortisone was concomitantly used. The use of sonography during the procedure led to significantly higher success compared with the procedures done without the adjunct use of this imaging modality, 99% and 94%, respectively ($P = .010$).

Calleja and colleagues[44] performed 25 trigger finger releases using percutaneous technique, immediately followed by open exploration, to determine how much of the A1 pulley had been released. All patients in this series had complete relief of triggering symptoms after the percutaneous procedure before the open procedure was performed. Only 24% of these digits had complete release of the A1 pulley after the minimally invasive approach; 15 of 25 had incomplete, superficial tendon injuries that were not clinically significant.

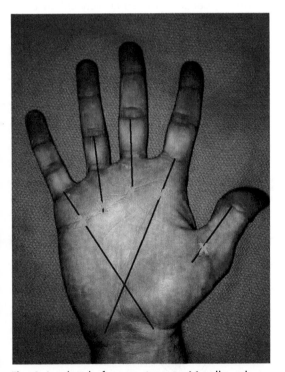

Fig. 4. Landmarks for percutaneous A1 pulley release. The Xs mark the proximal edge of the A1 pulley. Thumb: the intersection between the longitudinal axis of the thumb and the proximal digital crease. Index finger: the intersection between the proximal palmar crease and a line that connects the center of the proximal digital crease and the radial border of the pisiform. Long finger: the intersection between the proximal digit crease and the distal palmar crease. Ring finger: the intersection between the proximal digit crease and the distal palmar crease. Small finger: the intersection between the distal palmar crease and a line that connects the center of the proximal digital crease and the scaphoid tubercle. (*Courtesy of* Juan M. Giugale, MD, Pittsburgh, PA.)

PEDIATRIC TRIGGER DIGIT

The pathology, natural progression, and management of pediatric trigger fingers and trigger thumbs differ significantly from their adult counterparts. Commonly, children are brought in by their parents, at approximately 2 years of age, with the observation that a child has a flexed posture of the thumb or an inability to extend the thumb at the interphalangeal joint. Careful examination of the contralateral hand should be performed because 25% of children have bilateral involvement.[45] A nodule is usually present and palpable on the FPL tendon. This is termed, *Notta nodule*, after the physician who first described it.[46]

The etiology behind pediatric trigger fingers and thumbs remains largely unknown. Microscopic analysis of biopsied A1 pulleys and Notta nodules from pediatric thumbs have depicted large amounts of mature collagen and fibroblasts without evidence of infectious, inflammatory, or degenerative changes.[47] It is this fibrous proliferation that results in a discrepancy in the size of the FPL and the A1 pulley, leading to clinical symptoms of triggering. Recent evidence has failed to support the belief that pediatric trigger finger is a congenital condition.[48,49] The term, *congenital trigger finger*, is now considered a misnomer and the trigger finger in this patient population is considered an acquired pathology.[50]

The etiology of pediatric trigger finger, a much less common condition than trigger thumb, seems more complex and multifactorial. Nodularity of the FDS and FDP, constriction of the A1-A3 pulleys, and proximal decussation of the FDS are causes of triggering.[51] Trigger finger, in this age group, has been associated with congenital metabolic and inflammatory disorders, but a majority of cases are idiopathic. There is no consensus regarding the natural history of this condition available in the literature.

Surgical intervention of pediatric trigger thumb is not always necessary because the natural history is that a majority of cases resolve, albeit over a long period of time. A review of 26 pediatric trigger thumbs found that only 12% resolved by 6 months, which increased to 73% by 12 months after presentation.[45] A more recent review of 71 pediatric trigger thumb found that 63% resolved without intervention, but the median time to resolution was 48 months.[52] It is unclear whether disease severity, age, or any other variables affect the likelihood of symptom resolution. Therapy, passive extension exercises, and splinting have been conservative treatments, which have shown improvement in symptoms and increased range of motion at the interphalangeal joint, but whether these modalities are superior to mere observation is also unclear.[53,54] It is the authors' practice to recommend surgical intervention in the toddler population, especially if a fixed, flexion deformity is present, because it is an unlikely cohort to be compliant with splinting and therapy.

Surgery is usually performed under general anesthesia in this patient population. When performing open surgical release of a trigger thumb,

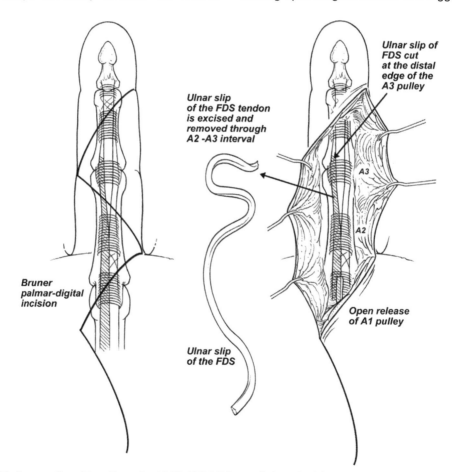

Fig. 5. FDS slip resection. (*From* Ryzewicz M, Wolf JM. Trigger digits: principles, management, and complications. J Hand Surg Am 2006;31:142, with permission.)

a transverse incision is made along the MCP crease. Blunt dissection is carried out to the level of the A1 pulley with caution because the digital nerve crosses the A1 pulley obliquely at this level. Sharp incision of the A1 pulley is carefully performed to avoid accidental release of the oblique pulley proximally, which could lead to bowstringing of the FPL tendon. The Notta nodule of the FPL tendon is palpable during the procedure but does not need to be excised. Surgical intervention has been found to have a high rate of success, more than 95%, with low rate of complications (2%–4%).[45,55] Failure and need for further surgical intervention are attributed to inadequate release of the A1 pulley.

Because the cause of finger triggering in children is more variable than merely a thickened A1 pulley, the outcomes of conservative treatment are unpredictable and the recommended surgical intervention is more involved. Cardon and colleagues[56] demonstrated that adjunct procedures, such as A3 pulley release and/or FDS slip resection, decreased disease recurrence and increased the likelihood of symptom resolution. Many investigators now advocate routine FDS slip resection in addition to A1 pulley release.[51,57] The FDS slip that appears thickened or nodular should be resected (**Fig. 5**). If neither appears diseased, 1 of the 2 slips should be arbitrarily excised. The surgeon should also examine the A2 and A3 pulleys and carefully incise these structures if there is evidence of constriction. Caution must be maintained because over-release of the A2 pulley may lead to bowstringing of the flexor tendons.

SUMMARY

Trigger finger is a common condition affecting both the adult and pediatric populations. A mismatch between the flexor tendons and the overlying tendon sheath causes a spectrum of symptoms from painful catching to fixed flexion contractures. Treatment differs between the 2 age groups. In adults, surgical intervention is usually recommended after a failure of conservative measures, including corticosteroid injections. Surgical intervention can be performed open or percutaneously, with similar reported success. In pediatrics, trigger thumb surgical release is similar to that of adults, but trigger finger procedures are more involved and address the multiple factors that could contribute to the pathology. Further investigation is needed to determine the cohort of patients that is more likely to require surgical intervention, preventing the need for prolonged conservative measures that may take months or years to alleviate symptoms.

REFERENCES

1. Strom L. Trigger finger in diabetes. J Med Soc N J 1977;74:951–4.
2. Sungpet A, Suphachatwong C, Kawinwonggowit V. Trigger digit and BMI. J Med Assoc Thai 1999;82:1025–7.
3. Hueston JT, Wilson WF. The aetiology of trigger finger: explained on the basis of intratendinous architecture. Hand 1972;4:257–60.
4. Sampson SP, Badalamente MA, Hurst LC, et al. Pathobiology of the human A1 pulley in trigger finger. J Hand Surg 1991;16A:714–21.
5. Lundin AC, Eliasson P, Aspenberg P. Trigger finger and tendinosis. J Hand Surg Br 2011;37(3):233–6.
6. Guerini H, Pessis E, Theumann N, et al. Sonographic appearance of trigger fingers. J Ultrasound Med 2008;27:1407–13.
7. Miyamoto H, Miura T, Isayama H, et al. Stiffness of the first annular pulley in normal and trigger fingers. J Hand Surg Am 2011;36:1486–91.
8. Quinnell R. Conservative management of trigger finger. Practitioner 1980;224:187–90.
9. Freiberg A, Mulholland RS, Levine R. Nonoperative treatment of trigger fingers and thumbs. J Hand Surg Am 1989;14:553–8.
10. Colbourn J, Heath N, Manary S, et al. Effectiveness of splinting for the treatment of trigger finger. J Hand Ther 2008;21:336–43.
11. Rogers JA, McCarthy JA, Tiedman JJ. Functional distal interphalangeal joint splinting for trigger finger in laborers: a review and cadaver investigation. Orthopaedics 1998;21:305–10.
12. Tarbhai K, Hannah S, von Schroeder HP. Trigger finger treatment: a comparison of 2 splint designs. J Hand Surg Am 2012;37:243–9.
13. Evans RB, Hunter JM, Burkhalter W. Conservative management of the trigger finger: a new approach. J Hand Ther 1988;1:59–68.
14. Murphy D, Failla JM, Koniuch MP. Steroid versus placebo injection for trigger finger. J Hand Surg Am 1995;20:628–31.
15. Castellanos J, Munoz-Mahamud E, Dominguez E, et al. Long-term effectiveness of corticosteroid injections for trigger finger and thumb. J Hand Surg Am 2015;40(1):121–6.
16. Fleisch SB, Spindler KP, Lee DH. Corticosteroid injections in the treatment of trigger finger: a level I and II systematic review. J Am Acad Orthop Surg 2007;15:166–71.
17. Rozental T, Zurakowski D, Blazar P. Trigger finger: prognostic indicators of recurrence following corticosteroid injection. J Bone Joint Surg Am 2008;90:1665–72.
18. Newport ML, Lane LB, Stuchin SA. Treatment of trigger finger by steroid injection. J Hand Surg Am 1990;15(5):748–50.

19. Ring D, Lozano-Calderon S, Shin R, et al. A prospective randomized controlled trial of injection of dexamethasone versus triamcinolone for idiopathic trigger finger. J Hand Surg Am 2008; 33:516–22.

20. Fowler JR, Ogrich L, Evangelista P, et al. Assessing injection techniques in the treatment of trigger finger. Mod Plast Surg 2012;2:83–6.

21. Kamhim M, Engel J, Heim M. The fate of injected trigger fingers. Hand 1983;15:218–20.

22. Taras JS, Laurel NJ, Raphael JS, et al. Corticosteroid injections for trigger digits: is intrasheath injection necessary? J Hand Surg Am 1998;23: 717–22.

23. Fitzgerald BT, Hofmeister EP, Fan RA, et al. Delayed flexor digitorum superficialis and pofundus ruptures in a trigger finger after a steroid injection: a case report. J Hand Surg 2005;30(3):479–82.

24. Wang AA, Hutchinson DT. The effect of corticosteroid injection for trigger finger on blood glucose level in diabetic patients. J Hand Surg Am 2006; 31:979–81.

25. Shakeel H, Ahmad S. Steroid injection versus NSAID injection for trigger finger: a comparative study of early outcomes. J Hand Surg Am 2012; 37:1319–23.

26. Turowski GA, Zdankiewicz PD, Thomson JG. The results of surgical treatment of trigger finger. J Hand Surg Am 1997;22:145–9.

27. Bruijnzeel H, Neuhaus V, Fostvedt S, et al. Adverse events of open A1 pulley release for idiopathic trigger finger. J Hand Surg Am 2012;37(8): 1650–6.

28. Lange-Riess D, Schuh R, Hönle W, et al. Long-term results of surgical release of trigger finger and trigger thumb in adults. Arch Orthop Trauma Surg 2009;129(12):1617–9.

29. Will R, Lubahn J. Complications of open trigger release. J Hand Surg Am 2010;35:594–6.

30. Thorpe AP. Results of surgery for trigger finger. J Hand Surg Br 1988;13:199–201.

31. Carrozzella J, Stern PJ, Von Kuster LC. Transection of radial digital nerve of the thumb during trigger release. J Hand Surg Am 1989;14:198–200.

32. Peterson WW, Manske PR, Bollinger BA, et al. Effect of pulley excision on flexor tendon biomechanics. J Orthop Res 1986;4:96–101.

33. Favre Y, Kinnen L. Resection of the flexor digitorum superficialis for trigger finger with proximal interphalangeal joint positional contracture. J Hand Surg Am 2012;37:2269–72.

34. Viet DL, Tsionos I, Boulouednine M, et al. Trigger finger treatment by ulnar superficialis slip resection. J Hand Surg Br 2004;29(4):368–73.

35. Wheen DJ, Tonkin MA, Green J, et al. Long-term results following digital flexor tenosynovectomy in rheumatoid arthritis. J Hand Surg Am 1995;20: 790–4.

36. Lorthioir J. Surgical treatment of trigger-finger by a subcutaneous method. J Bone Joint Surg Am 1958;40:793–5.

37. Saldana MJ. Trigger digits: diagnosis and management. J Am Acad Orthop Surg 2001;9:246–52.

38. Ryzewicz M, Wolf JM. Trigger digits: principles, management, and complications. J Hand Surg Am 2006;31:135–46.

39. Fiorini HJ, Santos JB, Hirakawa CK, et al. Anatomical Study of the A1 pulley: length and location by means of cutaneous landmarks on the palmar surface. J Hand Surg Am 2011;36:464–8.

40. Cebesoy O, Karakurum G, Kose KC, et al. Percutaneous release of the trigger thumb: is it safe, cheap and effective? Int Orthop 2007; 31(3):345–9.

41. Ragoowansi R, Acornley A, Khoo CT. Percutaneous trigger finger release: the "lift-cut" technique. Br J Plast Surg 2005;58(6):817–21.

42. Ha KI, Park MJ, Ha CW. Percutaneous release of trigger digits. J Bone Joint Surg Br 2001;83(1):75–7.

43. Zhao JG, Kan SL, Zhao L, et al. Percutaneous first annular pulley release for trigger digits: a systematic review and meta-analysis of current evidence. J Hand Surg 2014;39(11):2192–202.

44. Calleja H, Tanchuling A, Alagar D, et al. Anatomic Outcome of percutaneous release among patients with trigger finger. J Hand Surg Am 2010;35: 1671–4.

45. Dinham JM, Meggitt BF. Trigger thumbs in children: a review of the natural history and indications for treatment in 105 patients. J Bone Joint Surg Br 1974;56(1):153–5.

46. Clapham PJ, Chung KC. A historical perspective of the Notta's node in trigger fingers. J Hand Surg Am 2009;34(8):1518–22.

47. Buchman MT, Gibson TW, McCallum D, et al. Transmission electron microscopic pathoanatomy of congenital trigger thumb. J Pediatr Orthop 1999; 19(3):411–2.

48. Kikuchi N, Ogino T. Incidence and development of trigger thumb in children. J Hand Surg Am 2006; 31(4):541–3.

49. Moon WN, Suh SW, Kim IC. Trigger digits in children. J Hand Surg Br 2001;26(1):11–2.

50. Shah AS, Bae DS. Management of Pediatric Trigger Thumb and trigger finger. J Am Acad Orthop Surg 2012;20:206–13.

51. Bae DS, Sodha S, Waters PM. Surgical treatment of the pediatric trigger finger. J Hand Surg Am 2007; 32(7):1043–7.

52. Baek GH, Kim JH, Chung MS, et al. The natural history of pediatric trigger thumb. J Bone Joint Surg Am 2008;90(5):980–5.

53. Watanabe H, Hamada Y, Toshima T, et al. Conservative treatment for trigger thumb in children. Arch Orthop Trauma Surg 2001;121(7): 388–90.

54. Nemoto K, Nemoto T, Terada N, et al. Splint therapy for trigger thumb and finger in children. J Hand Surg Br 1996;21(3):416–8.

55. Dunsmuir RA, Sherlock DA. The outcome of treatment of trigger thumb in children. J Bone Joint Surg Br 2000;82(5):736–8.

56. Cardon LJ, Ezaki M, Carter PR. Trigger finger in children. J Hand Surg Am 1999;24(6):1156–61.

57. Tordai P, Engkvist O. Trigger fingers in children. J Hand Surg Am 1999;24(6):1162–5.

Use of High-Speed X ray and Video to Analyze Distal Radius Fracture Pathomechanics

Christina Gutowski, MD, MPH[a], Kurosh Darvish, PhD[b],
Frederic E. Liss, MD[c], Asif M. Ilyas, MD[c],
Christopher M. Jones, MD[c],*

KEYWORDS

- Distal radius fracture • High-speed X ray • Video X ray • Fracture biomechanics • Wrist guard

KEY POINTS

- Distal radius fractures are common injuries, especially in the pediatric and elderly populations, that account for significant morbidity and mortality.
- The combination of high-speed x-ray and video imaging has been used in other areas of medicine to investigate physiologic movement, joint kinematics, and fracture propagation. This type of recording system has not been used in the study of distal radius fracture pathomechanics.
- This imaging technique proved feasible with a drop tower apparatus consisting of a potted cadaver forearm, weights dropped to simulate a fall onto an outstretched hand, 2 identical video recorders, an x-ray source, and an image intensifier.
- In the presented pilot study, when impacted, the distal radius was found to shift in a volar direction with respect to the proximal carpal row, with the carpus also hyperextending. In elderly wrists, failure of the distal radius began as compressive failure on the dorsal cortex followed by tensile failure of the volar cortex. In younger wrists, both cortices tended to fail simultaneously.
- As a proof of concept, this study confirms that future studies with larger cadaveric samples can be analyzed with high-speed X ray and video to better understand distal radius fracture pathomechanics.

INTRODUCTION

Distal radius fractures are among the most common injuries treated by orthopedists[1] and the most frequently diagnosed fracture in women.[2] In fact, healthy women who are 60 years of age have a 17% chance of sustaining a fracture of the distal radius.[2] The incidence of this injury has increased significantly over the last several decades, a trend noted both domestically and internationally.[3–5] Distal radius fractures result in considerable pain and loss of productivity, often require surgical treatment, and are an indicator of increased risk of other fractures.[6] A 2011 report estimated that $170 million was paid by Medicare in 2007 toward treatment of distal radius fractures,

Disclosure: None of the authors of this article have any conflicts of interest or relationships to disclose. Nothing of benefit was received by any of the authors in the production of this article.

[a] Department of Orthopaedic Surgery, Thomas Jefferson University, 1025 Walnut Street, Room 516, College Building, Philadelphia, PA 19107, USA; [b] Department of Mechanical Engineering, Temple University, 1947 North 12th Street, Philadelphia, PA 19122, USA; [c] Department of Orthopaedic Surgery, Rothman Institute, Thomas Jefferson University, 925 Chestnut Street, Philadelphia, PA 19107, USA

* Corresponding author.

E-mail addresses: christopher.jones@rothmaninstitute.com; gunnar@mmk.su.se

orthopedic.theclinics.com

and the future burden to Medicare will approach $240 million if trends in utilization of internal fixation continue as anticipated.[7] These fractures are also a common injury in the pediatric population,[8] accounting for 25% of all fractures in this age group.[9] The estimated cost associated with treating pediatric distal radius fractures is upwards of $2 billion per year in the United States.[10] Given the high incidence of distal radius fractures in the young and old alike, and the significance as both a personal injury and a public health concern, further understanding of the biomechanical mechanism of this fracture is essential. Moreover, improving our understanding of failure mechanisms of the distal radius might enable us to develop both improved treatments and preventative or protective devices.

The failure sequence of the distal radius during a typical fall on an outstretched hand is not well described in the literature. Ulrich and colleagues[11] (1999) used high-resolution images captured by a micro–computed tomography scanner and micro-finite element analysis techniques to calculate stress and strain on areas of the distal radius at the tissue level and quantify load transfer through the trabecular network. However, this in vivo study did not simulate an actual fracture to the distal radius; only subfailure loads were applied to the bone through the scaphoid or lunate. In other anatomic locations, the bony sequence of injury is better understood. In the cervical spine, for example, axial loading has long been considered to be the force behind the mechanism of vertebral burst fracture. Both in vivo and in vitro laboratory experimental studies as well as finite element modeling can subsequently predict areas of the vertebral body where failure is likely to begin and propagate when exposed to a given load.[12] No study exists that investigates the failure mechanism of the distal radius to this extent.

There are several published research studies that have evaluated the effectiveness of wrist guards in protecting against distal radius fractures.[13] They use a variety of test setups to simulate an impact across the wrist by using force-measuring platforms and strain gauges to calculate the force applied to the distal radius. These studies were conducted both with the wrist bare and while wearing a protective guard. Investigations using both cadavers and human subjects suggest that various forms of wrist guards can be helpful in reducing momentum and allowing for a higher impulse to be applied to the wrist/brace construct before distal radius failure.[14–17] Although these biomechanical data points can provide valuable support for wrist guard utilization, they do not provide direct information regarding the biomechanics of force transmission across the wrist and forearm during a fall.

In order to better understand the sequence of events, specifically the relative motion and failure sequence that occurs during a distal radius fracture, the authors think that high-speed imaging techniques, combined x-ray and video imaging, offer promise. These techniques have been used in other fields, although the literature is scarce regarding their use in orthopedic trauma, especially in investigating distal radius fractures. For example, in veterinary medicine, a high-speed x-ray system was described by Snelderwaard and colleagues[18] to analyze the rapid projection of a small animal's tongue to capture prey during a feeding experiment. Techniques of imaging fluid movement[19] and the motion of artificial heart valves[20] have also been described by using high-speed modern video systems.

In orthopedic sports medicine and arthroplasty, dynamic fluoroscopy has been investigated to elucidate joint kinematics in vivo in attempt to understand the weight-bearing forces, shear stresses, and relative motion of the joint.[21,22] To the best of the authors' knowledge, combined high-speed X ray and video has not been used to investigate fracture pathomechanics. The objective of the current report is to serve as a proof-of-concept demonstration, evaluating the feasibility of combined high-speed x-ray and video imaging techniques applied to a fracture model. Specifically, the authors sought to investigate the fracture mechanism of the distal radius from a typical fall on an outstretched hand and the effectiveness of various wrist guard designs.

EXPERIMENTAL DESIGN

Eight fresh-frozen cadaveric arms were thawed at room temperature for 24 hours. The elbow was disarticulated, and all soft tissues were removed from the proximal forearm. The proximal radius and ulna were potted using R1 FastCast (Goldenwest Manufacturing, Grass Valley, CA) urethane casting resin. The forearms were positioned vertically in an impact testing apparatus with the wrist preloaded in extension (**Fig. 1**). The impact force, provided by a 45-kg drop weight, was transferred to the arm via a load transfer plate assembly that restricted motion to the vertical direction using guide shafts. A rigid weight stopper prevented excessive compression of the arm. Weight was dropped on bare cadaver wrists as well as those protected by one of 3 wrist guard designs.

The drop test was photographed with high-speed video and X ray using a mechanical trigger

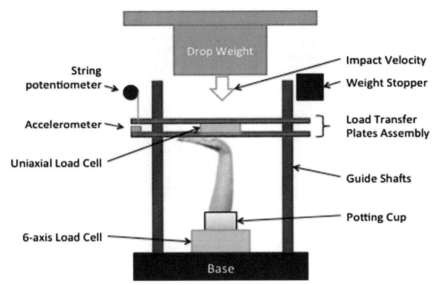

Fig. 1. Drop tower assembly, using potted cadaver forearm.

on the drop test apparatus (**Fig. 2**). The x-ray equipment consisted of a source radiating in the medial-lateral direction (150 kVP, Varian Medical Systems, Palo Alto, CA, USA) and a 550-mm image intensifier (VJ Technologies, Inc, Bohemia, NY, USA), which captured dynamic lateral x-ray images of the distal forearm and hand during impact

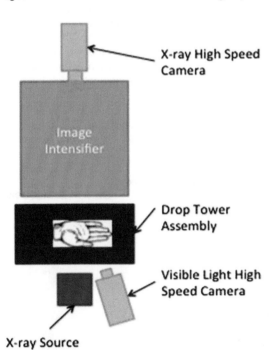

Fig. 2. Recording system assembled around drop tower assembly, including x-ray source, image intensifier, video camera for x-ray images, and video camera for visible light images.

loading. This machine captured images at 1000 frames per second (fps). Two high-speed video acquisition systems (Memrecam GX-1, nac Image Technology, Simi Valley, CA, USA) were positioned adjacent to the radiation source to record a video of the wrist setup viewed from the lateral direction as well as the dynamic lateral x-ray images. Images were also recorded at 1000 fps. All image data were stored in a hard drive and later analyzed with the Quicktime (Apple software) 7 video player using the zoom feature and image processing functions to best visualize the region of interest. Images were analyzed on a frame-by-frame basis to characterize the fracture sequence.

Impact force was measured using 2 load cells. Displacement and acceleration of the load transfer plate was measured with a string potentiometer and accelerometer, respectively. Strain in the distal radius and ulna was measured using strain gage rosettes. These measurement devices allowed for more traditional biomechanical data to be captured, consistent with those data described by previous studies, although these are not the focus of this report.

Three types of wrist guards were used, including a prototype created by the researchers. The two commercially available wrist guards were the Seirus Jam Master II (Seirus, San Diego, CA, USA), incorporating both volar and dorsal protective plates meant to be worn above a ski/snowboard glove, and the Dakine volar wrist guard (Dakine, Hood River, OR, USA), which is lower profile and consists of an aluminum volar plate. The prototype design included a viscoelastic foam core and thin rigid shell on the volar side of a neoprene sleeve (**Fig. 3**). The

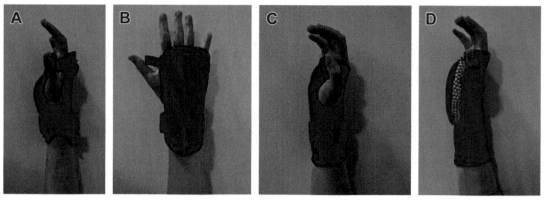

Fig. 3. Three wrist guard designs. From left: Seirus Jam Master II (*A*, *B*), Dakine wrist guard (*C*), and prototype design (*D*).

appropriate size guard was secured to the cadaver hand for impact tests. The high-speed x-ray images and videos were studied for patterns of relative motion and location/sequence of fracture development. Each forearm was first tested with nondestructive loads at approximately 30% of the anticipated failure load with and without the wrist guards. Destructive tests were then performed alternating between wrist guard type and no guard.

EARLY RESULTS AND FUTURE DIRECTION

A better understanding of the pathomechanics of distal radius fractures can be gleaned by studying the videos of dynamic wrist motion when exposed to axial load, resulting eventually in fracture of the distal radius. In the authors' study of 8 cadaver forearms, in both protected and unprotected wrists, the common failure mechanism occurred through axial compression of the extended carpus, causing the radius to shift slightly in a volar direction relative to the proximal carpal row and

the proximal carpal row to hyperextend (**Figs. 4** and **5**). The authors measured the radiocapite angle using a goniometer to quantify the proximal carpal row hyperextension. From preload to failure the capitate extended from 42° to 55° on average. In several videos, the capitate seemed to abut the dorsal radial rim and possibly transfer the load directly to the dorsal cortex of the radius.

Being a proof-of-concept analysis, the authors' study lacked power to make definitive conclusions on the sequence of failure during fracture; however, it seemed that in older cadavers, failure occurred first in the dorsal cortex followed by tension failure of the volar cortex, whereas in younger cadavers, both cortices failed simultaneously. When studying the wrist braces, it was noted that the volar brace tended to slide proximally down the wrist, affording less impact absorbance against axial load as compared with the prototype brace, which did not migrate from its intended position. The authors also noted that the volar splint seemed to function by transferring a portion of the wrist extension

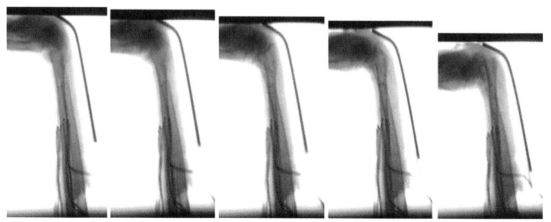

Fig. 4. Sequential frames of high-speed video X ray of impact onto potted cadaver wrist, protected with Dakine volar wrist guard.

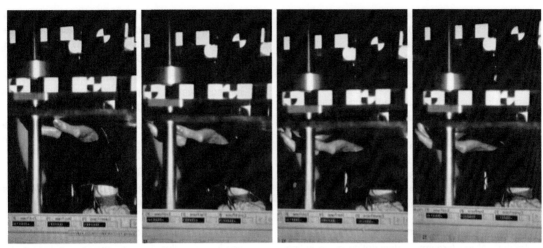

Fig. 5. Sequential frames of high-speed video impact onto potted cadaver wrist, protected with Dakine volar wrist guard.

load through the rigid support to the forearm straps, bypassing the wrist. Transferring the impact force proximally to protect the distal radius did potentially risk the development of a proximal fracture, which occurred in the midradial shaft and at the bone-potting cement interface in 2 specimens. Also, analyzing the high-speed video data provided other insights helpful in optimizing the guard design. For example, it was noted that the viscoelastic cushion, which was designed to fully compress to absorb the maximal force, only compressed a fraction of its thickness. Video analysis could be used to evaluate the compressibility and effectiveness of other types and thicknesses of material, including layered composites, which otherwise might be challenging to estimate their material properties.

Qualitative observations made from studying the high-speed video and X rays combined with quantitative analysis of strain gauge and load cell data can offer valuable insight into the distinct biomechanical failure sequence that occurs in distal radius fractures. By understanding this to a greater extent, personal protective devices can be enhanced to optimize effectiveness. It is the authors' belief that this pilot study offers sound proof of concept and support for this imaging technique to be used in larger studies of orthopedic trauma and specifically for distal radius fractures in the future.

REFERENCES

1. Lidstrom A. Fractures of the distal end of the radius. A clinical and statistical study of the end results. Acta Orthop Scand 1959;41(Suppl):1–118.

2. Lauritzen JP, Schwarz P, Lund B, et al. Changing incidence and residual lifetime risk of common osteoporosis-related fractures. Osteoporos Int 1993;3:127–32.

3. Melton L, Amadio P, Crowson C, et al. Long-term trends in the incidence of distal forearm fractures. Osteoporos Int 1998;8:341–8.

4. Alffram PA, Bauer GC. Epidemiology of fractures of the forearm. A biomechanical investigation of bone strength. J Bone Joint Surg Am 1962;44-A:105–14.

5. Bengner U, Johnell O. Increasing incidence of forearm fractures. A comparison of epidemiologic patterns 25 years apart. Acta Orthop Scand 1985;56: 158–60.

6. Mallmin H, Ljunghall S, Persson I, et al. Risk factors for fractures of the distal forearm: a population-based case-control study. Osteoporos Int 1994;49: 298–304.

7. Shauver MJ, Yin H, Banerjee M, et al. Current and future national costs to Medicare for the treatment of distal radius fracture in the elderly. J Hand Surg Am 2011;36:1282–7.

8. Cooper C, Dennison EM, Leufkens HGM, et al. Epidemiology of childhood fractures in Britain: a study using the general practice research database. J Bone Miner Res 2004;19(12):1976–81.

9. Nellans KW, Kowalski E, Chung KC. The epidemiology of distal radius fractures. Hand Clin 2012; 28(2):113–25.

10. Ryan LM, Teach SJ, Searcy K, et al. Epidemiology of pediatric forearm fractures in Washington, DC. J Trauma 2010;69(4-S):S200–5.

11. Ulrich D, van Rietbergen B, Laib A, et al. Load transfer analysis of the distal radius from in-vivo high-resolution CT imaging. J Biomech 1999;32:821–8.

12. Bozic KJ, Keyak JH, Skinner HB, et al. Three-dimensional finite element modeling of a cervical vertebra:

an investigation of burst fracture mechanism. J Spinal Disord 1994;7(2):102–10.

13. Kim S, Lee SK. Snowboard wrist guards- use, efficacy, and design. A systematic review. Bull NYU Hosp Jt Dis 2011;69(2):149–57.

14. Greenwald R, Janes P, Swanson S, et al. Dynamic impact response of human cadaveric forearms using a wrist brace. Am J Sports Med 1998;26(6):825–30.

15. Hwang I, Kim K, Kaufman K, et al. Biomechanical efficiency of wrist guards as a shock isolator. J Biomech Eng 2006;128(2):229–34.

16. Staebler M, Moore D, Akelman E, et al. The effect of wrist guards on bone strain in the distal forearm. Am J Sports Med 1999;27(4):500–6.

17. Cheng S, Rajaratnam K, Raskin K, et al. "Splint-top" fracture of the forearm: a description of an in-line skating injury associated with the use of protective wrist splints. J Trauma 1995;39(6):1194–7.

18. Snelderwaard PC, DeGroot JH, Deban SM. Digital video combined with conventional radiography creates an excellent high-speed x-ray video system. J Biomech 2002;35:1007–9.

19. Mishima K, Hibiki T, Nishihara H. Visualization and measurement of two-phase flow by using neutron radiography. Nucl Eng Des 1997;43:25–35.

20. Naemura K, Ohta Y, Fujimoto T, et al. Comparison of closing dynamics of mechanical prosthetic heart valves. ASAIO J 1997;43:401–4.

21. Stiehl JB, Komistek RD, Dennis DS, et al. Fluoroscopic analysis of kinematics after posterior cruciate retaining knee arthroplasty. J Bone Joint Surg Br 1995;77-B:884–9.

22. Li G, Van de Velde SK, Bingham JT. Validation of a non-invasive fluoroscopic imaging technique for the measurement of dynamic knee joint motion. J Biomech 2008;41:1616–22.

Oncology

Preface
Targeted Chemotherapy for Sarcoma and New Insights on Paget Disease

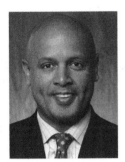

Felasfa M. Wodajo, MD
Editor

In the oncology section of this issue of *Orthopedic Clinics of North America*, we learn about Paget disease, a common skeletal disorder. In the review, "Paget Disease of Bone," Dr Al-Rashid and his colleagues from the Orthopaedic Oncology Service at Massachusetts General Hospital discuss the pathophysiology and treatment of Paget disease. The authors cover the possible genetic and environmental causes of the disease, appropriate diagnostic use of laboratory and imaging studies, current recommendations for medical therapy, and considerations for orthopedic surgeons operating on patients with Paget disease.

In "Targeted Chemotherapy in Bone and Soft-Tissue Sarcoma," the authors review the most commonly targeted pathways in sarcoma and a selection of targeted therapies showing initial promise or approaching clinical use. Dr Harwood and his colleagues from the Arthur James Cancer Hospital at The Ohio State University start by reviewing the unsatisfactory state of current systemic therapy options for the most common bone and soft tissue sarcomas. They then review the major and minor pathways involved in sarcomagenesis, which have yielded potential targets for therapy. For some of these pathways, such as Hedgehog and IGF, inhibition of tumor growth has been demonstrated in vitro. Other targets, such as mTOR and VEGF, have agents that have progressed to phase II and even phase III trials, with response seen in multiple sarcoma subtypes.

Felasfa M. Wodajo, MD
Musculoskeletal Tumor Surgery
Inova Fairfax Hospital
8305 Arlington Boulevard, Suite 400
Fairfax, VA 22031, USA

E-mail address:
wodajo@sarcoma.md

orthopedic.theclinics.com

Paget Disease of Bone

Mamun Al-Rashid, MD, FRCS (Orth)[a,b], Dipak B. Ramkumar, MD[c],
Kevin Raskin, MD[a], Joseph Schwab, MD, MS[a], Francis J. Hornicek, MD, PhD[a],
Santiago A. Lozano-Calderón, MD, PhD[a,b],*

KEYWORDS

- Paget disease of bone • Paget • Bone turnover • Bisphosphonates • SQSTM1
- Arthroplasty in Paget disease • Fracture fixation of pagetic bone • Paget sarcoma

KEY POINTS

- Paget disease of bone (PDB) is characterized by accelerated remodeling of bone. The disease is characterized by focal areas of excessive bone resorption and areas of abundant new bone formation.
- Early disease is characterized by primarily excessive bone resorption, mediated by osteoclasts. In later stages, osteoblastic activity predominates leading to focal areas of bone deposition leading to osseous thickening, sclerosis, and replacement of bone marrow with vascular and fibrous tissue.
- Familial and sporadic subtypes have been reported. Familial subtypes are often associated with a mutation in the SQSTM1 gene.
- Clinically the disease may be present as monostotic or polyostotic variants. The most common presenting symptom is poorly localized bone pain. Additionally, patients may also present with pathologic stress fractures, secondary osteoarthritis in juxtaposed joints, or bony enlargement causing compression of neural elements in the spine or skull.
- The mainstay of medical management involves the use of bisphosphonates, which is especially true for patients with symptoms of bone pain. Surgical indications include fixation of a fracture through pagetic bone, prophylactic fixation of an impending fracture, total joint arthroplasty in severe arthritis of the juxtaposed joints, spinal decompression to relieve compression of neural elements, or osteotomies used to correct severe, progressive deformity. The most devastating sequelae of long-standing Paget disease is its malignant transformation to Paget sarcoma, a secondary osteosarcoma with poor prognosis.

INTRODUCTION

Paget disease was first described in 1877 by Sir James Paget, a physician at St Bartholomew's Hospital in London, England. Sir Paget described a series of middle-aged patients who presented with aberrant bony structure.[1] As he followed these patients, he went on to notice progressively worsening bony deformities at multiple sites of involvement. Some of his patients went on to develop bone sarcomas that ultimately led to their demise.[1] Over the last 137 years, how much has our understanding of this disease evolved? Are we, as clinicians, better adept in the screening, earlier identification, assessment, and treatment of this disease?

[a] Orthopaedic Oncology Service, Department of Orthopaedic Surgery, Massachusetts General Hospital, Harvard Medical School, 55 Fruit Street, Boston, MA 02114, USA; [b] Orthopaedic Oncology Service, Department of Orthopaedic Surgery, Beth Israel Deaconess Medical Center, Harvard Medical School, 330 Brookline Avenue, Boston, MA 02215, USA; [c] Department of Orthopaedic Surgery, Dartmouth-Hitchcock Medical Center, Lebanon, NH 03766, USA
* Corresponding author. Orthopaedic Oncology Service, Department of Orthopaedic Surgery, Massachusetts General Hospital, 55 Fruit Street, Boston, MA 02114.
E-mail address: slozanocalderon@mgh.harvard.edu

Orthop Clin N Am 46 (2015) 577–585
http://dx.doi.org/10.1016/j.ocl.2015.06.008

This review aims to provide a synopsis of our current understanding and discusses the progress made, the controversies, and the current medical and surgical principles of treatment. We now know this condition is the result of disordered bone remodeling, as opposed to James Paget's initial perception of this being an osteitis or inflammation of the bone. This disease results from an uncoupling of the normal equilibrium of bone formation and resorption. Subsequently, the normal architecture of the affected bone is replaced by disorganized bony tissue that is structurally weaker and is, over time, subject to stress deformities and pathologic fractures.[2–4] In the long-term, a subset of patients with Paget disease of bone (PDB) will undergo malignant transformation, developing Paget sarcoma, a biologically malignant neoplasia, usually an osteosarcoma, with a poor prognosis.

NATURAL HISTORY AND EPIDEMIOLOGY

Anthropological analyses of skeletal remains indicate that PDB first appeared in Western European populations during the Roman period.[5] Multiple prevalence surveys carried out since the 1970s have demonstrated that PDB becomes more prevalent with increased age and that men are more frequently affected when compared with women. Additionally, geographic differences also exist, with PDB being more common in the United Kingdom and other Western European nations and less prevalent in Scandinavia, Eastern Europe, and Asia.[6] Follow-up prevalence studies have revealed a gradual decline in prevalence of PDB since the 1970s, with some studies indicating rates almost 50% less.[7,8] PDB typically presents in middle-aged and older populations. It can arise as a monostotic or polyostotic disease, with more recent epidemiologic studies favoring the monostotic variety as being more common.[9] The pagetic lesion typically expands in size without treatment, and serial radiographs often demonstrate marginal expansion in size (approximately 0.8 cm per year) in the setting of a radiographic evidence of lysis and sclerosis, concurring with the microscopic findings of increased bone turnover (both bone resorption and bone formation).[10]

CAUSE AND GENETICS

Both genetic and environmental factors have been implicated in the development of PDB. Historical review of patients and families with PDB has revealed both familial and sporadic subtypes. Hocking and colleagues[11] and Laurin and colleagues[12]

first posited in 2002 that the familial subtype of PDB was strongly associated with mutations in the sequestosome 1 or p62 gene, SQSTM1. This gene encodes a ubiquitously expressed protein found in the nucleus and cytoplasm of most cells and has been associated with multiple cellular activities, including nuclear factor kappa B signaling, modulation of potassium channels, control of transcription, autophagy, and sequestration and subsequent degradation of ubiquinated proteins.[9] In bone specifically, it is still unclear as to the inhibition of which of these activities results in the metabolic derangements manifested in the phenotype of PDB.

SQSTM1 mutations were noted in approximately 20% to 40% of familial PDB and up to 5% of sporadic cases of PDB. In a follow-up study in 2004, Hocking and colleagues[13,14] reported that patients with SQSTM1 mutations experience more severe phenotypes of PDB, including evidence of earlier onset and manifestations of disease at multiple skeletal sites.

Penetrance studies of SQSTM1 mutations, however, imply that the genetic mutation alone is not necessarily responsible for manifestation of PDB. Although penetrance of SQSTM1 mutations was originally estimated to be greater than 80% at 70 years of age in observational studies in families in which the disease was highly expressed, several studies have failed to find manifestations of PDB in appropriately aged mutation carriers.[9,15]

In addition to the potential genetic underpinnings of PDB described earlier, an alternative cause has been proposed, a potential infection with paramyxoviruses. This theory stemmed from the observation that paramyxoviral-like nuclear inclusions are commonly present in osteoclasts in pagetic bone. Some studies have reported detection of viral mRNA or protein based on biotechnological amplification methods in samples obtained from patients with PDB and have comparatively failed to find similar mRNA or protein in controls.[16,17] Yet other studies have also failed to detect viral RNA or protein. Similarly, live paramyxovirus has never been isolated from diseased tissue.[18,19]

PATHOLOGY AND PATHOPHYSIOLOGY

Fundamentally, PDB is characterized by accelerated remodeling of bone. Microscopically, the disease is a mixture of focal areas of excessive bone resorption and areas of abundant new bone formation with replacement of normal bone marrow with vascular and fibrous tissue.[20] The progression of the disease has been categorized into phases based on radiographic and histologic criteria. Early in the disease, excessive bone resorption predominates in focal regions with high concentrations of osteoclasts. These osteoclasts are usually multinucleated and actively resorb bone. After this phase, increased bone formation is noted, with increased concentrations of hyperactive osteoblasts, with bone formation rates increased 6- to 7-fold over the basal steady state.[21,22] The bone deposition is somewhat disorganized rather than following a smooth, lamellar pattern. As the rapid bone formation phase starts to predominate in more advanced stages of PDB, the lesions become more sclerotic, leading to thickening of bone and subsequent replacement of the bone marrow with vascular and fibrous tissue. The presence of woven bone and marrow fibrosis is also seen in other high bone turnover conditions. As a result, these histologic changes are often considered epiphenomena to an underlying high bone-remodeling rate and not pathognomonic for PDB. Please see **Fig. 1**.

CLINICAL PRESENTATION

Paget disease can often be silent or asymptomatic until secondary abnormalities from progressive disease become apparent. Among the symptomatic group, the most common presentation is poorly localized bone pain. Typically the pain is constant, present at rest, and worst at night. Secondary causes include pathologic stress fractures through abnormally enlarged, weak, and deformed pagetic bone and secondary osteoarthritis in adjacent joints usually resulting from bony deformity and altered biomechanical forces. In the skull, bony enlargement can cause nerve compression leading to deafness; in the spine, bony deformity and exuberant bone growth can cause symptoms related to spinal stenosis and/or radicular compression. Studies have demonstrated that

the level of bone pain is directly proportional to the level of disease activity.[23,24]

Serum Markers

Physiologic markers of bone turnover can be elevated in patients with PDB and appropriately confirm the sequence of phases undergone by the pathologic bone. Studies have measured the level of alkaline phosphatase, a marker of osteoblastic activity, as well as N-telopeptide of type I collagen, a marker of osteoclastic activity, and found them to be correspondingly elevated during the bone formation and bone resorption phases of PDB.[25] Measurements of total serum alkaline phosphatase (ALP) concentration are used to assess the activity of PDB and to monitor the effects of antiresorptive treatment. Bone-specific alkaline phosphatase, procollagen type-I N-terminal propeptide, provides good correlation with disease activity but has not been shown to offer any clinically significant benefit over measuring total ALP in routine practice.[26] However, in patients with coexisting liver disease, procollagen type-1 N-terminal propeptide concentrations provide a more specific reflection of disease activity.

Imaging

The radiographic features of PDB can mirror the histologic stages. During the osteoclastic phase, which is the first stage of disease, lytic features are seen on radiographs, classically described in long bones as an advancing V-shaped lesion or "blade of a grass" appearance.[27] In the mixed stages of disease, when osteoclastic as well as osteoblastic processes are occurring, this can manifest radiologically as mixed areas of lysis and sclerosis. In the final stages of disease, usually a sclerotic pattern predominates. However, it is important to note that all 3 histologic processes

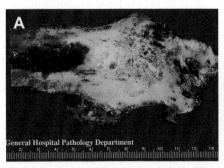
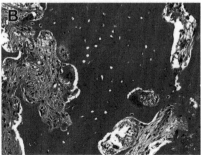

General Hospital Pathology Department

Fig. 1. (A) Gross resection specimen of a patient with PDB. The cortex is thickened and bony trabeculae are coarse, irregular, and thickened. (B) Histologic specimen demonstrating thickened bony trabeculae with the characteristic mosaic pattern and osteoclastic and osteoblastic activity (hematoxylin-eosin, original magnification ×10). (*Courtesy of* Dr G. Petur Nielsen, Massachusetts General Hospital.)

may be present in the same bone at the same time. Additionally, the radiographs may also show evidence of long bone bowing deformity, including coxa vara deformity of the femoral neck. Presence of stress fractures radiologically manifest as incomplete fissure fractures on the tension side of the bone with associated deformity.

Radioisotope bone scans may be used as a screening tool for the assessment of polyostotic involvement. It is important to note, however, that the bone scan can be negative in the early osteolytic stages of PDB because of low metabolic activity and consequent decreased uptake of the radioisotope.[27]

Lastly, the use of computed tomography scans and MRI may aid in further evaluation of patients with clinical findings concerning for fracture but concomitant negative radiographs, preoperative planning for arthroplasty or corrective osteotomies, and in the biopsy planning in patients with findings concerning for Paget sarcoma.

MEDICAL MANAGEMENT OF PAGET DISEASE

The principal indications for medical treatment of Paget disease are to relieve symptoms of bone pain and prevent complications arising from unchecked destruction of healthy bone and abnormal overgrowth of pagetic bone. This approach for treatment is particularly applicable to the subset of the Paget population with skull base involvement at risk of deafness or spinal cord compromise caused by bone overgrowth or at risk of fracture caused by the involvement of weight-bearing bones.[23,24] Other medical indications for treatment include optimization of bone turnover to reduce vascularity in patients undergoing elective surgery, such as joint arthroplasty. In such cases, decreased vascularity of pagetic bone can help reduce intraoperative blood loss.[28] Finally, antiresorptive treatment may also be appropriate in patients with polyostotic Paget disease with hypercalcemia as a means of treating the underlying cause of the electrolyte derangement.

The long-term efficacy of prophylactic treatment of asymptomatic patients with PDB is still not clear. Some investigators report no reduction in complications or clinical benefits in randomized controlled trials comparing asymptomatic patients with PDB receiving bisphosphonate treatment to normalize bone turnover markers versus those patients being treated for symptomatic disease.[29] Other studies report that patients who have undergone long-term treatment with bisphosphonates, for an average of 12 years, whose bone turnover rates had not normalized, had higher complications.[30] Therefore, some investigators advocate that the

potential of these antiresorptive medications to reduce disease progression, bone deformity, and related complications is significant enough to treat this asymptomatic subset of patients with antiresorptive treatment.[28] However, sufficient data are still lacking as most studies have a relatively short-term follow-up to realize the true long-term benefits of prophylactic treatment in asymptomatic patients. In symptomatic patients, there exists an established consensus on the choice of medical treatment options, which essentially includes bisphosphonates and calcitonin.

Bisphosphonates

Bisphosphonates are currently the mainstay medical treatment for Paget disease. They are synthetic analogues of inorganic pyrophosphate and bind to hydroxyapatite in bone. Modern bisphosphonates all broadly share similar pharmacologic properties, including selective skeletal uptake, binding to hydroxyapatite crystals, and resulting in suppression of osteoclast-mediated bone resorption. Both the degree of reduction in bone turnover and normalization of bone ALP levels (used to monitor disease activity) depend on the potency of agent and the dose and duration of treatment.[23] Various randomized controlled trials comparing the effects of different bisphosphonates in Paget disease have failed to show an overall significant benefit of one class over another.[31–33] In one study, Reid and colleagues[34] did report, however, that zoledronic acid had a better pain reduction rate and higher quality of life in patients with Paget disease.

There are different modalities of bisphosphonate treatment administration to patients with Paget disease, each with its own advantages and disadvantages. The choice of intravenous administration (as in zoledronic acid) can be better for compliance. The side effect of this modality is that it can provoke transient flulike symptoms in 10% to 15% of patients. Some of the bisphosphonates taken orally may require fasting after dosing to allow adequate absorption. The side effects include dyspepsia and/or diarrhea. Other long-term effects of bisphosphonates reported are uveitis, skin rashes, renal impairment, osteonecrosis of the mandible, and subtrochanteric stress fractures.[35]

Calcitonin

Calcitonins, because of their innate ability to reduce bone resorption, were first licensed for use in the treatment of PDB in the mid 1970s.[36] Calcitonin has been routinely administrated as a subcutaneous injection. Symptomatic improvement of bone pain occurs typically within 2 to 3 weeks; a decrease in activity of disease, as indicated by the reduction of baseline serum alkaline phosphatase, is noted after 3 to 6 months of treatment.[28] The potency of its antiresorptive effect is significantly less than comparable bisphosphonates. Moreover, its duration of effect is considerably shorter in comparison. Side effects of calcitonins include nausea, vomiting, diarrhea, and pain at the site of injection. Therefore, given these limitations, calcitonins are not recommended as the first-line treatment of PDB. It can be considered specifically in the subset of patients who cannot tolerate bisphosphonates and, therefore, is useful as an adjunct or as second-line treatment.

SURGICAL MANAGEMENT OF PAGET DISEASE

The surgical challenges of Paget disease arise on account of the primary disease process resulting in poor quality, fragile, and highly vascular bone, which can lead to large perioperative bleeding. Intramedullary fibrosis and, hence, difficulty for insertion of intramedullary devices may also play a role. Lastly, bony enlargement and deformity and possible altered biomechanical stresses leading to degenerative changes increase the challenges of surgical treatment.[28] It is debatable, however, as to whether the incidence of osteoarthritis is increased in PDB. There are published reports[37–39] in the literature suggesting that there is an association by reporting increased acceleration of osteoarthritis in joints juxtaposed to the pagetic bone.[39] Conversely, other investigators have found no difference in rates of osteoarthritis.[40] The limitation with the available published data is the relatively small sample sizes of PDB patient populations studied making it difficult to arrive at statistically sound conclusions. Nevertheless, for the orthopedic surgeon, it is important to understand the pathophysiology, pattern of bony involvement, and progression of this disease while planning and executing surgical procedures.

Surgical indications include fracture fixation through pagetic bone, realignment surgery to correct deformity in the major weight-bearing bones, prevention of impending fractures, joint replacement in severe arthritis in pagetic bone, spinal decompression to relieve pagetic bony compression of nerve roots and spinal canal stenosis, and radical resection and reconstruction for malignant transformation in pagetic bone.

Preoperative Assessment and Optimization of Pagetic Patients Before Surgery

Pagetic bone is highly vascular; thus, operating on highly active pagetic bone poses a significant risk of perioperative blood loss. It is, therefore, important to start bisphosphonate therapy at least 6 weeks before surgery.[3,41] The authors would recommend comanaging such patients with an endocrinologist with experience in the medical management of this condition. Usually the serum ALP trend is a useful marker of disease activity, and some investigators have suggested that a 50% reduction to pretreatment levels is a good measure of control.[3] It is important, however, to remember that, although serum ALP is increased in 95% of patients with Paget disease, a normal level does not exclude the diagnosis because patients with monostotic disease or those with metabolically inactive disease may have normal levels of ALP. Procollagen type-1 N-terminal propeptide and bone-specific ALP are other useful markers that can be used in the assessment, as previously discussed.[35]

Fixation of Fracture Through Pagetic Bone

The key principles of fracture fixation apply to fixation of fractures in pagetic bone. The surgeon should, wherever possible, use load-sharing devices to allow earlier weight bearing to mitigate the additional risk of further osteopenia in pagetic bone. In general, intramedullary devices spanning the entire diseased segment of bone and allowing for fixation into healthier segments of bone may allow for greater stability of the construct.[42]

It is important to obtain preoperative imaging in multiple planes to assess the suitability of intramedullary fixation, as severe bony deformity may preclude the use of these devices. In these situations, using long locking plates should be considered to improve stability. At the authors' institution, they have found that a 90/90 double locking plate construct, using an anteroposterior and lateral plating, can often be used in such situations. This construct similarly allows for increased stability and also early weight bearing. Please see **Fig. 2**.

It is also worth noting that studies reviewing nonoperative management of fractures in PDB report high nonunion rates.[43,44] In contrast, other studies have suggested that fracture healing is not compromised in patients with PDB.[45] In the authors' experience, they have found overall better outcomes with surgical fixation of these fractures, reducing nonunion rates and also facilitating earlier rehabilitation. Thorough assessment of the medical comorbidities, patients' baseline function, and the nature and characteristics of the fracture should be part of the decision-making algorithm.

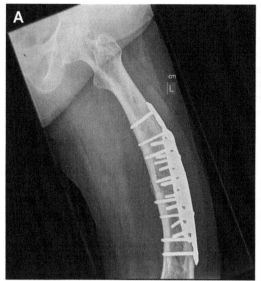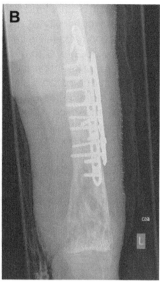

Fig. 2. (*A, B*) Anteroposterior projection x-ray radiographs of the left femur demonstrating the use of the 90/90 double locking plate construct in a patient with a stress fracture through pagetic bone.

Osteotomy

The main indications for osteotomy in PDB include correction of severe progressive deformity in symptomatic patients. Where the bony deformity precludes the insertion of a joint replacement prosthesis, extra-articular osteotomy may need to be done as a staged procedure to first correct the deformity and then proceed with joint reconstruction. It is important to ensure adequate preoperative imaging and planning in order to thoroughly appreciate the plane of the deformity. Many deformities are multiplanar and require multiple osteotomies for correction. For these complex deformities, Taylor spatial frame external fixators can be used to correct multiplanar deformities. Some investigators suggest better outcomes can be expected with osteotomies done at metaphyseal levels versus diaphyseal locations.[44]

Total Hip Arthroplasty

Several studies have concluded that total joint arthroplasty in the setting of osteoarthritis in pagetic patients improves pain, brings reduction of symptoms, and improves functional outcomes.[46,47] The specific issues with pagetic bone are the poor bone quality, deformity, increased perioperative bleeding risks, and fixation of prosthesis to bone.

When considering a total hip arthroplasty, on the acetabular side, the specific issues are protrusio and sclerotic bone. The sclerosis can make reaming challenging, and some investigators recommend the use of high-speed burrs to aid bone preparation.[47] The use of medial bone graft, large

hemispherical cups with screw fixation, and lateral offset acetabular liners have all been suggested as adjuncts to address optimization of cup positioning and achieving a satisfactory hip center of rotation. In some situations, antiprotrusio cages may be needed.

The femoral issues include coxa vara and avoiding a varus malposition. Thus, preoperative long leg films are particularly useful in templating. Considerations during planning should be given to trochanteric osteotomy for adequate exposure. Customized implants may be required to accommodate the deformity versus performing realignment osteotomy for deformity correction.

When considering fixation of the prosthesis to bone, there are proponents of both cemented and uncemented fixation, with both groups reporting good outcomes.[48–50] Nonetheless, failure rates with revision being the end point have been reported in up to 15% of cases following the use of cemented components.[48,51,52] Some reports have suggested that implant failures are correlated with activity of Paget disease reflected by the levels of ALP.[48]

Total Knee Arthroplasty

Although a smaller group of studies have looked at total knee arthroplasty in patients with PDB, they generally report a satisfactory outcome for these patients.[46,53,54] This subset of patients poses significant technical challenges to which the orthopedic surgeon must be aware of. Firstly, getting an extensile exposure is important, as different series have reported patellar tendon avulsions on account of soft tissue/collateral ligament tightness and enlarged, thickened patellas.[55] Therefore, careful, sequential exposure, protection of the patellar tendon, earlier patellar debridement/cutting, and extensile exposures may be helpful.[53]

The deformities to contend with are distal femoral varus angulation and excessive anterior tibial bowing. Several investigators have noted that with such femoral deformities, the use of intramedullary guides have led to malpositioning of the femoral component in a flexed and varus alignment. To counteract this, they recommended the use of extramedullary guides for preparation of femur.[46] On the tibial side, excessive anterior tibial bowing risks disproportionate anterior bone resection; therefore, increasing the posterior slope during tibial resection may mitigate this.

Because of the bony expansion of the pagetic bone on either the femoral or tibial side, prosthesis mismatch can occur.[53,54] It is important to recognize this on preoperative templating and planning and choose prosthetic systems that allow matching of different sized femoral and tibial components.

In terms of implant failures in total knee arthroplasty, there are limited data, which reveals no significantly increased rate of loosening with the use of cemented implants, when compared with the general population.[53]

Spinal Involvement

Paget disease of the spine may manifest as bony overgrowth of the neural arch and vertebral body expansion. These processes can lead to narrowing of the spinal canal and neural foramina. In addition, there may be soft tissue hypertrophy and ossification of the anterior/posterior longitudinal ligaments and the ligament flavum. The net clinical manifestations can be radiculopathy or myelopathy from spinal stenosis.

Symptomatic patients many need surgical decompression. As with any other anatomic regions of the body affected by Paget disease, preoperative medical treatment and disease control is important to minimize bleeding risks.

Pagetic Sarcoma

The most devastating sequela of long-standing Paget disease is its malignant transformation to Paget sarcoma. The Massachusetts General Hospital's series of patients with Paget sarcoma had a survival rate of 14% at 2.5 years.[56] Mankin and Hornicek[56] report that these pagetic sarcomas are more malignant than the other connective tissue tumors and more patients present with metastatic disease. They surmise that the increased

vascularity of the pagetic bone may partially be responsible for this. Malignant transformation is thought to be more common in patients with polyostotic disease. New symptoms of severe pain with destructive bony changes and soft tissue mass should alert the clinician to possible malignant transformation.

Most Paget sarcomas are histologically osteosarcomas, but any type of high-grade bone or soft tissue sarcoma is possible. The unifying feature is the high-grade nature of the tumor and the poor outcome, regardless of whether patients present with metastatic disease or not. Most of these patients are elderly with multiple medical comorbidities; depending on the polyostotic extent, some patients may even exhibit some cardiac dysfunction. The latter makes administration of chemotherapy challenging, and these patients often develop metastatic disease leading to death.

SUMMARY

The current understanding of Paget disease of bone has vastly changed since Sir James Paget described the first case in 1877. With advances in molecular biology and genetics, the pathophysiology and cause of the disease have been better elucidated. Medical management of this condition with bisphosphonates and occasionally calcitonin continues to remain the mainstay of treatment. Surgical indications include fractures through pagetic bone, need to correct deformity in the major long bones, prophylactic treatment of impending fractures through pagetic bone, joint arthroplasty in severe arthritis, and spinal decompression in cases of bony compression of neural elements. Advances in surgical technique, especially with the use of 90/90 plating and locked plating techniques, have now allowed for early return to function and mobilization. Despite medical and surgical intervention, a small subset of patients with PDB develops Paget sarcoma, an osteosarcoma with poor prognosis.

ACKNOWLEDGMENTS

The authors would like to extend their sincerest gratitude to Dr G. Petur Nielsen of the Department of Pathology, Massachusetts General Hospital, for his assistance in providing imaging of the histologic and gross pathologic specimens of Paget disease of bone.

REFERENCES

1. Coppes-Zantinga AR, Coppes MJ. Sir James Paget (1814–1889): a great academic Victorian. J Am Coll Surg 2000;191(1):70–4.

2. Kaplan FS, Singer FR. Paget's disease of bone: pathophysiology and diagnosis. Instr Course Lect 1993;42:417–24.

3. Kaplan FS, Singer FR. Paget's disease of bone: pathophysiology, diagnosis, and management. J Am Acad Orthop Surg 1995;3(6):336–44.

4. Merkow RL, Lane JM. Paget's disease of bone. Orthop Clin North Am 1990;21(1):171–89.

5. Mays S. Archaeological skeletons support a Northwest European origin for Paget's disease of bone. J Bone Miner Res 2010;25(8):1839–41.

6. Cooper C, Dennison E, Schafheutle K, et al. Epidemiology of Paget's disease of bone. Bone 1999; 24(5):3S–5S.

7. Cooper C, Schafheutle K, Dennison E, et al. The epidemiology of Paget's disease in Britain: is the prevalence decreasing? J Bone Miner Res 1999; 14(2):192–7.

8. Poor G, Donath J, Fornet B, et al. Epidemiology of Paget's disease in Europe: the prevalence is decreasing. J Bone Miner Res 2006;21(10):1545–9.

9. Cundy T, Reid IR. Reprint: Paget's disease of bone. Clin Biochem 2012;45(12):970–5.

10. Renier JC, Audran M. Progression in length and width of pagetic lesions, and estimation of age at disease onset. Rev Rhum Engl Ed 1997;64(1):35–43.

11. Hocking LJ, Lucas GJ, Daroszewska A, et al. Domain-specific mutations in sequestosome 1 (SQSTM1) cause familial and sporadic Paget's disease. Hum Mol Genet 2002;11(22):2735–9.

12. Laurin N, Brown JP, Morissette J, et al. Recurrent mutation of the gene encoding sequestosome 1 (SQSTM1/p62) in Paget disease of bone. Am J Hum Genet 2002;70(6):1582–8.

13. Hocking LJ, Lucas GJA, Daroszewska A, et al. Novel UBA domain mutations of SQSTM1 in Paget's disease of bone: genotype phenotype correlation, functional analysis, and structural consequences. J Bone Miner Res 2004;19(7):1122–7.

14. Chung PY, Beyens G, Guañabens N, et al. Founder effect in different European countries for the recurrent P392L SQSTM1 mutation in Paget's disease of bone. Calcif Tissue Int 2008;83(1):34–42.

15. Bolland MJ, Tong PC, Naot D, et al. Delayed development of Paget's disease in offspring inheriting SQSTM1 mutations. J Bone Miner Res 2007;22(3): 411–5.

16. Friedrichs WE, Reddy SV, Bruder JM, et al. Sequence analysis of measles virus nucleocapsid transcripts in patients with Paget's disease. J Bone Miner Res 2002;17(1):145–51.

17. Mee AP, Dixon JA, Hoyland JA, et al. Detection of canine distemper virus in 100% of Paget's disease samples by in situ-reverse transcriptase-polymerase chain reaction. Bone 1998;23(2):171–5.

18. Matthews BG, Afzal MA, Minor PD. Failure to detect measles virus RNA in bone cells from patients with Paget's disease. J Clin Endocrinol Metab 2008; 93(4):1398–401.

19. Ralston SH, Afzal MA, Helfrich MH, et al. Multicenter blinded analysis of RT-PCR detection methods for paramyxoviruses in relation to Paget's disease of bone. J Bone Miner Res 2007;22(4):569–77.

20. Roodman GD, Windle JJ. Paget disease of bone. J Clin Invest 2005;115(2):200–8.

21. Parfitt AM. Targeted and nontargeted bone remodeling: relationship to basic multicellular unit origination and progression. Bone 2002;30(1):5–7.

22. Langston AL, Ralston SH. Management of Paget's disease of bone. Rheumatology 2004;43(8):955–9.

23. Bolland MJ, Cundy T. Paget's disease of bone: clinical review and update. J Clin Pathol 2013;66(11): 924–7.

24. Lozano-Calderon SA, Colman MW, Raskin KA, et al. Use of bisphosphonates in orthopedic surgery: pearls and pitfalls. Orthop Clin North Am 2014; 45(3):403–16.

25. Alvarez L, Peris P, Pons F, et al. Relationship between biochemical markers of bone turnover and bone scintigraphic indices in assessment of Paget's disease activity. Arthritis Rheum 1997;40(3):461–8.

26. Reid IR, Davidson JS, Wattie D, et al. Comparative responses of bone turnover markers to bisphosphonate therapy in Paget's disease of bone. Bone 2004; 35(1):224–30.

27. Whitehouse RW. Paget's disease of bone. Semin Musculoskelet Radiol 2002;6:313–22.

28. Merlotti D, Gennari L, Martini G, et al. Current options for the treatment of Paget's disease of the bone. Open Access Rheumatol Res Rev 2009;1(1): 108–20.

29. Langston AL, Campbell MK, Fraser WD, et al. Randomized trial of intensive bisphosphonate treatment versus symptomatic management in Paget's disease of bone. J Bone Miner Res 2010;25(1):20–31.

30. Meunier PJ, Vignot E. Therapeutic strategy in Paget's disease of bone. Bone 1995;17(5):S489–91.

31. Miller PD, Brown JP, Siris ES, et al. A randomized, double-blind comparison of risedronate and etidronate in the treatment of Paget's disease of bone. Am J Med 1999;106(5):513–20.

32. Roux C, Gennari C, Farrerons J, et al. Comparative prospective, double-blind, multicenter study of the efficacy of tiludronate and etidronate in the treatment of Paget's disease of bone. Arthritis Rheum 1995;38(6):851–8.

33. Siris E, Weinstein RS, Altman R, et al. Comparative study of alendronate versus etidronate for the treatment of Paget's disease of bone. J Clin Endocrinol Metab 1996;81(3):961–7.

34. Reid IR, Miller P, Lyles K, et al. Comparison of a single infusion of zoledronic acid with risedronate for Paget's disease. N Engl J Med 2005;353(9): 898–908.

35. Ralston SH, Langston AL, Reid IR. Pathogenesis and management of Paget's disease of bone. Lancet 2008;372(9633):155–63.

36. Brandi ML. Current treatment approaches for Paget's disease of bone. Discov Med 2010;10(52): 209–12.

37. Altman RD, Collins B. Musculoskeletal manifestations of Paget's disease of bone. Arthritis Rheum 1980;23(10):1121–7.

38. Hadjipavlou A, Lander P, SroLovltz H. Pagetic arthritis pathophysiology and management. Clin Orthop Relat Res 1986;208:15–9.

39. Helliwell PS. Osteoarthritis and Paget's disease. Rheumatology 1995;34(11):1061–3.

40. Guyer PB, Dewbury KC. The hip joint in Paget's disease (Paget's "coxopathy"). Br J Radiol 1978; 51(608):574–8.

41. Siris ES, Lyles KW, Singer FR, et al. Medical management of Paget's disease of bone: indications for treatment and review of current therapies. J Bone Miner Res 2006;21(S2):P94–8.

42. Cornell CN. Internal fracture fixation in patients with osteoporosis. J Am Acad Orthop Surg 2003;11(2): 109–19.

43. Bradley CM, Nade S. Outcome after fractures of the femur in Paget's disease. Aust N Z J Surg 1992; 62(1):39–44.

44. Parvizi J, Frankle MA, Tiegs RD, et al. Corrective osteotomy for deformity in Paget disease. J Bone Joint Surg Am 2003;85(4):697–702.

45. Ludkowski P, Wilson-Macdonald J. Total arthroplasty in Paget's disease of the hip: a clinical review and review of the literature. Clin Orthop Relat Res 1990; 255:160–7.

46. Gabel GT, Rand JA, Sim FH. Total knee arthroplasty for osteoarthrosis in patients who have Paget disease of bone at the knee. J Bone Joint Surg Am 1991;73(5):739–44.

47. Parvizi J, Schall DM, Lewallen DG, et al. Outcome of uncemented hip arthroplasty components in patients with Paget's disease. Clin Orthop Relat Res 2002;403:127–34.

48. Guyen O, Vaz G, Vallese P, et al. Total hip arthroplasty and Paget's bone disease. J Bone Joint Surg Br 2005;87(Suppl II):134. Available online at: http://www.bjjprocs.boneandjoint.org.uk/content/87-B/SUPP_II/134.1.

49. Parvizi J, Klein GR, Sim FH. Surgical management of Paget's disease of bone. J Bone Miner Res 2006; 21(S2):P75–82.

50. Sochar DH, Porter ML. Charnley low-friction arthroplasty for Paget's disease of the hip. J Arthroplasty 2000;15(2):210–9.

51. McDonald DJ, Sim FH. Total hip arthroplasty in Paget's disease. A follow-up note. J Bone Joint Surg Am 1987;69(5):766–72.

52. Lusty PJ, Walter WL, Walter WK, et al. Cementless hip arthroplasty in Paget's disease at medium-term follow-up (average of 6.7 years). J Arthroplasty 2007;22(5):692–6.

53. Lee GC, Sanchez-Sotelo J, Berry DJ. Total knee arthroplasty in patients with Paget's disease of bone at the knee. J Arthroplasty 2005;20(6):689–93.

54. Cameron HU. Total knee replacement in Paget's disease. Orthop Rev 1989;18(2):206–8.

55. Vail TP, Callaghan JJ. Total knee replacement with patella magna and pagetoid patella. Orthopedics 1995;18(12):1174.

56. Mankin HJ, Hornicek FJ. Paget's sarcoma: a historical and outcome review. Clin Orthop Relat Res 2005;438:97–102.

Targeted Chemotherapy in Bone and Soft-Tissue Sarcoma

Jared L. Harwood, MD, John H. Alexander, MD,
Joel L. Mayerson, MD*, Thomas J. Scharschmidt, MD

KEYWORDS

• Targeted • Chemotherapy • Sarcoma • Bone • Tumor

KEY POINTS

- The evolution of our medical knowledge regarding sarcoma is explored, with special emphasis on its application to targeted chemotherapy as a treatment modality.
- The basic science behind sarcomatogenesis is discussed to identify common links among disparate tumor types. These common links offer targets that are being increasingly studied as novel treatments in sarcoma.
- The most common targets and pathways are discussed with relevant updates and clinical trials.

INTRODUCTION

Bone sarcomas and soft-tissue sarcomas (STS) encompass a heterogeneous group of human cancers that derive from the embryonic mesoderm. The diversity of sarcomas, with respect to histology, natural history, therapeutic sensitivities, and metastatic potential, stems in part from the diversity of mesodermic tissue, which includes bone, cartilage, adipose, muscle, vasculature, and hematopoietic. In the orthopedic literature, sarcomas tend to be broadly categorized as either of bone or soft tissue in origin. However, recent genomic and molecular discoveries (**Table 1**) have enabled us to reclassify these tumors and expand our therapeutic breadth to include optimized (and often personalized) cytotoxic chemotherapeutic regimens, radiopharmaceuticals, oncolytic viruses, immune-modulating therapies, and—the focus of this review—targeted chemotherapeutic agents. Although the mainstay of therapy for localized sarcoma remains surgical resection, neoadjuvant and adjuvant chemotherapy, and radiation, play an essential role in both local and systemic control.

The effect of chemotherapy has been most profound in the management of localized primary bone sarcomas, including osteosarcoma and Ewing sarcoma (ES). Link and colleagues[1] conducted one of the first randomized controlled trials showing the benefit of adjuvant chemotherapy in patients with localized osteosarcoma. At 2 years, patients who received chemotherapy had improved relapse-free survival of 66% compared with 17%; however, because of the short duration, they were unable to show an improvement in overall survival. Similar results were demonstrated by Eilber and colleagues[2] in 1987, recently validated with long-term follow-up showing a durable improvement in overall survival with adjuvant chemotherapy.[3] In the decades following, clinical research has focused primarily on optimizing adjuvant cytotoxic regimens,[4–8] including the initiation of neoadjuvant chemotherapy.[9,10] Current National Comprehensive Cancer Network guidelines

Department of Orthopaedics, The Ohio State University, 725 Prior Hall, 376 West 10 Avenue, Columbus, OH 43210, USA
* Corresponding author.
E-mail address: Joel.Mayerson@osumc.edu

Orthop Clin N Am 46 (2015) 587–608
http://dx.doi.org/10.1016/j.ocl.2015.06.011
0030-5898/15/$ – see front matter © 2015 Elsevier Inc. All rights reserved.

Table 1
Molecular characterization of STS with specific genetic alterations

Genetic Aberration	Histotype	Translocation[a]	Genes Involved[b]
Chromosomal Translocations (10%–15%)			
Aberrant transcription	Myxoid liposarcoma	t(12;16) (q13;p11)	*FUS-DDIT3EWSR1-DDIT3*
		t(12;22) (q13;q11–q12)	
	Synovial sarcoma	t(X;18) (p11;q11)	*SS18-SSX1*
		t(X;18) (p11;q11)	*SS18-SSX2*
	ASPS	t(X;17) (p11.2;q25)	*ASPL-TFE3*
	Low-grade ESS	t(7;17) (p15;q21)	*JAZF1-SUZ12*
	Ewing sarcoma/PNET	t(11;22) (q24;q12)	*EWSR1-FLI1*
		t(21;22) (q22;q12)	*EWSR1-ERG*
	DSRCT	t(11;22) (p13;q12)	*WT1-EWSR1*
	Clear-cell sarcoma	t(12;22) (q13;q12)	*ATF1-EWSR1*
	Alveolar	t(2;13) (p36;q14)	*PAX3-FOXO1*
	rhabdomyosarcoma	t(1;13) (p36;q14)	*PAX7-FOXO1*
	IMT	t(2;19) (p23;p13.1)	*TPM4-ALK*
		t(1:2) (q22–23;p23)	*TPM3-ALK*
	Low-grade fibromyxoid	t(7;16) (q32–34;p11)	*FUS-CREB3L2*
	sarcoma	t(11;16) (p11;p11)	*FUS-CREB3L1*
Fusion (increased expression of kinase)	Dermatofibrosarcoma	t(17;22) (q22;q13)	*COL1A1-PDGFB*
Chimeric (ligand independent kinase activation)	Infantile fibrosarcoma	t(12;15) (p13;q25)	*ETV6-NTRK3*
Oncogenic Mutations (20%)			
Activating	GIST	NA	*c-KIT, PDGFA, BRAF*
	MRCLS	NA	*PI3CA*
Inactivating	MPNST	NA	*NF-1*
	Rhabdoid tumors	NA	*INI1*
	PEComa family	NA	*TSC1/2*
Gene Amplification (10%–15%)			
NA	WDLS/DDLS	NA	*MDM2*
			CDK4
			c-JUN
	Intimal sarcomas	NA	*MDM2*
			CDK4

Abbreviations: DDLS, dedifferentiated liposarcoma; DSRCT, desmoplastic small round cell tumor; ESS, endometrial stromal tumor; GIST, gastrointestinal stromal tumor; IMT, inflammatory myofibroblastic tumor; MPNST, malignant peripheral nerve sheath tumor; MRCLS, myxoid round cell liposarcoma; NA, not available/applicable; EComa, perivascular epithelioid cell tumor; PNET, primitive neuroectodermal tumor; WDLS, well-differentiated liposarcoma.

[a] Translocations with a prevalence of greater than 5% are included.

[b] Sarcomas with specific genetic alterations (40%–50%). The approximate percentage of STS made up by the specified genomic group is shown in parentheses. Sarcoma with complex genomics (50%–60%) comprises the following: leiomyosarcoma, myofibrosarcoma, pleomorphic liposarcoma, pleomorphic rhabdomyosarcoma, undifferentiated pleomorphic sarcoma.

From Linch M, Miah AB, Thway K, et al. Systemic treatment of soft-tissue sarcoma—gold standard and novel therapies. Nat Rev Clin Oncol 2014;11(4):189; with permission.

recommend 1 of 4 first-line regimens including cisplatin/doxorubicin, high-dose methotrexate/cisplatin/doxorubicin with or without ifosfamide, or ifosfamide/cisplatin/epirubicin.[11] Despite the relative success in the treatment of nonmetastatic osteosarcoma, progression-free survival (PFS) and overall survival in metastatic osteosarcoma remains poor and an area that demands innovation.[12–15]

Similarly to osteosarcoma, ES of bone has a predilection for adolescents and a tendency to have subclinical micrometastases at the time of presentation.[16,17] More specifically, analysis of a large cohort of ES patients demonstrated that 18.4% presented with metastatic disease.[18] The addition of chemotherapy to the treatment algorithm in ES similarly revolutionized treatment outcomes in localized ES.[19] After further studies optimizing sequencing and timing of the chemo-therapeutic agents,[20–23] current treatment regi-mens involve neoadjuvant chemotherapy with a combination of vincristine, doxorubicin, cyclo-phosphamide, ifosfamide, and etoposide, fol-lowed by surgery and adjuvant chemotherapy with or without radiation.[24] This treatment strategy results in a 5-year relapse-free and overall survival of 52% to 78% in localized ES,[19–21,25,26] with out-comes closely tied to the histologic response to neoadjuvant therapy and the presence of metasta-tic disease.[18,22,27–30] Unfortunately, as with osteo-sarcoma, despite the optimization of cytotoxic regimens the 10-year overall survival in patients with metastatic ES is only 27% to 39%.[16,31–34]

Chondrosarcoma, a heterogeneous group of malignant cartilaginous tumors most commonly seen in the adult population, has traditionally been considered both chemoresistant and radia-tion resistant. At present, surgical resection is the primary treatment modality; however, in patients with high-grade/metastatic disease or certain his-tologic subtypes adjuvant therapy may be consid-ered,[35] underscoring the importance of novel targeted therapies in high-risk patients. STS are traditionally considered to be chemoresistant tu-mors, and therapy relies heavily on surgical resec-tion[36] and, if a high-grade lesion, localized radiation to improve local control.[37–39] The 5-year survival of nonmetastatic high-grade STS of the extremity is approximately 70%, with local recur-rence having the greatest effect on survival.[40] However, in the setting of metastatic high-grade extremity STS, survival is dismal, with 3-year survival rates less than 20%.[41] There are, how-ever, certain groups of patients that do benefit from systemic chemotherapy. Meta-analysis of doxorubicin-based adjuvant chemotherapy has demonstrated an improvement in time to recur-rence and overall recurrence-free survival, an ef-fect that was more significant in extremity STS. Unfortunately, this improvement in recurrence rate did not translate into an increased overall survival.[42] Additional studies and a recent meta-analysis have supported the use of high-dose ifos-famide as an additional first-line agent.[43–45]

Further evaluation of specific histologic sub-types has shown a small number of STS that are particularly responsive to adjuvant chemotherapy. The ANGIOTAX study, a phase II clinical trial investigating the effect of paclitaxel in patients with metastatic or unresectable angiosarcoma, demonstrated a modest clinical benefit. With the addition of paclitaxel the PFS at 2 months was 74%, however, this was not a durable response with only a 24% PFS at 6 months and an overall 18-month survival of 21%.[46] In patients with

liposarcoma, doxorubicin remains the agent of choice; interestingly the myxoid liposarcoma variant is particularly sensitive to cytotoxic regi-mens.[47] Finally, historical data show that synovial cell sarcoma is sensitive to high-dose ifosfamide therapy,[48] a finding that was further supported by a large retrospective analysis of patients with STS treated in the European Organization for Research and Treatment of Cancer (EORTC)/Soft Tissue and Bone Sarcoma Group.[49] A common constraint with the aforementioned regimens is discontinuation secondary to dosing limitations with long-term therapy, possibly leading to relapse with poor outcomes.[50] In a 2011 review by Patriki-dou and colleagues,[36] several key limitations with the use of adjuvant chemotherapy in STS were dis-cussed. Specifically, the lack of homogenous sub-type studies attributable to the rarity of STS and the need for subtype targeted therapy was highlighted.

In conclusion, current systemic treatment stra-tegies are marginally effective for most bone sar-comas and STS, underscoring the need for more effective and individualized regimens. **Table 2** lists several relevant completed and ongoing clinical trials and studies.

BASIC SCIENCE

Sarcomatogenesis, as with most human cancers, is characterized by changes on a genomic level that manifest as phenotypic changes including self-sufficient growth, insensitivity to growth inhib-itory signals, elusion of apoptosis, unlimited repli-cative potential, angiogenesis, tissue invasion, and metastasis[51] (**Fig. 1**). In recent decades, the development of genomic sequencing techniques has transformed our understanding of human dis-ease, with particular emphasis on its effect in oncology and tumorigenesis. In particular, sequencing has been instrumental in identifying key pathways and the development of chemother-apeutic agents targeting these aberrant pathways in tumor cells.

The most well-known and first of its kind to be approved by the Food and Drug Administration (FDA) is the tyrosine kinase inhibitor, imatinib. Initially developed to target the BCR-ABL fusion protein in chronic myeloid leukemia, it has since been found to have activity against the KIT tyro-sine kinase receptor present in gastrointestinal stromal tumors, leading to a partial response in at least 47.5% of patients, with 80% of patients able to tolerate maintenance therapy for more than 9 months.[52,53] Personalization of chemother-apeutic regimens and the identification of prog-nostic biomarkers have become more readily

Table 2
Current and recently completed clinical trials

Trial/Reference	Date	Phase	Tumor	Mechanism of Action/Target	Agent(s) Tested	Route/Frequency	Number Treated	Results
NCT01524926/ (Schöffski,[176] 2012)	—	II	AKT and/or MET altered tumors to include alveolar soft-part sarcoma, clear cell sarcoma, and alveolar rhabdomyosarcoma (≥15 y old)	Alk/MET	Crizotinib	PO/daily	582 (estimate)	Recruiting
NCT00093080 (Chawla et al,[177] 2012)	2004	II	Metastatic/unresectable soft-tissue or bone sarcoma	mTOR inhibitor	Ridaforolimus	IV/daily	212	28.8% achieved clinical benefit response (CR, PR, or SD for >16 wk)
(Yoo et al,[178] 2013)	—	II	Metastatic or recurrent bone and STS after the failure of anthracycline- and ifosfamide-containing regimens	mTOR inhibition	Everolimus	PO/daily	38	28.9% reached 16-wk PFS. Median PFS was 1.9 mo and median OS was 5.8 mo
NCT01614795 (Wagner,[179] 2015, #8372)	2012	II	STS (1–30 y old)	IGF-1R + mTOR	Cixutumumab + Temsirolimus	IV/weekly	43	No responses. 16% PF at 12 wk
NCT01016015 (Schwartz et al,[180] 2013)	2009	II	STS (1–30 y old)	IGF-1R + mTOR	Cixutumumab + Temsirolimus	IV/weekly	174	Combination therapy with clinical activity. 39% were PF at 12 wk. IGF-1R expression not predictive of outcome
NCT00831844 (Weigel,[181] 2014)	2009	II	Solid tumors (7–30 y old)	IGF-1R	Cixutumumab	IV/weekly	114	Limited activity noted. 4.4% with PR. 12.3% with SD
NCT00563680 (Tap et al,[182] 2012)	2007–2012	II	Ewing family tumors, DSRCTs (≥16 y old)	IGF-1R monoclonal antibody	Ganitumab	—	38	ORR was primary end point and seen in 6% of patients. CBR (seen in 17% of patients) and safety were secondary end points. 49% had SD. 63% experienced adverse events

Study	Phase	Year	Tumor type	Target/Mechanism	Drug	Route	N	Results
NCT00642941 (Pappo et al,[183] 2014)	II	2007–2010	Recurrent/refractory rhabdomyosarcoma, osteosarcoma, and synovial sarcoma (≥2 y old)	IGF-1R monoclonal antibody	R1507	IV/weekly	228	ORR was 2.5%. Partial responses were seen in 4 patients. 4 patients had >50% reduction in tumor size that lasted <4 wk. Median PFS was 5.7 wk. Median OS was 11 mo
NCT00385203 (Judson et al,[184] 2014)	II	2006–2009	GIST + STS progressing on imatinib/sunitinib	VEGF	Cediranib	Daily	34	Some activity noted by ^{18}FDG-PET in 5 patients, but no statistical reduction in SUV_{max} across the cohort. 4 of 6 patients with ASPS saw confirmed and durable partial responses
NCT00942877 (Kummar et al,[185] 2013)	II	2009	ASPS	VEGFR inhibitor	Cediranib	PO/daily	43	Partial response seen in 35% of patients. SD seen in 60%. Disease control rate of 84% at 24 wk
NCT00288015 (Agulnik et al,[186] 2013)	II	2006	Angiosarcoma and epithelioid hemangioendotheliomas	VEGF antibody	Bevacizumab	IV	32	Therapy was well tolerated in 15 patients with SD at 26 wk
NCT00070109 (Baruchel et al,[187] 2012)	II	2008–2013	Recurrent rhabdomyosarcoma, ES, and nonrhabdomyosarcoma STS	Unknown, suspect superoxide-induced apoptosis	Trabectedin	IV/every 3 wk	50	1 RMS patient had PR; 1 with RMS, 1 with SCS, and 1 with ES had SD at 2, 3, and 15 cycles
NCT01189253 (Butrynski,[188] 2015), EORTC	III	2011	Advanced/metastatic-related sarcomas	Unknown, suspect superoxide-induced apoptosis	Trabectedin vs doxorubicin-based chemotherapy (DXCT)	IV/every 3 wk	121	PFS and survival curves with no significant differences between arms. Response rate was higher in DXCT arm
(Cesne et al,[189] 2013)	II	—	Recurrent/advanced STS	Unknown, suspect superoxide-induced apoptosis	Trabectedin	—	350	Pooled analysis of 5 phase II studies. RR (10.1% in younger, 9.6% in older), PFS (2.5 vs 3.7 mo), and OS (13 vs 14 mo) did not differ among young and elderly cohorts

(continued on next page)

Table 2
(continued)

Trial/Reference	Date	Phase	Tumor	Mechanism of Action/Target	Agent(s) Tested	Route/ Frequency	Number Treated	Results
NCT01303094 (Le Cesne et al,[190] 2015, #71639)	2011	II	Advanced STS (≥18 y old)	Unknown, suspect superoxide-induced apoptosis	Trabectedin	IV/every 3 wk	178	91 patients (51%) had not progressed. Of these 53 were randomly assigned to continuation (C) vs interruption (I). PFS at 6 mo was 51.9% in the C group and 23.1% in the I group
NCT00928525 (Grignani,[191] 2011)	—	II	Chondrosarcoma	COL1A1-PDGFB	Imatinib	IM	26	PFS at 4 mo was 35%, median OS was 11 mo. No long-lasting disease-free progression or clinical benefit was observed. Temporary dose reduction required in 60%
(Ugurel et al,[192] 2014)	—	II	Dermatofibrosarcoma protuberans	COL1A1-PDGFB	Imatinib	Daily	16	Primary end point was response with secondary end points as safety, tumor relapse, and response biomarkers. Median therapy duration was 3.1 mo. Median tumor shrinkage was 31.5%. CR of 7.1%, PR of 50%, 35.7% SD, and 7.1% PD was seen. Neoadjuvant use was efficacious and well tolerated
(Sugiura et al,[193] 2010)	—	II	Metastatic unresectable or refractory KIT+/PDGFR+ sarcoma (12–75 y old)	Multitargeted tyrosine kinase inhibitor	Imatinib	Daily	22	1 PR (4.5%). 50% PFS at 61 d

Trial (Reference)	Years	Phase	Indication	Mechanism	Drug	Route	N	Results
NCT01209598 (Dickson,[194] 2013)	2010–current	II	CDK-4-amplified liposarcoma (≥18 y old)	CDK4/CDK6 inhibitor	PD0332991	PO/daily	29	At 12 wk, PFS was 66%, exceeding the 40% needed to consider the study positive
NCT00023998 (Ebb,[195] 2012)	2001–current	II	HER2+ osteosarcoma	Monoclonal antibody that interferes with HER2/neu receptor	Trastuzumab + chemotherapy	—	96 received chemotherapy (41 of these were HER+ and received trastuzumab)	Outcomes were poor. No significant difference between HER2− and HER2+ patients (EFS at 30 mo of 32% in both groups, OS 50% and 59%, respectively)
NCT00217620 (Von Mehren, Demetri,[196] 2012)	—	II	STS	Multitargeted tyrosine kinase inhibitor	Sorafenib	BID	37	No responses in any of the cohorts. Median PFS was 3 mo. Median OS was 17 mo
NCT00889057 (Grignani et al,[197] 2012)	2008–2011	II	Osteosarcoma (15–75 y old)	Multitargeted tyrosine kinase inhibitor	Sorafenib	BID	35	PFS at 4 mo was 46%. Median PFS was 4 mo. Median OS of 7 mo. CBR 29%. PR in 8%. Minor response in 6%. SD in 34%. PR/SD >6 mo in 17%
NCT01804374/ SERIO (Aglietta,[198] 2015)	2011–2014	II	Unresectable advanced and metastatic osteosarcoma (≥18 y old)	Multitargeted tyrosine kinase inhibitor/mTOR	Sorafenib + Everolimus	Daily	38	Dose reduction/interruptions were required in 66%. 6-mo PFS was 45%, shy of the 50% threshold to call the study positive
NCT00297258 (Sleijfer et al,[199] 2009)	2005–2012	II	STS	Multitargeted tyrosine kinase inhibitor	Pazopanib	PO/daily	148	Primary end point of PFS at 12 wk and secondary end points of response, safety, and OS were reached in leiomyosarcoma, synovial sarcoma, and other cohorts. End points were not reached in the adipocytic STS cohort

Abbreviations: ASPS, alveolar soft-part sarcoma; BID, twice daily; CBR, clinical benefit rate; CR, complete response; EFS, event-free survival; ES, Ewing sarcoma; FDG, fluorodeoxyglucose; GIST, gastrointestinal stromal tumor; IM, intramuscular; IV, intravenous; ORR, overall response rate; OS, overall survival; PD, progressive disease; PF, progression free; PFS, progression-free survival; PO, by mouth; PR, partial response; RMS, rhabdomyosarcoma; RR, response rate; SCS, synovial cell sarcoma; SD, stable disease; STS, soft-tissue sarcoma; SUV$_{max}$, standardized uptake value; VEGF, vascular endothelial growth factor; VEGFR, vascular endothelial growth factor receptor.

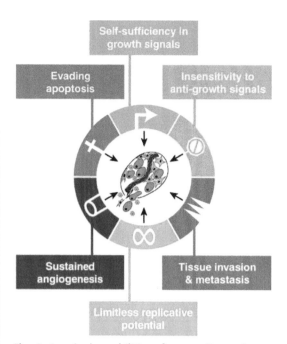

Fig. 1. Acquired capabilities of cancer. Research suggests that most, if not all cancers have acquired the same set of functional capabilities during their development, albeit through various mechanistic strategies. (*From* Hanahan D, Weinberg RA. The hallmarks of cancer. Cell 2000;100:58.)

available since the development of next-generation sequencing programs.[54,55] Although still in its nascence, this method has led to the development of a flurry of potential targeted therapeutics.[56]

A variety of genetic aberrations and, thus, therapeutic targets have been identified in bone sarcomas and STS. Based on genomic studies, Linch and colleagues[57] proposed the concept of 2 broad categories of sarcomas. The first group consists of sarcomas that contain specific chromosomal translocations producing chimeric fusion proteins, oncogenic mutations, and gene amplifications, as are commonly seen in ES, synovial cell sarcoma, clear-cell sarcoma, alveolar soft-part sarcoma, alveolar rhabdomyosarcoma, and myxoid liposarcoma, among others. The second category includes tumors that develop consistent with the traditional view of oncogenesis, with the progressive accumulation of mutations leading to loss of tumor-suppressor function and gain-of-function oncogenes. In osteosarcoma the latter paradigm prevails, as evidenced by the complex karyotypes seen in conventional high-grade osteosarcomas.[58]

With roughly 150 different subtypes of STS and bone sarcomas,[59] research on viable targets in chemotherapy has yielded approximately 140

potential gene targets that seem to drive cancer formation and progression.[60] These genes represent several molecular functions, the most common of which are kinases, with a significant proportion of these thought to be targetable (**Fig. 2**).

MAJOR PATHWAYS
p53 and Rb

There is strong evidence supporting the role of TP53 and RB1 in the development of osteosarcoma (**Figs. 3** and **4**, **Table 2**). Li-Fraumeni syndrome is characterized by germline mutations in p53 and is associated with high rates of osteosarcoma.[61] Similarly, in heritable retinoblastoma increased rates of osteosarcoma and leiomyosarcoma are observed in comparison with nonheritable counterparts.[62,63] A high incidence of somatic TP53 and RB1 mutations are also observed in sporadic osteosarcoma.[63–65] In chondrosarcoma, 96% of central high-grade tumors show alterations of the Rb pathway, leading to a loss of the tumor suppressor CDKN2A/p16 among other common mutations.[66] Abnormal p53 expression is not limited to bone sarcomas and is also a predictor for decreased survival in well-differentiated STS.[67] In addition, several other genetic syndromes including Rothmund-Thomson, Werner, Bloom, and RAPADILINO syndromes, which cause mutations in genes belonging to the RecQ DNA helicase family, have been shown to be associated with increased rates of osteosarcoma.[58,68] These common abnormalities are potential therapeutic targets.

Murine Double Minute

Closely related to p53 in oncogenesis is the murine double minute (MDM)2 proto-oncogene whose gene product promotes degradation of p53 via the ubiquitination pathway. The MDM family of proteins is involved in p53 degradation and is upregulated in many tumor types, especially parosteal osteosarcoma. Inactivation of p53 disrupts checkpoint responses to DNA damage, leading to the accumulation of additional oncogenic mutations. MDM2 is amplified in a wide variety of bone sarcomas and STS.[69] In particular, its amplification is very characteristic of well-differentiated and dedifferentiated liposarcoma.[47] MDM4 also binds to p53 and is amplified in ES in comparison with benign counterparts.[69]

In liposarcoma, the therapeutic agents RG7112 and MI-219 are small-molecule inhibitors of MDM2-p53, and have been tested with activity noted.[70,71] Nutlin-3 is an MDM2 antagonist that works to activate p53 and create a stabilizing effect

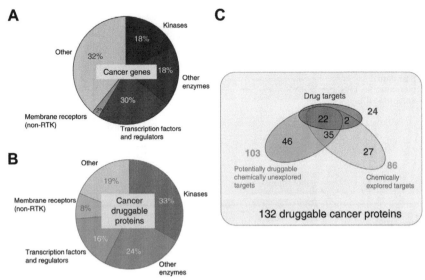

Fig. 2. The cancer genome and druggable cancer genome landscapes. (*A*) Functional classes of the protein products of 140 cancer genes that are activated by intragenic mutation to drive oncogenesis. Kinases account for 18% while enzymes as a whole comprise 36%. (*B*) Functional classes of 132 druggable cancer proteins from among the 479 cancer genes assessed, whereby kinases account for the higher proportion of 57%. RTK, receptor tyrosine kinase. (*C*) Druggable cancer proteins that are assigned as such because they are already drug targets (24 proteins, set shown in purple), have published active drug-like small molecules (86, set shown in green), or have 3-dimensional (3D) structures containing strictly druggable cavities (103, set shown in blue). A group of 46 proteins have druggable 3D structures but have few or no published compounds, and are therefore of considerable immediate interest for drug discovery. (*From* Workman P, Al-Lazikani B, Clarke PA. Genome-based cancer therapeutics: targets, kinase drug resistance and future strategies for precision oncology. Curr Opin Pharmacol 2013;13:487; with permission.)

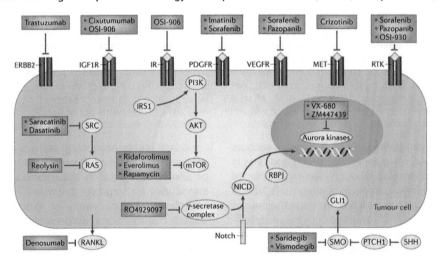

Nature Reviews | Cancer

Fig. 3. Molecular targets and associated drugs identified for therapeutic intervention in osteosarcoma. Therapeutic targets include specific cell surface receptor tyrosine kinases (RTKs): ERBB2, insulin-like growth factor 1 receptor (IGF1R), insulin receptor (IR), platelet-derived growth factor receptor (PDGFR), vascular endothelial growth factor receptor (VEGFR), and hepatocyte growth factor (HGF) receptor (also known as MET). Alternatively, pan-RTK inhibitors, such as sorafenib, pazopanib, and OSI-930, could be used. Other potential targets include PI3K, insulin receptor substrate 1 (IRS1), AKT, mTOR, sonic hedgehog (SHH), smoothened (SMO), Patched 1 (PTCH1), glioma-associated oncogene homologue 1 (GLI1), Notch, Notch intracellular domain (NICD), and recombination signal binding protein for immunoglobulin κJ region (RBPJ). Aberrant activation of these signaling molecules and pathways in osteosarcoma may promote tumor cell proliferation, survival, migration, angiogenesis, and metastasis. (*From* Kansara M, Teng MW, Smyth MJ, et al. Translational biology of osteosarcoma. Nat Rev Cancer 2014;14:728; with permission.)

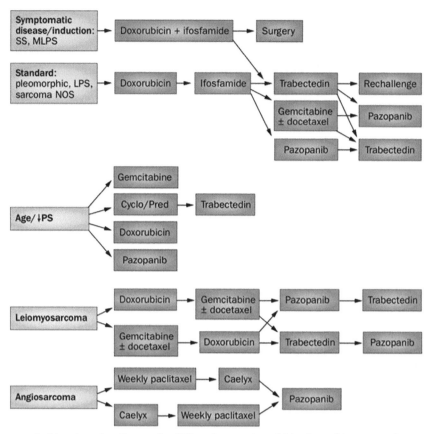

Fig. 4. Recommended treatment pathways for STS and examples of histology-driven paradigms. Where treatments appear in a vertical column, there is no hierarchy of which agent should be used in preference to another. For the high age or low performance status (PS) group, only 2 lines of therapy are presented. Further therapy lines, however, would be considered contingent based on PS and patient factors. Cyclo, cyclophosphamide; LPS, liposarcoma; MLS, myxoid liposarcoma; NOS, not otherwise specified; Pred, prednisolone; PS, performance status; SS, synovial sarcoma. (*From* Linch M, Miah AB, Thway K, et al. Systemic treatment of soft-tissue sarcoma—gold standard and novel therapies. Nat Rev Clin Oncol 2014;11:190; with permission.)

on the malignant potential in malignancies such as ES.[72] However, resistance has been noted, and is postulated to develop through overexpression of MDMX. Thus, new compounds such as RO-5963 target both MDM2 and MDMX to inhibit their effect on p53 activity.[73,74] Several of these small-molecule MDM antagonists are currently undergoing phase I trials (NCT01877382, NCT01462175, and NCT01164033), with 1 follow-up study being conducted with RO5045337, a Nutlin-3 analogue (NCT01677780).

Wnt

The Wnt pathway, which plays an important role in limb development and osteoblastic differentiation,[75] is inactivated in human osteosarcoma. This inactivation prevents the degradation of β-catenin, leading to downstream cellular proliferation.[76–78] Wnt/β-catenin signaling occurs via both canonical and noncanonical pathways. Numerous participants in these pathways have been found to be abnormal in a variety of sarcomas, and may be candidates for targeted therapies.[79,80] Given the complexity and necessity of Wnt signaling for normal cell functions, some worry that targeting it may lead to significant detriment to normal cell function. That being said, targets on the extracellular (Wif-1, Dkk, sFRPs, and monoclonal antibodies), intracellular (APC), and nuclear (β-catenin/Tcf-mediated transactivation, c-Myc, c-Met, cyclin D1, and survivin) levels have been proposed as options.[81] Finally, in a noncanonical pathway, Wnt activates cell growth via activation of mammalian target of rapamycin (mTOR) (see later discussion).[82]

FHL2 is a multifunctional adaptor protein that can act as an oncoprotein or a tumor suppressor, depending on which tissue expresses the gene. In osteosarcoma, FHL2 silencing reduces

Wnt/β-catenin signaling, which in turn leads to reduced cell proliferation, apoptosis, cell invasion, migration, tumorigenesis, and metastasis.[83]

Notch

Notch signaling is similar to the Wnt pathway in that it is a key regulator of tissue development. The Notch family consists of transmembrane receptors that when activated form an intracellular complex, which when cleaved translocates to the nucleus. In the nucleus, Notch influences gene transcription leading to cell proliferation, differentiation, and apoptosis. More specifically, it has been shown to influence proliferation of immature osteoblasts and prevent their maturation.[84] Recent studies have shown that Notch signaling may play a role in metastasis, drug resistance, and poor prognosis in osteosarcoma.[85]

Hedgehog

The Hedgehog (Hh) pathway regulates the proliferation and differentiation of tissues and organs during development, especially chondrocytes.[86] The ligands signal through the PTCH (patched) receptor to relieve its inhibition of the SMO (smoothened) receptor, which results in the activation of glioma-associated oncogene (Gli), a zinc finger transcription factor, leading to increased gene transcription.[87] The effect of hedgehog activation is not limited to chondrosarcoma. Gli is overexpressed in rhabdomyosarcoma, ES, and osteosarcoma, indicating a potential role in the pathogenesis of these tumors.[88]

In osteosarcoma IPI-926, an Hh inhibitor, was found to decrease xenograft tumor size and weight, especially in metastatic osteosarcoma cell lines.[87]

RUNX

RUNX is a family of transcription factors that regulates the differentiation, survival, and growth of tissues; more specifically, RUNX2 regulates osteogenesis. RUNX2 is a downstream product of many of the aforementioned pathways, including Wnt and Indian Hh. In osteosarcoma, RUNX2 is often constitutively activated. Similarly to other pathways, this increased expression translates to greater metastatic potential. In addition, RUNX2 seems to be intimately related to Rb and p53, and in their absence RUNX2 expression is increased.[89]

MET

Additional genes involved in mesenchymal cell differentiation have been implicated in the development of osteosarcoma and other sarcomas. MET, an oncogene tyrosine kinase receptor, is activated by hepatocyte growth factor during development and is overexpressed in undifferentiated pleomorphic sarcoma (previously known as malignant fibrous histiocytoma), rhabdomyosarcoma, synovial sarcoma, epithelioid sarcoma, and peripheral nerve sheath tumors. More specifically, the fusion of ASPL and MET in alveolar soft-part sarcoma and the t(12:22) fusion gene in clear-cell sarcoma have been shown to increase MET transcription.[57] In undifferentiated pleomorphic sarcoma, abnormal expression of c-MET and its downstream effector, p-MEK pathway, is seen in 38% and 37% of a large sample population, respectively.[90] MET expression has also been associated with more aggressive phenotypes and poor prognosis in sarcoma.[91,92] In addition, it has been shown to play an important role in osteosarcoma. In vitro and in vivo studies have shown that primary osteoblasts, when exposed to elevated levels of MET as seen in osteosarcoma, develop a malignant phenotype.[93]

Wagner and colleagues[94] used a selective competitive MET inhibitor, tivantinib (ARQ197), in 47 patients, and demonstrated a partial response in 1 patient with clear-cell sarcoma and stable disease (SD) in 60%.

Mammalian Target of Rapamycin

mTOR is an intracellular serine/threonine kinase involved in the phosphatidylinositol 3-kinase (PI3K)/AKT signaling cascade and several other receptor tyrosine kinases (RTKs), including insulin growth factor (IGF). The mTOR pathway is abnormally activated in sarcomas including, but not limited to, osteosarcoma.[95] In human cancers the activation of the mTOR signaling may occur by a variety of means. The receptors may be constitutively activated, as seen in osteosarcoma cell lines with poor prognosis,[96] or downstream effectors of mTOR may be altered in a way that leads to increased mTOR pathway activity.[97]

Everolimus, an mTOR inhibitor, was evaluated in the phase I/II trial C2485,[97] followed by 2 randomized phase III trials. The EXIST-1 trial, a randomized phase III double-blind, placebo-controlled study (Examining Everolimus In a Study of TSC), evaluated the activity and safety of everolimus in 117 patients with tuberous sclerosis complex (TSC)-associated subependymal giant cell astrocytoma (SEGA). The EXIST-2 trial was a randomized, double-blind, placebo-controlled trial that assessed the response rate of 118 patients on everolimus with at least 1 angiomyolipoma (AML) and a definite diagnosis of TSC-related or sporadic lymphangioleiomyomatosis. The response rate at 6 months of treatment was significantly higher in the everolimus group when compared with the placebo group (42% vs 0%, respectively; P<.0001). Time to AML progression was also statistically significantly longer in patients on everolimus (P<.0001).[98,99] Everolimus is currently used in the treatment of advanced renal cell cancer (FDA approval 2009), tuberous sclerosis–associated SEGA (FDA approval 2010), unresectable pancreatic neuroendocrine tumors (FDA approval 2011), and HR-positive/HER2-negative breast cancer (FDA approval in 2012).[100]

Demetri and colleagues[101] performed a large, randomized placebo-controlled phase III trial (Sarcoma Multicenter Clinical Evaluation of the Efficacy of Ridaforolimus or SUCCEED trial) that evaluated the mTOR inhibitor ridaforolimus to assess the maintenance of disease in patients with advanced sarcomas. A total of 702 patients received ridaforolimus and demonstrated a mild, but significant median PFS of 17.7 weeks versus 14.6 weeks with placebo. In addition, there was a mean 1.3% decrease in target lesion size versus 10.3% increase with placebo. In 2012 ridaforolimus failed to receive FDA approval. The FDA response letter cited the need for additional clinical trials to prove its safety and efficacy.

Insulin Growth Factor Pathway

The IGF signaling system, specifically IGF-2, is known to play an important role in many mesenchymal tumors.[102] In normal physiologic states, IGF signaling regulates growth and development via activation of tyrosine kinase receptors and downstream pathways including Ras/Raf/MEK/ERK, PI3k, AKT, and mTOR, ultimately leading to increased mitosis and survival.[103] In particular, IGF-1/-2 and IGF receptors are overexpressed secondary to induced transcription by ES fusion proteins[104] and the effect of ES fusion proteins to decrease levels of IGFBP3,[105] a carrier protein that antagonizes IGF-1 action. Of clinical relevance, the activation of the IGF pathway is associated with decreased PFS and overall survival in patients with ES.[106] A similar induction of IGF-2 expression is noted in synovial sarcoma, a finding supported by increased IGF-2 expression in human lung fibroblasts expressing the SYT-SSX1 and SYT-SSX2 fusion oncogenes, and upregulation of IGF-2 in clinical samples.[107] Interestingly the IGF pathway activity has also been implicated in pediatric rhabdomyosarcoma[108]; however, whereas IGF-R1 and IGF-PB3 expression was elevated in all subtypes, IGF-2 was shown to be associated with translocation-negative subtypes in particular.[109] Van de Luijtgaarden and colleagues[110] showed that not only is the IGF pathway overexpressed in osteosarcoma, but that chemotherapy leads to a reduction in the expression of IGF-1 and downstream effectors, a fact that influences the efficacy of targeted therapies based on timing in conjunction with cytotoxic agents. In addition, downstream blockade of mTOR leads to feedback activation of AKT via the IGF receptor. This finding may explain why IGF and mTOR inhibitors seem to be synergistic. Regardless, the IGF pathway plays an important role in sarcomatogenesis, making it an appealing target for future therapies.

Monoclonal antibodies against IGF-1R have shown a response in at least 60% of cases in xenograft models.[111] The IGF pathway has been studied extensively in ES, with some significant response rates in approximately 15% of cases, suggesting that there is a subset of patients who are more likely to respond. Several studies have looked into targeting IGF-1R with drugs such as R1507, figitumumab, and cixutumumab, and in combination with rapamycin (mTORC1 inhibitor). Resistance has been a problem, as resistant cells have maintained IGF-1R but have downregulated its expression. Instead, these cells upregulate IGF-2 and insulin receptor A, with enhanced mitogen-activate protein kinase signaling and less reliance on AKT activation.[112] Silencing of EWS-FLI1 using antisense DNA, siRNA, and dominant negatives such as cytarabine, markedly impairs ES cell growth.[113] Agents such as YK-4-2709[114] and mithramycin[115] target EWS-FLI1 directly.

Ezrin

Ezrin, an ezrin-radixin-moesin protein, functions to link the membrane and cytoskeletal actin to promote cell mobility, cell-cell and cell-matrix adherence, signal transduction, and RTKs activation.[116–120] Interesting research has shown that ezrin overexpression promotes metastasis via numerous pathways, including loss of intercellular adhesions via decreased E-cadherin surface localization,[119] increased cell survival,[121] and amplified metastatic signal transduction.[122] This increased metastatic potential and decreased survival has been observed in rhabdomyosarcoma,[123] ES,[124] high-grade STS,[125,126] pleomorphic malignant fibrous histiocytoma,[127] myxofibrosarcoma,[128] chondrosarcoma,[129] and osteosarcoma.[121,130–133]

Given the functional characteristics of ezrin, targeting is expected to prevent metastatic progression but not to have an appreciable effect on the primary tumor.[134] NSC305787 and NSC668394 are 2 small molecules that directly bind to ezrin that have demonstrated statistically significant reduction in tumor growth in organ cultures at 7 days.[135]

Interleukin-11Rα

Interleukin (IL)-11, a cytokine produced by bone marrow mesenchymal cells, has an effect on hematopoietic, adipocytic, epithelial, osseous, and cartilaginous tissues.[136] IL-11 stimulates cell migration via a PI3K/AKT and nuclear factor (NF)-κβ–dependent pathway, ultimately leading to increased expression of the cell adhesion molecule, ICAM-1.[137] The effect of IL-11 has been observed in a wide variety of human cancers. With respect to sarcomas, IL-11 expression is increased in patients with chondrosarcoma in comparison with primary chondrocytes. In addition, IL-11Rα is highly expressed in osteosarcoma, and seems to play an important role in angiogenesis and metastasis in these patients.[138] Finally, IL-11R-α is also expressed on the cell surface of osteosarcoma pulmonary metastases. Therefore, studies investigating the utility of IL-11 pathway inhibitors may play a role in retarding metastasis.

Signal Transducer and Activator of Transcription 3

Signal transducer and activator of transcription (STAT), in particular STAT3, is a DNA-binding transcription factor that functions as a downstream effector of membrane-bound receptors. Interestingly these receptors include epidermal growth factor receptor, platelet-derived growth factor receptor (PDGFR), IL-6 and IL-11 receptors, and many natural and synthetic molecules including carcinogens. Activation of STAT-3 occurs via receptor kinases, Src, Janus-activated kinases, and ERK (extracellular signal-regulated kinase). The activation of STAT3 is known to cause many cellular changes including suppression of apoptosis, proliferation, invasion, angiogenesis, and metastasis, leading to initiation and promotion of tumorigenesis.[139] Chen and colleagues[140] demonstrated increased activity of STAT3 in 19% of osteosarcoma, 27% of rhabdomyosarcoma, and 15% of a wide variety of other STS patient samples with microarray immunohistochemical staining. The role of STAT3 in STS was further supported by additional analysis of patient samples showing more constitutive STAT3 expression in malignant tumors when compared with benign controls, although the study was limited by the lack of traditional tissue-type classifications of samples.[141] Finally, the role of STAT3 in cellular growth and inhibition of apoptosis in osteosarcoma cell lines has been supported by Wang and colleagues,[142] indicating that STAT3

inhibitors may play a role in a wide variety of human sarcomas.

In the study by Wang and colleagues,[142] inhibition of STAT3 signaling with STAT3 inhibitor S31 to 201 patients suppressed osteosarcoma cell growth and induced apoptosis in a time-dependent and dose-dependent manner. A phase I trial (NCT00955812) was completed in 2012 that involved 30 patients who were treated with a STAT3 inhibitor, OPB-31121. No responses were observed and, even though twice-daily administration was feasible, its pharmacokinetics were unfavorable, with high intersubject variability and much lower concentrations than those seen in mouse models.[143]

Vascular Endothelial Growth Factor

Tumor growth and cellular survival depends on the continued supply of nutrients and oxygen to the rapidly dividing cells. In hypoxic environments, increased expression of HIF-1α leads to increased expression of vascular endothelial growth factor (VEGF), a primary initiator of angiogenesis.[144,145] The critical role of VEGF in tumor angiogenesis makes it an intriguing target for drug development. The effects of VEGF are not limited to angiogenesis, as it also plays a role in cellular migration, survival, and proliferation, and increased vascular permeability.[145] VEGF overexpression is observed in many human sarcomas including chondrosarcoma,[146] synovial sarcoma,[147] ES,[148] rhabdomyosarcoma,[149] osteosarcoma,[150] and angiosarcoma.[151,152] Phase II clinical trials investigating the VEGF pathway as a target have delivered promising results. Kummar and colleagues[153] demonstrated a partial response in 35% and SD in 60% of patients with metastatic alveolar soft-part sarcoma receiving cediranib. Impressively, the disease control rate was 84% at 24 weeks. Agulnik and colleagues[154] conducted a phase II trial evaluating bevacizumab in patients with unresectable angiosarcoma or epithelioid hemangioendothelioma and showed that the drug was well tolerated, with SD in 47% of patients at 26 weeks.

Other Growth Factors and Their Receptor Tyrosine Kinases

RTKs play a pivotal role in the cellular response to environmental stimuli, including, but not limited to, growth factors. RTK stimulation or constitutive activation is implicated in the development of a myriad of human cancers. Early studies demonstrated elevated serum levels of VEGF and basic fibroblast growth factor (FGF), potent stimulators of angiogenesis, in patients with STS.[155,156]

Moreover, FGF signaling is abnormally expressed in subtypes of chondrosarcoma with increased expression of FGFR-3.[157] In addition, PDGFR-β, AXL, and C-X-C chemokine receptor 4 are overexpressed in myxoid liposarcoma.[158] Similarly, PDGFR-α may play a critical role in synovial sarcoma.[159] Furthermore, in dermatofibrosarcoma protuberans (DFSP), the COL1A1–PDGF-β fusion gene is highly expressed in most patients,[160,161] and places the production of PDGF-β under the control of the promoter region for the COL1-α1 gene.[162] The importance of PDGF is not limited to STS. A recent study by Takagi and colleagues[163] demonstrated that PDGF released by platelets in response to platelet-osteosarcoma cell interactions induced proliferation of osteosarcoma cell lines.

Early trials with imatinib, including the Imatinib Target Exploration Consortium Study B2225, showed a 100% response rate in locally advanced DFSP cases. Combined analysis of the EORTC trial 62,027 and Southwest Oncology Group trial S0345 found a clinical benefit rate greater than 70%, a median time to progression of 1.7 years, and a 1-year overall survival of 87.5%.[164]

Kasper and colleagues[165] reported the combined results of a phase II/III (PALETTE) trial involving 118 and 246 patients with STS, respectively, who were treated with pazopanib, a multitargeted tyrosine kinase inhibitor. Combined median survival was 11.7 months, 36% of patients had a PFS greater than 6 months, and 34% had an overall survival longer than 18 months. Median follow-up was 2.3 years, with 22.1% of patients being declared both long-term responders and survivors. Of note, 3.5% of patients were able to remain on pazopanib for longer than 2 years, indicating significant tolerability.[166]

Chimeric Transcription Factors

Many sarcomas have been found to have highly specific chromosomal translocations, which seem to play a crucial role in tumorigenesis, and in certain tumor types their presence plays a prognostic role.[167] Common fusion oncogenes have been discussed with respect to their effector mechanisms; however, there are several other human sarcomas associated with pathognomonic fusion proteins that may serve as potential therapeutic targets. The previously mentioned liposarcoma variants, myxoid and round cell liposarcoma, are characterized by the chimeric fusion protein FUS-CHOP, t(12;16).[168] The FUS-CHOP protein functions as an abnormal transcription factor blocking adipocytic differentiation.[169] Another common fusion oncogene is ASPL-TFE3, t(x;17), consistently found

in alveolar soft-part sarcoma, which functions as a transcription factor for a myriad of genes. In particular, it deregulates expression of c-Met, AKT, and mTOR-complex 1, among others.[170,171] Finally, alveolar rhabdomyosarcoma is characterized by the presence of the PAX3/7-FKHR fusion gene. This fusion product increases NF-κβ pathway activity, which ultimately inhibits myogenic differentiation.[172]

B-Cell Lymphoma 2

Apoptosis in cancer is regulated by interactions between members of the B-cell lymphoma 2 (Bcl-2) protein family. Bcl-2 and parathyroid hormone-related protein have been shown to play a critical role in the malignant transformation of osteochondroma into peripheral chondrosarcoma. By comparison, this is a late finding in high-grade central chondrosarcomas.[173] Furthermore, Bcl-2 contributes to chemoresistance in chondrosarcoma cell lines, a process that was reversible in vitro with Bcl-2 inhibitors.[174] These data support the investigation of Bcl-2 inhibitors in chondrosarcoma, a traditionally chemoresistant tumor.

Furthermore, Bcl2, Bcl-xL, and myeloid cell leukemia 1 (Mcl1) are prosurvival molecules that regulate apoptosis in cancer cells that can be subdivided into 2 functionally distinct classes. These 2 classes include Bcl-2-associated and the BH3-only proteins.

Two BH3 mimetics, ABT-263 and ABT-737, have been shown to induce apoptosis in chondrosarcoma xenografts,[175] although human studies in sarcoma have yet to be undertaken. ABT-199 is a potent Bcl-2 inhibitor for which a phase I trial is recruiting patients with refractory multiple myeloma (NCT01794520).

SUMMARY

The pathways and oncogenes discussed herein, and their downstream effectors, play a crucial role in the development of human sarcoma and provide a glimmer of hope in the development of targeted therapies. These developing therapies are adding to the armamentarium of the clinician and are broadening the horizon for the gold-standard treatment of STS. In response to the recent advances in molecular genetics, potential targets continued to be discovered at a prodigious rate. As more pieces of the puzzle become available, clinicians must take a step back and continue to piece the puzzle together to gain a better overall understanding of the complex molecular interactions present in normal and pathologic tissues.

REFERENCES

1. Link MP, Goorin AM, Miser AW, et al. The effect of adjuvant chemotherapy on relapse-free survival in patients with osteosarcoma of the extremity. N Engl J Med 1986;314:1600–6.

2. Eilber F, Giuliano A, Eckardt J, et al. Adjuvant chemotherapy for osteosarcoma: a randomized prospective trial. J Clin Oncol 1987;5:21–6.

3. Bernthal NM, Federman N, Eilber FR, et al. Long-term results (>25 years) of a randomized, prospective clinical trial evaluating chemotherapy in patients with high-grade, operable osteosarcoma. Cancer 2012;118:5888–93.

4. Bramwell VH, Burgers M, Sneath R, et al. A comparison of two short intensive adjuvant chemotherapy regimens in operable osteosarcoma of limbs in children and young adults: the first study of the European Osteosarcoma Intergroup. J Clin Oncol 1992;10:1579–91.

5. Souhami RL, Craft AW, Van der Eijken JW, et al. Randomised trial of two regimens of chemotherapy in operable osteosarcoma: a study of the European Osteosarcoma Intergroup. Lancet 1997;350:911–7.

6. Lewis IJ, Nooij MA, Whelan J, et al. Improvement in histologic response but not survival in osteosarcoma patients treated with intensified chemotherapy: a randomized phase III trial of the European Osteosarcoma Intergroup. J Natl Cancer Inst 2007;99:112–28.

7. Le Deley MC, Guinebretière JM, Gentet JC, et al. SFOP OS94: a randomised trial comparing preoperative high-dose methotrexate plus doxorubicin to high-dose methotrexate plus etoposide and ifosfamide in osteosarcoma patients. Eur J Cancer 2007; 43:752–61.

8. Collins M, Wilhelm M, Conyers R, et al. Benefits and adverse events in younger versus older patients receiving neoadjuvant chemotherapy for osteosarcoma: findings from a meta-analysis. J Clin Oncol 2013;31:2303–12.

9. Bacci G, Picci P, Ruggieri P, et al. Primary chemotherapy and delayed surgery (neoadjuvant chemotherapy) for osteosarcoma of the extremities. The Istituto Rizzoli experience in 127 patients treated preoperatively with intravenous methotrexate (high versus moderate doses) and intraarterial cisplatin. Cancer 1990;65:2539–53.

10. Ferrari S, Ruggieri P, Cefalo G, et al. Neoadjuvant chemotherapy with methotrexate, cisplatin, and doxorubicin with or without ifosfamide in nonmetastatic osteosarcoma of the extremity: an Italian sarcoma group trial ISG/OS-1. J Clin Oncol 2012;30: 2112–8.

11. National Comprehensive Cancer Network. NCCN Clinical Practice Guidelines in Oncology: Bone Cancer. Version 1. 2015. Available online at: http://www.nccn.org/professionals/physician_gls/pdf/bone.pdf. Accessed 28 July, 2015.

12. Bacci G, Briccoli A, Rocca M, et al. Neoadjuvant chemotherapy for osteosarcoma of the extremities with metastases at presentation: recent experience at the Rizzoli Institute in 57 patients treated with cisplatin, doxorubicin, and a high dose of methotrexate and ifosfamide. Ann Oncol 2003;14:1126–34.

13. Navid F, Willert JR, McCarville MB, et al. Combination of gemcitabine and docetaxel in the treatment of children and young adults with refractory bone sarcoma. Cancer 2008;113:419–25.

14. Goorin AM, Harris MB, Bernstein M, et al. Phase II/III trial of etoposide and high-dose ifosfamide in newly diagnosed metastatic osteosarcoma: a pediatric oncology group trial. J Clin Oncol 2002;20: 426–33.

15. Berger M, Grignani G, Ferrari S, et al. Phase 2 trial of two courses of cyclophosphamide and etoposide for relapsed high-risk osteosarcoma patients. Cancer 2009;115:2980–7.

16. Esiashvili N, Goodman M, Marcus RBJ. Changes in incidence and survival of Ewing sarcoma patients over the past 3 decades: Surveillance Epidemiology and End Results data. J Pediatr Hematol Oncol 2008;30:425–30.

17. Herzog CE. Overview of sarcomas in the adolescent and young adult population. J Pediatr Hematol Oncol 2005;27:215–8.

18. Cotterill SJ, Ahrens S, Paulussen M, et al. Prognostic factors in Ewing's tumor of bone: analysis of 975 patients from the European Intergroup Cooperative Ewing's Sarcoma Study Group. J Clin Oncol 2000;18:3108–14.

19. Nesbit MEJ, Gehan EA, Burgert EO Jr, et al. Multimodal therapy for the management of primary, nonmetastatic Ewing's sarcoma of bone: a long-term follow-up of the First Intergroup study. J Clin Oncol 1990;8:1664–74.

20. Burgert EOJ, Nesbit ME, Garnsey LA, et al. Multimodal therapy for the management of nonpelvic, localized Ewing's sarcoma of bone: intergroup study IESS-II. J Clin Oncol 1990;8:1514–24.

21. Evans RG, Nesbit ME, Gehan EA, et al. Multimodal therapy for the management of localized Ewing's sarcoma of pelvic and sacral bones: a report from the second intergroup study. J Clin Oncol 1991;9:1173–80.

22. Paulussen M, Ahrens S, Dunst J, et al. Localized Ewing tumor of bone: final results of the cooperative Ewing's Sarcoma Study CESS 86. J Clin Oncol 2001;19:1818–29.

23. Grier HE, Krailo MD, Tarbell NJ, et al. Addition of ifosfamide and etoposide to standard chemotherapy for Ewing's sarcoma and primitive neuroectodermal tumor of bone. N Engl J Med 2003; 348:694–701.

24. Maheshwari AV, Cheng EY. Ewing sarcoma family of tumors. J Am Acad Orthop Surg 2010;18: 94–107.

25. Granowetter L, Womer R, Devidas M, et al. Dose-intensified compared with standard chemotherapy for nonmetastatic Ewing sarcoma family of tumors: a Children's Oncology Group Study. J Clin Oncol 2009;27:2536–41.

26. Womer RB, West DC, Krailo MD, et al. Randomized controlled trial of interval-compressed chemotherapy for the treatment of localized Ewing sarcoma: a report from the Children's Oncology Group. J Clin Oncol 2012;30:4148–54.

27. Oberlin O, Patte C, Demeocq F, et al. The response to initial chemotherapy as a prognostic factor in localized Ewing's sarcoma. Eur J Cancer Clin Oncol 1985;21:463–7.

28. Bacci G, Ferrari S, Bertoni F, et al. Prognostic factors in nonmetastatic Ewing's sarcoma of bone treated with adjuvant chemotherapy: analysis of 359 patients at the Istituto Ortopedico Rizzoli. J Clin Oncol 2000;18:4–11.

29. Lin PP, Jaffe N, Herzog CE, et al. Chemotherapy response is an important predictor of local recurrence in Ewing sarcoma. Cancer 2007; 109:603–11.

30. Wunder JS, Paulian G, Huvos AG, et al. The histological response to chemotherapy as a predictor of the oncological outcome of operative treatment of Ewing sarcoma. J Bone Joint Surg Am 1998;80: 1020–33.

31. Paulussen M, Ahrens S, Burdach S, et al. Primary metastatic (stage IV) Ewing tumor: survival analysis of 171 patients from the EICESS studies. European Intergroup Cooperative Ewing Sarcoma Studies. Ann Oncol 1998;9:275–81.

32. Miser JS, Krailo MD, Tarbell NJ, et al. Treatment of metastatic Ewing's sarcoma or primitive neuroectodermal tumor of bone: evaluation of combination ifosfamide and etoposide—a Children's Cancer Group and Pediatric Oncology Group study. J Clin Oncol 2004;22:2873–6.

33. Magnan H, Goodbody CM, Riedel E, et al. Ifosfamide dose-intensification for patients with metastatic Ewing sarcoma. Pediatr Blood Cancer 2015; 62(4):594–7.

34. Hamilton SN, Carlson R, Hasan H, et al. Long-term outcomes and complications in pediatric Ewing sarcoma. Am J Clin Oncol 2015. [Epub ahead of print].

35. Gelderblom H, Hogendoorn PC, Dijkstra SD, et al. The clinical approach towards chondrosarcoma. Oncologist 2008;13:320–9.

36. Patrikidou A, Domont J, Cioffi A, et al. Treating soft tissue sarcomas with adjuvant chemotherapy. Curr Treat Options Oncol 2011;12:21–31.

37. Cormier JN, Pollock RE. Soft tissue sarcomas. CA Cancer J Clin 2004;54:94–109.

38. Pisters PW, Harrison LB, Leung DH, et al. Long-term results of a prospective randomized trial of adjuvant brachytherapy in soft tissue sarcoma. J Clin Oncol 1996;14:859–68.

39. Yang JC, Chang AE, Baker AR, et al. Randomized prospective study of the benefit of adjuvant radiation therapy in the treatment of soft tissue sarcomas of the extremity. J Clin Oncol 1998;16: 197–203.

40. Eilber FC, Rosen G, Nelson SD, et al. High-grade extremity soft tissue sarcomas: factors predictive of local recurrence and its effect on morbidity and mortality. Ann Surg 2003;237:218–26.

41. Kang S, Kim HS, Kim S, et al. Post-metastasis survival in extremity soft tissue sarcoma: a recursive partitioning analysis of prognostic factors. Eur J Cancer 2014;50:1649–56.

42. Adjuvant chemotherapy for localised resectable soft-tissue sarcoma of adults: meta-analysis of individual data. Sarcoma Meta-analysis Collaboration. Lancet 1997;350:1647–54.

43. Buesa JM, López-Pousa A, Martín J, et al. Phase II trial of first-line high-dose ifosfamide in advanced soft tissue sarcomas of the adult: a study of the Spanish Group for Research on Sarcomas (GEIS). Ann Oncol 1998;9:871–6.

44. Casali PG, Blay JY. Soft tissue sarcomas: ESMO Clinical Practice Guidelines for diagnosis, treatment and follow-up. Ann Oncol 2010;21(Suppl 5): v198–203.

45. Pervaiz N, Colterjohn N, Farrokhyar F, et al. A systematic meta-analysis of randomized controlled trials of adjuvant chemotherapy for localized resectable soft-tissue sarcoma. Cancer 2008; 113:573–81.

46. Penel N, Bui BN, Bay JO, et al. Phase II trial of weekly paclitaxel for unresectable angiosarcoma: the ANGIOTAX Study. J Clin Oncol 2008;26: 5269–74.

47. Kollar A, Benson C. Current management options for liposarcoma and challenges for the future. Expert Rev Anticancer Ther 2014;14:297–306.

48. Rosen G, Forscher C, Lowenbraun S, et al. Synovial sarcoma. Uniform response of metastases to high dose ifosfamide. Cancer 1994;73: 2506–11.

49. Sleijfer S, Ouali M, van Glabbeke M, et al. Prognostic and predictive factors for outcome to first-line ifosfamide-containing chemotherapy for adult patients with advanced soft tissue sarcomas: an exploratory, retrospective analysis on large series from the European Organization for Research and Treatment of Cancer-Soft Tissue and Bone Sarcoma Group (EORTC-STBSG). Eur J Cancer 2010;46:72–83.

50. Leahy M, Garcia Del Muro X, Reichardt P, et al. Chemotherapy treatment patterns and clinical

outcomes in patients with metastatic soft tissue sarcoma. The SArcoma treatment and Burden of Illness in North America and Europe (SABINE) study. Ann Oncol 2012;23:2763–70.

51. Hanahan D, Weinberg RA. The hallmarks of cancer. Cell 2000;100:57–70.

52. van Oosterom AT, Judson I, Verweij J, et al. Safety and efficacy of imatinib (STI571) in metastatic gastrointestinal stromal tumours: a phase I study. Lancet 2001;358:1421–3.

53. Waller CF. Imatinib mesylate. Recent Results Cancer Res 2014;201:1–25.

54. Cronin M, Ross JS. Comprehensive next-generation cancer genome sequencing in the era of targeted therapy and personalized oncology. Biomark Med 2011;5:293–305.

55. Roukos DH, Ku CS. Clinical cancer genome and precision medicine. Ann Surg Oncol 2012;19:3646–50.

56. Workman P, Al-Lazikani B, Clarke PA. Genome-based cancer therapeutics: targets, kinase drug resistance and future strategies for precision oncology. Curr Opin Pharmacol 2013;13:486–96.

57. Linch M, Miah AB, Thway K, et al. Systemic treatment of soft-tissue sarcoma-gold standard and novel therapies. Nat Rev Clin Oncol 2014;11:187–202.

58. Kansara M, Teng MW, Smyth MJ, et al. Translational biology of osteosarcoma. Nat Rev Cancer 2014;14:722–35.

59. Jo VY, Fletcher CD. WHO classification of soft tissue tumours: an update based on the 2013 (4th) edition. Pathology 2014;46:95–104.

60. Vogelstein B, Papadopoulos N, Velculescu VE, et al. Cancer genome landscapes. Science 2013;339:1546–58.

61. Ognjanovic S, Olivier M, Bergemann TL, et al. Sarcomas in TP53 germline mutation carriers: a review of the IARC TP53 database. Cancer 2012;118:1387–96.

62. MacCarthy A, Bayne AM, Brownbill PA, et al. Second and subsequent tumours among 1927 retinoblastoma patients diagnosed in Britain 1951-2004. Br J Cancer 2013;108:2455–63.

63. Toguchida J, Ishizaki K, Sasaki MS, et al. Preferential mutation of paternally derived RB gene as the initial event in sporadic osteosarcoma. Nature 1989;338:156–8.

64. Chen X, Bahrami A, Pappo A, et al. Recurrent somatic structural variations contribute to tumorigenesis in pediatric osteosarcoma. Cell Rep 2014;7:104–12.

65. Wunder JS, Gokgoz N, Parkes R, et al. TP53 mutations and outcome in osteosarcoma: a prospective, multicenter study. J Clin Oncol 2005;23:1483–90.

66. van Oosterwijk JG, Anninga JK, Gelderblom H, et al. Update on targets and novel treatment options for high-grade osteosarcoma and chondrosarcoma. Hematol Oncol Clin North Am 2013;27:1021–48.

67. Hieken TJ, Das Gupta TK. Mutant p53 expression: a marker of diminished survival in well-differentiated soft tissue sarcoma. Clin Cancer Res 1996;2:1391–5.

68. Hayden JB, Hoang BH. Osteosarcoma: basic science and clinical implications. Orthop Clin North Am 2006;37:1–7.

69. Ito M, Barys L, O'Reilly T, et al. Comprehensive mapping of p53 pathway alterations reveals an apparent role for both SNP309 and MDM2 amplification in sarcomagenesis. Clin Cancer Res 2011;17:416–26.

70. Ray-Coquard I, Blay JY, Italiano A, et al. Effect of the MDM2 antagonist RG7112 on the P53 pathway in patients with MDM2-amplified, well-differentiated or dedifferentiated liposarcoma: an exploratory proof-of-mechanism study. Lancet Oncol 2012;13:1133–40.

71. Shangary S, Qin D, McEachern D, et al. Temporal activation of p53 by a specific MDM2 inhibitor is selectively toxic to tumors and leads to complete tumor growth inhibition. Proc Natl Acad Sci U S A 2008;105:3933–8.

72. Pishas KI, Al-Ejeh F, Zinonos I, et al. Nutlin-3a is a potential therapeutic for Ewing sarcoma. Clin Cancer Res 2011;17:494–504.

73. Frith AE, Hirbe AC, Van Tine BA. Novel pathways and molecular targets for the treatment of sarcoma. Curr Oncol Rep 2013;15:378–85.

74. Graves B, Thompson T, Xia M, et al. Activation of the p53 pathway by small-molecule-induced MDM2 and MDMX dimerization. Proc Natl Acad Sci U S A 2012;109:11788–93.

75. Hartmann C, Tabin CJ. Dual roles of Wnt signaling during chondrogenesis in the chicken limb. Development 2000;127:3141–59.

76. Hoang BH. Wnt, osteosarcoma, and future therapy. J Am Acad Orthop Surg 2012;20:58–9.

77. Cai Y, Mohseny AB, Karperien M, et al. Inactive Wnt/beta-catenin pathway in conventional high-grade osteosarcoma. J Pathol 2010;220:24–33.

78. Kansara M, Tsang M, Kodjabachian L, et al. Wnt inhibitory factor 1 is epigenetically silenced in human osteosarcoma, and targeted disruption accelerates osteosarcomagenesis in mice. J Clin Invest 2009;119:837–51.

79. Mandal D, Srivastava A, Mahlum E, et al. Severe suppression of Frzb/sFRP3 transcription in osteogenic sarcoma. Gene 2007;386:131–8.

80. Vijayakumar S, Liu G, Rus IA, et al. High-frequency canonical Wnt activation in multiple sarcoma subtypes drives proliferation through a TCF/beta-catenin target gene, CDC25A. Cancer Cell 2011;19:601–12.

81. Lin CH, Ji T, Chen CF, et al. Wnt signaling in osteosarcoma. Adv Exp Med Biol 2014;804:33–45.

82. Yang Q, Guan KL. Expanding mTOR signaling. Cell Res 2007;17:666–81.

83. Brun J, Dieudonné FX, Marty C, et al. FHL2 silencing reduces Wnt signaling and osteosarcoma tumorigenesis in vitro and in vivo. PLoS One 2013; 8:e55034.

84. Tao J, Jiang MM, Jiang L, et al. Notch activation as a driver of osteogenic sarcoma. Cancer Cell 2014; 26:390–401.

85. Mu X, Isaac C, Greco N, et al. Notch signaling is associated with ALDH activity and an aggressive metastatic phenotype in murine osteosarcoma cells. Front Oncol 2013;3:143.

86. Samuel AM, Costa J, Lindskog DM. Genetic alterations in chondrosarcomas - keys to targeted therapies? Cell Oncol (Dordr) 2014;37:95–105.

87. Lo WW, Wunder JS, Dickson BC, et al. Involvement and targeted intervention of dysregulated Hedgehog signaling in osteosarcoma. Cancer 2014;120:537–47.

88. Kelleher FC, Cain JE, Healy JM, et al. Prevailing importance of the hedgehog signaling pathway and the potential for treatment advancement in sarcoma. Pharmacol Ther 2012;136:153–68.

89. Martin JW, Zielenska M, Stein GS, et al. The Role of RUNX2 in osteosarcoma oncogenesis. Sarcoma 2011;2011:282745.

90. Lahat G, Zhang P, Zhu QS, et al. The expression of c-Met pathway components in unclassified pleomorphic sarcoma/malignant fibrous histiocytoma (UPS/MFH): a tissue microarray study. Histopathology 2011;59:556–61.

91. Scotlandi K, Baldini N, Oliviero M, et al. Expression of Met/hepatocyte growth factor receptor gene and malignant behavior of musculoskeletal tumors. Am J Pathol 1996;149:1209–19.

92. Wallenius V, Hisaoka M, Helou K, et al. Overexpression of the hepatocyte growth factor (HGF) receptor (Met) and presence of a truncated and activated intracellular HGF receptor fragment in locally aggressive/malignant human musculoskeletal tumors. Am J Pathol 2000;156:821–9.

93. Patane S, Avnet S, Coltella N, et al. MET overexpression turns human primary osteoblasts into osteosarcomas. Cancer Res 2006;66:4750–7.

94. Wagner AJ, Goldberg JM, Dubois SG, et al. Tivantinib (ARQ 197), a selective inhibitor of MET, in patients with microphthalmia transcription factor-associated tumors: results of a multicenter phase 2 trial. Cancer 2012;118:5894–902.

95. Egas-Bejar D, Anderson PM, Agarwal R, et al. Theranostic profiling for actionable aberrations in advanced high risk osteosarcoma with aggressive biology reveals high molecular diversity: the human fingerprint hypothesis. Oncoscience 2014;1: 167–79.

96. Wang YH, Han XD, Qiu Y, et al. Increased expression of insulin-like growth factor-1 receptor is correlated with tumor metastasis and prognosis in patients with osteosarcoma. J Surg Oncol 2012; 105:235–43.

97. Krueger DA, Care MM, Holland K, et al. Everolimus for subependymal giant-cell astrocytomas in tuberous sclerosis. N Engl J Med 2010;363:1801–11.

98. Franz DN, Belousova E, Sparagana S, et al. Everolimus for subependymal giant cell astrocytoma in patients with tuberous sclerosis complex: 2-year open-label extension of the randomised EXIST-1 study. Lancet Oncol 2014;15:1513–20.

99. Bissler JJ, Kingswood JC, Radzikowska E, et al. Everolimus for angiomyolipoma associated with tuberous sclerosis complex or sporadic lymphangioleiomyomatosis (EXIST-2): a multicentre, randomised, double-blind, placebo-controlled trial. Lancet 2013;381:817–24.

100. Pazdur R, et al. FDA Approval for everolimus. 2013. Available at: http://www.cancer.gov/about-cancer/ treatment/drugs/fda-everolimus. Accessed June 23, 2015.

101. Demetri GD, Chawla SP, Ray-Coquard I, et al. Results of an international randomized phase III trial of the mammalian target of rapamycin inhibitor ridaforolimus versus placebo to control metastatic sarcomas in patients after benefit from prior chemotherapy. J Clin Oncol 2013;31:2485–92.

102. Rikhof B, de Jong S, Suurmeijer AJ, et al. The insulin-like growth factor system and sarcomas. J Pathol 2009;217:469–82.

103. Steigen SE, Schaeffer DF, West RB, et al. Expression of insulin-like growth factor 2 in mesenchymal neoplasms. Mod Pathol 2009;22:914–21.

104. Cironi L, Riggi N, Provero P, et al. IGF1 is a common target gene of Ewing's sarcoma fusion proteins in mesenchymal progenitor cells. PLoS One 2008;3:e2634.

105. Mora J, Rodríguez E, de Torres C, et al. Activated growth signaling pathway expression in Ewing sarcoma and clinical outcome. Pediatr Blood Cancer 2012;58:532–8.

106. van de Luijtgaarden AC, Versleijen-Jonkers YM, Roeffen MH, et al. Prognostic and therapeutic relevance of the IGF pathway in Ewing's sarcoma patients. Target Oncol 2013;8:253–60.

107. Sun Y, Gao D, Liu Y, et al. IGF2 is critical for tumorigenesis by synovial sarcoma oncoprotein SYT-SSX1. Oncogene 2006;25:1042–52.

108. Ayalon D, Glaser T, Werner H. Transcriptional regulation of IGF-I receptor gene expression by the PAX3-FKHR oncoprotein. Growth Horm IGF Res 2001;11:289–97.

109. Makawita S, Ho M, Durbin AD, et al. Expression of insulin-like growth factor pathway proteins in rhabdomyosarcoma: IGF-2 expression is associated

with translocation-negative tumors. Pediatr Dev Pathol 2009;12:127–35.

110. van de Luijtgaarden AC, Roeffen MH, Leus MA, et al. IGF signaling pathway analysis of osteosarcomas reveals the prognostic value of pAKT localization. Future Oncol 2013;9:1733–40.

111. Kolb EA, Kamara D, Zhang W, et al. Kamara D, Zhang W, R1507, a fully human monoclonal antibody targeting IGF-1R, is effective alone and in combination with rapamycin in inhibiting growth of osteosarcoma xenografts. Pediatr Blood Cancer 2010;55:67–75.

112. Rainusso N, Wang LL, Yustein JT. The adolescent and young adult with cancer: state of the art—bone tumors. Curr Oncol Rep 2013;15:296–307.

113. Stegmaier K, Wong JS, Ross KN, et al. Signature-based small molecule screening identifies cytosine arabinoside as an EWS/FLI modulator in Ewing sarcoma. PLoS Med 2007;4:e122.

114. Erkizan HV, Kong Y, Merchant M, et al. A small molecule blocking oncogenic protein EWS-FLI1 interaction with RNA helicase A inhibits growth of Ewing's sarcoma. Nat Med 2009;15:750–6.

115. Grohar PJ, Woldemichael GM, Griffin LB, et al. Identification of an inhibitor of the EWS-FLI1 oncogenic transcription factor by high-throughput screening. J Natl Cancer Inst 2011;103:962–78.

116. Gautreau A, Poullet P, Louvard D, et al. Ezrin, a plasma membrane-microfilament linker, signals cell survival through the phosphatidylinositol 3-kinase/Akt pathway. Proc Natl Acad Sci U S A 1999;96:7300–5.

117. Louvet-Vallee S. ERM proteins: from cellular architecture to cell signaling. Biol Cell 2000;92: 305–16.

118. Bretscher A, Edwards K, Fehon RG. ERM proteins and merlin: integrators at the cell cortex. Nat Rev Mol Cell Biol 2002;3:586–99.

119. Pujuguet P, Del Maestro L, Gautreau A, et al. Ezrin regulates E-cadherin-dependent adherens junction assembly through Rac1 activation. Mol Biol Cell 2003;14:2181–91.

120. Geissler KJ, Jung MJ, Riecken LB, et al. Regulation of Son of sevenless by the membrane-actin linker protein ezrin. Proc Natl Acad Sci U S A 2013;110: 20587–92.

121. Khanna C, Wan X, Bose S, et al. The membrane-cytoskeleton linker ezrin is necessary for osteosarcoma metastasis. Nat Med 2004;10:182–6.

122. Hunter KW. Ezrin, a key component in tumor metastasis. Trends Mol Med 2004;10:201–4.

123. Yu Y, Davicioni E, Triche TJ, et al. The homeoprotein six1 transcriptionally activates multiple protumorigenic genes but requires ezrin to promote metastasis. Cancer Res 2006;66:1982–9.

124. Krishnan K, Bruce B, Hewitt S, et al. Ezrin mediates growth and survival in Ewing's sarcoma through the AKT/mTOR, but not the MAPK, signaling pathway. Clin Exp Metastasis 2006;23:227–36.

125. Weng WH, Ahlen J, Astrom K, et al. Prognostic impact of immunohistochemical expression of ezrin in highly malignant soft tissue sarcomas. Clin Cancer Res 2005;11:6198–204.

126. Carneiro A, Bendahl PO, Åkerman M, et al. Ezrin expression predicts local recurrence and development of metastases in soft tissue sarcomas. J Clin Pathol 2011;64:689–94.

127. Kim MS, Cho WH, Song WS, et al. Prognostic significance of ezrin expression in pleomorphic malignant fibrous histiocytoma. Anticancer Res 2007;27: 1171–8.

128. Huang HY, Li CF, Fang FM, et al. Prognostic implication of ezrin overexpression in myxofibrosarcomas. Ann Surg Oncol 2010;17:3212–9.

129. Soderstrom M, Palokangas T, Vahlberg T, et al. Expression of ezrin, Bcl-2, and Ki-67 in chondrosarcomas. APMIS 2010;118:769–76.

130. Ogino W, Takeshima Y, Mori T, et al. High level of ezrin mRNA expression in an osteosarcoma biopsy sample with lung metastasis. J Pediatr Hematol Oncol 2007;29:435–9.

131. Ferrari S, Zanella L, Alberghini M, et al. Prognostic significance of immunohistochemical expression of ezrin in non-metastatic high-grade osteosarcoma. Pediatr Blood Cancer 2008;50:752–6.

132. Wang Z, He ML, Zhao JM, et al. Meta-analysis of associations of the ezrin gene with human osteosarcoma response to chemotherapy and prognosis. Asian Pac J Cancer Prev 2013;14: 2753–8.

133. Mu Y, Zhang H, Che L, et al. Clinical significance of microRNA-183/Ezrin axis in judging the prognosis of patients with osteosarcoma. Med Oncol 2014; 31:821.

134. Ren L, Khanna C. Role of ezrin in osteosarcoma metastasis. Adv Exp Med Biol 2014;804:181–201.

135. Bulut G, Hong SH, Chen K, et al. Small molecule inhibitors of ezrin inhibit the invasive phenotype of osteosarcoma cells. Oncogene 2012;31:269–81.

136. Schwertschlag US, Trepicchio WL, Dykstra KH, et al. Hematopoietic, immunomodulatory and epithelial effects of interleukin-11. Leukemia 1999; 13:1307–15.

137. Li TM, Wu CM, Huang HC, et al. Interleukin-11 increases cell motility and up-regulates intercellular adhesion molecule-1 expression in human chondrosarcoma cells. J Cell Biochem 2012;113:3353–62.

138. Lewis VO, Ozawa MG, Deavers MT, et al. The interleukin-11 receptor alpha as a candidate ligand-directed target in osteosarcoma: consistent data from cell lines, orthotopic models, and human tumor samples. Cancer Res 2009;69:1995–9.

139. Aggarwal BB, Kunnumakkara AB, Harikumar KB, et al. Signal transducer and activator of

transcription-3, inflammation, and cancer: how intimate is the relationship? Ann N Y Acad Sci 2009; 1171:59–76.

140. Chen CL, Loy A, Cen L, et al. Signal transducer and activator of transcription 3 is involved in cell growth and survival of human rhabdomyosarcoma and osteosarcoma cells. BMC Cancer 2007;7:111.

141. David D, Rajappan LM, Balachandran K, et al. Prognostic significance of STAT3 and phosphorylated STAT3 in human soft tissue tumors - a clinicopathological analysis. J Exp Clin Cancer Res 2011; 30:56.

142. Wang X, Goldstein D, Crowe PJ, et al. Impact of STAT3 inhibition on survival of osteosarcoma cell lines. Anticancer Res 2014;34:6537–45.

143. Bendell JC, Hong DS, Burris HA 3rd, et al. Phase 1, open-label, dose-escalation, and pharmacokinetic study of STAT3 inhibitor OPB-31121 in subjects with advanced solid tumors. Cancer Chemother Pharmacol 2014;74:125–30.

144. Kim KJ, Li B, Winer J, et al. Inhibition of vascular endothelial growth factor-induced angiogenesis suppresses tumour growth in vivo. Nature 1993; 362:841–4.

145. Takahashi H, Shibuya M. The vascular endothelial growth factor (VEGF)/VEGF receptor system and its role under physiological and pathological conditions. Clin Sci (Lond) 2005;109:227–41.

146. Lin CY, Hung SY, Chen HT, et al. Brain-derived neurotrophic factor increases vascular endothelial growth factor expression and enhances angiogenesis in human chondrosarcoma cells. Biochem Pharmacol 2014;91:522–33.

147. Wakamatsu T, Naka N, Sasagawa S, et al. Deflection of vascular endothelial growth factor action by SS18-SSX and composite vascular endothelial growth factor- and chemokine (C-X-C motif) receptor 4-targeted therapy in synovial sarcoma. Cancer Sci 2014;105:1124–34.

148. Katuri V, Gerber S, Qiu X, et al. WT1 regulates angiogenesis in Ewing Sarcoma. Oncotarget 2014;5:2436–49.

149. Miyoshi K, Kohashi K, Fushiujmi F, et al. Close correlation between CXCR4 and VEGF expression and frequent CXCR7 expression in rhabdomyosarcoma. Hum Pathol 2014;45:1900–9.

150. Yang J, Zhao L, Tian W, et al. Correlation of WWOX, RUNX2 and VEGFA protein expression in human osteosarcoma. BMC Med Genomics 2013;6:56.

151. Itakura E, Yamamoto H, Oda Y, et al. Detection and characterization of vascular endothelial growth factors and their receptors in a series of angiosarcomas. J Surg Oncol 2008;97:74–81.

152. Young RJ, Fernando M, Hughes D, et al. Angiogenic growth factor expression in benign and malignant vascular tumours. Exp Mol Pathol 2014;97: 148–53.

153. Kummar S, Allen D, Monks A, et al. Cediranib for metastatic alveolar soft part sarcoma. J Clin Oncol 2013;31:2296–302.

154. Agulnik M, Yarber JL, Okuno SH, et al. An open-label, multicenter, phase II study of bevacizumab for the treatment of angiosarcoma and epithelioid hemangioendotheliomas. Ann Oncol 2013;24:257–63.

155. Graeven U, Andre N, Achilles E, et al. Serum levels of vascular endothelial growth factor and basic fibroblast growth factor in patients with soft-tissue sarcoma. J Cancer Res Clin Oncol 1999;125:577–81.

156. Yoon SS, Segal NH, Olshen AB, et al. Circulating angiogenic factor levels correlate with extent of disease and risk of recurrence in patients with soft tissue sarcoma. Ann Oncol 2004;15:1261–6.

157. van Oosterwijk JG, Meijer D, van Ruler MA, et al. Screening for potential targets for therapy in mesenchymal, clear cell, and dedifferentiated chondrosarcoma reveals Bcl-2 family members and TGFbeta as potential targets. Am J Pathol 2013;182:1347–56.

158. Hoffman A, Ghadimi MP, Demicco EG, et al. Localized and metastatic myxoid/round cell liposarcoma: clinical and molecular observations. Cancer 2013;119:1868–77.

159. Ho AL, Vasudeva SD, Laé M, et al. PDGF receptor alpha is an alternative mediator of rapamycin-induced Akt activation: implications for combination targeted therapy of synovial sarcoma. Cancer Res 2012;72:4515–25.

160. Llombart B, Monteagudo C, Sanmartín O, et al. Dermatofibrosarcoma protuberans: a clinicopathological, immunohistochemical, genetic (COL1A1-PDGFB), and therapeutic study of low-grade versus high-grade (fibrosarcomatous) tumors. J Am Acad Dermatol 2011;65:564–75.

161. Walluks K, Chen Y, Woelfel C, et al. Molecular and clinicopathological analysis of dermatofibrosarcoma protuberans. Pathol Res Pract 2013;209: 30–5.

162. O'Brien KP, Seroussi E, Dal Cin P, et al. Various regions within the alpha-helical domain of the COL1A1 gene are fused to the second exon of the PDGFB gene in dermatofibrosarcomas and giant-cell fibroblastomas. Genes Chromosomes Cancer 1998;23:187–93.

163. Takagi S, Takemoto A, Takami M, et al. Platelets promote osteosarcoma cell growth through activation of the platelet-derived growth factor receptor-Akt signaling axis. Cancer Sci 2014; 105:983–8.

164. Rutkowski P, Van Glabbeke M, Rankin CJ, et al. Imatinib mesylate in advanced dermatofibrosarcoma protuberans: pooled analysis of two phase II clinical trials. J Clin Oncol 2010;28:1772–9.

165. Kasper B, Sleijfer S, Litière S, et al. Long-term responders and survivors on pazopanib for

advanced soft tissue sarcomas: subanalysis of two European Organisation for Research and Treatment of Cancer (EORTC) clinical trials 62043 and 62072. Ann Oncol 2014;25:719–24.

166. van der Graaf WT, Blay JY, Chawla SP, et al. Pazopanib for metastatic soft-tissue sarcoma (PALETTE): a randomised, double-blind, placebo-controlled phase 3 trial. Lancet 2012;379:1879–86.

167. de Souza RR, Oliveira ID, del Giúdice Paniago M, et al. Investigation of IGF2, Hedgehog and fusion gene expression profiles in pediatric sarcomas. Growth Horm IGF Res 2014;24:130–6.

168. Crozat A, Aman P, Mandahl N, et al. Fusion of CHOP to a novel RNA-binding protein in human myxoid liposarcoma. Nature 1993;363:640–4.

169. Rodriguez R, Tornin J, Suarez C, et al. Expression of FUS-CHOP fusion protein in immortalized/transformed human mesenchymal stem cells drives mixoid liposarcoma formation. Stem Cells 2013;31:2061–72.

170. Kobos R, Nagai M, Tsuda M, et al. Combining integrated genomics and functional genomics to dissect the biology of a cancer-associated, aberrant transcription factor, the ASPSCR1-TFE3 fusion oncoprotein. J Pathol 2013;229:743–54.

171. Reis H, Hager T, Wohlschlaeger J, et al. Mammalian target of rapamycin pathway activity in alveolar soft part sarcoma. Hum Pathol 2013;44:2266–74.

172. Charytonowicz E, Matushansky I, Doménech JD, et al. PAX7-FKHR fusion gene inhibits myogenic differentiation via NF-kappaB upregulation. Clin Transl Oncol 2012;14:197–206.

173. Bovee JV, van den Broek LJ, Cleton-Jansen AM, et al. Up-regulation of PTHrP and Bcl-2 expression characterizes the progression of osteochondroma towards peripheral chondrosarcoma and is a late event in central chondrosarcoma. Lab Invest 2000;80:1925–34.

174. van Oosterwijk JG, Herpers B, Meijer D, et al. Restoration of chemosensitivity for doxorubicin and cisplatin in chondrosarcoma in vitro: BCL-2 family members cause chemoresistance. Ann Oncol 2012;23:1617–26.

175. Morii T, Ohtsuka K, Ohnishi H, et al. BH3 mimetics inhibit growth of chondrosarcoma–a novel targeted-therapy for candidate models. Anticancer Res 2014;34:6423–30.

176. Schöffski P. CREATE: Cross-tumoral Phase 2 With Crizotinib. ClinicalTrials.gov Identifier NCT01524926. Available at: https://clinicaltrials.gov/ct2/show/NCT01524926?term=nct01524926&rank=1. Accessed July 28, 2015.

177. Chawla SP, Staddon AP, Baker LH, et al. Study of AP23573/MK-8669 (Ridaforolimus), A Mammalian Target of Rapamycin (mTOR) Inhibitor, in Participants With Advanced Sarcoma (MK-8669–018 AM1). ClinicalTrials.gov Identifier NCT00093080. Available at: https://clinicaltrials.gov/ct2/show/NCT00093080?term=NCT00093080&rank=1. Accessed July 28, 2015.

178. Yoo C, Lee J, Rha SY, et al. Multicenter phase II study of everolimus in patients with metastatic or recurrent bone and soft-tissue sarcomas after failure of anthracycline and ifosfamide. Invest New Drugs 2013;31(6):1602–8.

179. Wagner L. Cixutumumab and Temsirolimus in Treating Younger Patients With Recurrent or Refractory Sarcoma. ClinicalTrials.gov Identifier NCT01614795. Available at: https://clinicaltrials.gov/ct2/show/NCT01614795?term=nct01614795&rank=1. Accessed July 28, 2015.

180. Schwartz GK, Tap WD, Qin LX, et al. Temsirolimus and Cixutumumab in Treating Patients With Locally Advanced, Metastatic, or Recurrent Soft Tissue Sarcoma or Bone Sarcoma. ClinicalTrials.gov Identifier NCT01016015. Available at: https://clinicaltrials.gov/ct2/show/NCT01016015?term=NCT01016015&rank=1. Accessed July 28, 2015.

181. Weigel B. Cixutumumab in Treating Patients With Relapsed or Refractory Solid Tumors. ClinicalTrials.gov Identifier NCT00831844. Available at: https://clinicaltrials.gov/ct2/show/NCT00831844?term=NCT00831844&rank=1. Accessed July 28, 2015.

182. Tap WD, Demetri G, Barnette P, et al. A Phase 2 Study of AMG 479 in Relapsed or Refractory Ewing's Family Tumor and Desmoplastic Small Round Cell Tumors. ClinicalTrials.gov Identifier NCT00563680. Available at: https://clinicaltrials.gov/ct2/show/NCT00563680?term=00563680&rank=1. Accessed July 28, 2015.

183. Pappo AS, Patel SR, Crowley J, et al. A Study of R1507 in Patients With Recurrent or Refractory Sarcoma. ClinicalTrials.gov Identifier NCT00642941. Available at: https://clinicaltrials.gov/ct2/show/NCT00642941?term=00642941&rank=1. Accessed July 28, 2015.

184. Judson I, Scurr M, Gardner K, et al. The Biological Activity of Cediranib (AZD2171) in Gastro-Intestinal Stromal Tumours(GIST). ClinicalTrials.gov Identifier NCT00385203. Available at: https://clinicaltrials.gov/ct2/show/NCT00385203?term=00385203&rank=1. Accessed July 28, 2015.

185. Kummar S, Allen D, Monks A, et al. Phase II Study of Cediranib (AZD2171) in Patients With Alveolar Soft Part Sarcoma. ClinicalTrials.gov Identifier NCT00942877. Available at: https://clinicaltrials.gov/ct2/show/NCT00942877?term=00942877&rank=1. Accessed July 28, 2015.

186. Agulnik M. Bevacizumab in Treating Patients With Angiosarcoma. ClinicalTrials.gov Identifier NCT00288015. Available at: https://clinicaltrials.gov/ct2/show/NCT00288015?term=00288015&rank=1. Accessed July 28, 2015.

187. Baruchel S, Pappo A, Krailo M, et al. Trabectedin in Treating Young Patients With Recurrent or Refractory

Soft Tissue Sarcoma or Ewing's Family of Tumors. ClinicalTrials.gov Identifier: NCT00070109. Available at: https://clinicaltrials.gov/ct2/show/NCT 00070109?term=00070109&rank=1. Accessed July 28, 2015.

188. Butrynski JE. Doxorubicin Hydrochloride or Trabectedin in Treating Patients With Previously Untreated Advanced or Metastatic Soft Tissue Sarcoma. ClinicalTrials.gov Identifier NCT01189253. Available at: https://clinicaltrials.gov/ct2/show/NCT01189253?term=NCT01189253&rank=1. Accessed July 28, 2015.

189. Cesne AL, Judson I, Maki R, et al. Trabectedin is a feasible treatment for soft tissue sarcoma patients regardless of patient age: a retrospective pooled analysis of five phase II trials. Br J Cancer 2013; 109(7):1717–24.

190. Le Cesne A, Blay JY, Domont J, et al. Continuing vs Intermittent Trabectedin-regimen in Patients With Advanced Soft Tissue Sarcoma Experiencing Response or Stable Disease After the 6th Cycle (T-DIS). ClinicalTrials.gov Identifier: NCT01303094. Available at: https://clinicaltrials.gov/ct2/show/NCT 01303094?term=01303094&rank=1. Accessed July 28, 2015.

191. Grignani G. Imatinib in Patients With Desmoid Tumor and Chondrosarcoma (Basket 1). ClinicalTrials.gov Identifier: NCT00928525. Available at: https://clinicaltrials.gov/ct2/show/NCT00928525?term=grignani+imatinib&rank=1. Accessed July 28, 2015.

192. Ugurel S, Mentzel T, Utikal J, et al. Neoadjuvant imatinib in advanced primary or locally recurrent dermatofibrosarcoma protuberans: a multicenter phase II DeCOG trial with long-term follow-up. Clin Cancer Res 2014;20(2):499–510.

193. Sugiura H, Fujiwara Y, Ando M, et al. Multicenter phase II trial assessing effectiveness of imatinib mesylate on relapsed or refractory KIT-positive or PDGFR-positive sarcoma. J Orthop Sci 2010; 15(5):654–60.

194. Dickson M. PD0332991 in Patients With Advanced or Metastatic Liposarcoma. ClinicalTrials.gov Identifier: NCT01209598. Available at: https://clinicaltrials.gov/ct2/show/NCT01209598?term=NCT01209598&rank=1. Accessed July 28, 2015.

195. Ebb D. Chemotherapy With or Without Trastuzumab in Treating Patients With Metastatic Osteosarcoma. ClinicalTrials.gov Identifier: NCT00023998. Available at: https://clinicaltrials.gov/ct2/show/NCT 00023998?term=NCT00023998&rank=1. Accessed July 28, 2015.

196. Von Mehren M, Demetri GD. S0505 Sorafenib in Treating Patients With Advanced Soft Tissue Sarcomas. ClinicalTrials.gov Identifier: NCT00217620. Available at: https://clinicaltrials.gov/ct2/show/NCT 00217620?term=00217620&rank=1. Accessed July 28, 2015.

197. Grignani G. Sorafenib in Relapsed High Grade Osteosarcoma. ClinicalTrials.gov Identifier: NCT00889057. Available at: https://clinicaltrials.gov/ct2/show/NCT00889057?term=NCT00889057&rank=1. Accessed July 28, 2015.

198. Aglietta M. Phase II Open Label, Non-randomized Study of Sorafenib and Everolimus in Relapsed and Non-resectable Osteosarcoma (SERIO). ClinicalTrials.gov Identifier: NCT01804374. Available at: https://clinicaltrials.gov/ct2/show/NCT01804374?term=NCT01804374&rank=1. Accessed July 28, 2015.

199. Sleijfer S, Ray-Coquard I, Papai Z, et al. Pazopanib In Patients With Relapsed Or Refractory Soft Tissue Sarcoma. ClinicalTrials.gov Identifier: NCT00297258. Available at: https://clinicaltrials.gov/ct2/show/NCT00297258?term=NCT00297258&rank=1. Accessed July 28, 2015.

Index

Note: Page numbers of article titles are in **boldface** type.

orthopedic.theclinics.com

United States Postal Service

Statement of Ownership, Management, and Circulation
(All Periodicals Publications Except Requestor Publications)

1. Publication Title	2. Publication Number	3. Filing Date
Orthopedic Clinics of North America	9 5 0 - 9 2 0	9/18/15

4. Issue Frequency	5. Number of Issues Published Annually	6. Annual Subscription Price
Jan, Apr, Jul, Oct	4	$310.00

7. Complete Mailing Address of Known Office of Publication (Not printer) (Street, city, county, state, and ZIP+4®)

Elsevier Inc.
360 Park Avenue South
New York, NY 10010-1710

Contact Person
Stephen R. Bushing

Telephone (Include area code)
215-239-3688

8. Complete Mailing Address of Headquarters or General Business Office of Publisher (Not printer)

Elsevier Inc., 360 Park Avenue South, New York, NY 10010-1710

9. Full Names and Complete Mailing Addresses of Publisher, Editor, and Managing Editor (Do not leave blank)

Publisher (Name and complete mailing address)

Linda Belfus, Elsevier Inc., 1600 John F. Kennedy Blvd., Ste. 1800, Philadelphia, PA 19103-2899

Editor (Name and complete mailing address)

Jennifer Flynn-Briggs, Elsevier Inc., 1600 John F. Kennedy Blvd., Ste. 1800, Philadelphia, PA 19103-2899

Managing Editor (Name and complete mailing address)

Adrianne Brigido, Elsevier Inc., 1600 John F. Kennedy Blvd., Ste. 1800, Philadelphia, PA 19103-2899

10. Owner (Do not leave blank. If the publication is owned by a corporation, give the name and address of the corporation immediately followed by the names and addresses of all stockholders owning or holding 1 percent or more of the total amount of stock. If not owned by a corporation, give the names and addresses of the individual owners. If owned by a partnership or other unincorporated firm, give its name and address as well as those of each individual owner. If the publication is published by a nonprofit organization, give its name and address.)

Full Name	Complete Mailing Address
Wholly owned subsidiary of	1600 John F. Kennedy Blvd., Ste. 1800
Reed/Elsevier, US holdings	Philadelphia, PA 19103-2899

11. Known Bondholders, Mortgagees, and Other Security Holders Owning or Holding 1 Percent or More of Total Amount of Bonds, Mortgages, or Other Securities. If none, check box → ☐ None

Full Name	Complete Mailing Address
N/A	

12. Tax Status (For completion by nonprofit organizations authorized to mail at nonprofit rates) (Check one)
The purpose, function, and nonprofit status of this organization and the exempt status for federal income tax purposes:
☐ Has Not Changed During Preceding 12 Months
☐ Has Changed During Preceding 12 Months (Publisher must submit explanation of change with this statement)

13. Publication Title	14. Issue Date for Circulation Data Below
Orthopedic Clinics of North America	July 2015

PS Form 3526, July 2014 (Page 1 of 3 (Instructions Page 3)) PSN 7530-01-000-9931 PRIVACY NOTICE: See our Privacy policy in www.usps.com

---

15. Extent and Nature of Circulation		Average No. Copies Each Issue During Preceding 12 Months	No. Copies of Single Issue Published Nearest to Filing Date
a. Total Number of Copies (Net press run)		1005	864
b. Legitimate Paid and Or Requested Distribution (By Mail and Outside the Mail)	(1) Mailed Outside-County Paid/Requested Mail Subscriptions stated on PS Form 3541. (Include paid distribution above nominal rate, advertiser's proof copies and exchange copies)	336	195
	(2) Mailed In-County Paid/Requested Mail Subscriptions stated on PS Form 3541. (Include paid distribution above nominal rate, advertiser's proof copies and exchange copies)		
	(3) Paid Distribution Outside the Mails Including Sales Through Dealers And Carriers, Street Vendors, Counter Sales, and Other Paid Distribution Outside USPS®	230	249
	(4) Paid Distribution by Other Classes of Mail Through the USPS (e.g. First-Class Mail®)		
c. Total Paid and or Requested Circulation (Sum of 15b (1), (2), (3), and (4)) ▲		566	444
d. Free or Nominal Rate Distribution (By Mail and Outside the Mail)	(1) Free or Nominal Rate Outside-County Copies included on PS Form 3541	98	77
	(2) Free or Nominal Rate In-County Copies included on PS Form 3541		
	(3) Free or Nominal Rate Copies mailed at Other classes Through the USPS (e.g. First-Class Mail®)		
	(4) Free or Nominal Rate Distribution Outside the Mail (Carriers or Other means)		
e. Total Nonrequested Distribution (Sum of 15d (1), (2), (3) and (4)		98	77
f. Total Distribution (Sum of 15c and 15e) ▲		664	521
g. Copies not Distributed (See instructions to publishers #4 (page #3)) ▲		341	343
h. Total (Sum of 15f and g) ▲		1005	864
i. Percent Paid and/or Requested Circulation (15c divided by 15f times 100)		85.24%	85.22%

* If you are claiming electronic copies go to line 16 on page 3. If you are not claiming Electronic copies, skip to line 17 on page 3

16. Electronic Copy Circulation	Average No. Copies Each Issue During Preceding 12 Months	No. Copies of Single Issue Published Nearest to Filing Date
a. Paid Electronic Copies		
b. Total paid Print Copies (Line 15c) + Paid Electronic copies (Line 16a)		
c. Total Print Distribution (Line 15f) + Paid Electronic Copies (Line 16a)		
d. Percent Paid (Both Print & Electronic copies) (16b divided by 16c X 100)		

☐ I certify that 50% of all my distributed copies (electronic and print) are paid above a nominal price.

17. Publication of Statement of Ownership
If the publication is a general publication, publication of this statement is required. Will be printed in the __October 2015__ issue of this publication.

18. Signature and Title of Editor, Publisher, Business Manager, or Owner

Stephen R. Bushing – Inventory Distribution Coordinator

Date
September 18, 2015

I certify that all information furnished on this form is true and complete. I understand that anyone who furnishes false or misleading information on this form or who omits material or information requested on the form may be subject to criminal sanctions (including fines and imprisonment) and/or civil sanctions (including civil penalties).

PS Form 3526, July 2014 (Page 3 of 3)

Moving?

Make sure your subscription moves with you!

To notify us of your new address, find your **Clinics Account Number** (located on your mailing label above your name), and contact customer service at:

Email: journalscustomerservice-usa@elsevier.com

800-654-2452 (subscribers in the U.S. & Canada)
314-447-8871 (subscribers outside of the U.S. & Canada)

Fax number: 314-447-8029

Elsevier Health Sciences Division
Subscription Customer Service
3251 Riverport Lane
Maryland Heights, MO 63043

ELSEVIER

Printed and bound by CPI Group (UK) Ltd, Croydon, CR0 4YY

03/10/2024

01040381-0002